Homemaker/
Home Health Aide

Connie Campbell

408-767-7

408 244-1631

408 264-7968

0414*2140

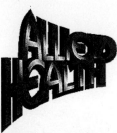

Homemaker/ Home Health Aide

Fifth Edition

Helen Huber, BA
Audree Spatz, MEd, BSN, RN

Revised by
The Center for Applied Gerontology,
Educational Division of
Council for Jewish Elderly

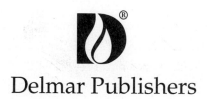

Delmar Publishers

an International Thomson Publishing company I T P®

Albany • Bonn • Boston • Cincinnati • Detroit • London • Madrid
Melbourne • Mexico City • New York • Pacific Grove • Paris • San Francisco
Singapore • Tokyo • Toronto • Washington

NOTICE TO THE READER

Cover Design: Brian Sullivan
Delmar Staff
Publisher: Susan Simpfenderfer
Acquisitions Editor: Dawn Gerrain
Developmental Editor: Marjorie A. Bruce/Debra Flis
Project Editor: Coreen Filson/Brooke Graves, Graves Editorial Service
Production Coordinator: John Mickelbank
Art and Design Coordinator: Vincent S. Berger
Editorial Assistant: Donna L. Leto

COPYRIGHT © 1998
By Delmar Publishers
a division of International Thomson Publishing Inc.

The ITP logo is a trademark under license.

Printed in the United States of America

For more information, contact:

Delmar Publishers
3 Columbia Circle, Box 15015
Albany, New York 12212-5015

International Thomson Publishing Europe
Berkshire House
168-173 High Holborn
London, WC1V 7AA
England

Thomas Nelson Australia
102 Dodds Street
South Melbourne, 3205
Victoria, Australia

Nelson Canada
1120 Birchmount Road
Scarborough, Ontario
Canada, M1K 5G4

International Thomson Editores
Campos Eliseos 385, Piso 7
Col Polanco
11560 Mexico D F Mexico

International Thomson Publishing GmbH
Konigswinterer Strasse 418
53227 Bonn
Germany

International Thomson Publishing Asia
221 Henderson Road
#05-10 Henderson Building
Singapore 0315

International Thomson Publishing—Japan
Hirakawacho Kyowa Building, 3F
2-2-1 Hirakawacho
Chiyoda-ku, Tokyo 102
Japan

Library of Congress Cataloging-in-Publication Data
Huber, Helen.
Homemaker/home health aide / Helen Huber, Audree Spatz.— 5th ed. / revised by Council for Jewish Elderly, Center for Applied Gerontology.
p.   cm.
Includes bibliographical references and index.
ISBN 0-8273-8084-4 (alk. paper)
1. Home health aides. 2. Visiting housekeepers. 3. Home nursing. I. Spatz, Audree. II. Center for Applied Gerontology. III. Title.
[DNLM: 1. Homemaker Services. 2. Home Health Aides. 3. Home Nursing. WY 115 H877h 1998]
RA645.3.H8 1998
649'.8—dc21
DNLM/DLC
for Library of Congress
97-12232
CIP

Summary Contents

Contents

Procedures

The video icon indicates procedures that can be found in Delmar's Home Care Aide videotape series, second edition.

Preface

INTRODUCTION

Homemaker/Home Health Aide, 5th edition, is a comprehensive textbook designed for use in basic home health aide training programs and also as a reference book in required continuous in-service courses for home health aides.

The book is divided into eight sections: Section 1, Becoming a Home Health Aide; Section 2, Stages of Human Development; Section 3, Preventing the Spread of Infectious Disease; Section 4, Understanding Health; Section 5, Body Systems and Common Disorders; Section 6, Clients Requiring Special Care; Section 7, Maternal/Infant Care; and Section 8, Employment. The practical application of procedures required by OBRA are integrated into each unit. The procedures are listed in a step-by-step format and are illustrated with photographs to show students the correct methods for performing tasks. Note: Not all procedures are allowed in all states. You should be aware of limits set by state guidelines.

The demand for home health aides is expected to increase due to changing health care patterns related to increasing health care costs. This text was designed to train new individuals entering the field to be caring, dedicated, and skilled paraprofessionals. Although the skills required today for home health aides are different compared to those required early in this century, when home health aides first provided care to clients in their homes, the goal has not changed: to give safe, competent care to the client.

THE FIFTH EDITION

The fifth edition has been reorganized to integrate the procedures with the theory throughout the text to enhance the learning process. The fifth edition now features full-color photographs and illustrations, key terms in color, and an all-new design to aid in the learning process. Additional features of this edition include:

- incorporation of new CDC infection control guidelines
- OBRA-recommended content that ensures competency and compliance with federal training standards
- emphasis on the role of the home health aide as a valuable member of the health care team
- expanded end-of-chapter review questions
- case study-type review questions for each unit to help promote critical thinking
- appendix of emergency procedures guidelines
- new procedures for:
  Caring for a Client During a Seizure
  Burping an Infant

SUPPLEMENTS

The instructional system/package has been revised to achieve two goals:

1. To assist students in learning essential information to permit them to function as home health care providers.
2. To assist instructors in planning and implementing their instructional approach for the most efficient use of time and resources.

Instructor's Guide

The revised Instructor's Guide provides the instructor with valuable resources to simplify the planning and implementation of the instructional program. The Instructor's Guide includes:

- Teaching tips and strategies
- Teaching resources
- Course syllabus
- Individual unit lesson plans
- Class activities
- Additional review questions with answers
- Case studies with questions for discussion
- Quizzes and final examination with answers
- Answers to text review questions
- Answers to application exercises in workbook
- Answers to crossword puzzles

- Answers to quizzes and case studies in workbook
- Transparency masters

Workbook

The revised student workbook provides additional questions, practice exercises, quizzes, and case studies. This material is designed to help the student master the text content and skills. The workbook content includes:

- Unit objectives and terms to define
- Expanded application exercises, including true/false, short answer/fill-in-the-blanks, matching, multiple choice, and documentation exercises
- Crossword puzzles
- Quizzes
- Case studies with questions

ABOUT THE AUTHOR

Council for Jewish Elderly (CJE) has at its core a deep and abiding commitment to Jewish communal values and the dignity of the older person. Through dedication to quality programs and services, CJE provides care for all older people and their families. CJE acknowledges and respects the individuality and independence of each person it serves.

CJE's range of services extends from assisting those who live in their own homes, but may need occasional physical or psychological support, to those who need the most protection and care in a long-term facility. Established in 1972, CJE has continually met the daily needs of the Chicago elderly. For additional information, contact CJE at (773) 508-1000, or point your browser to http://www.cje.net.

The **Center for Applied Gerontology** is the first practice-focused adult education program initiated by a social service agency in Chicago. Established in 1984 by Council for Jewish Elderly, the Center provides certified and accredited education and training for professionals and paraprofessionals in the gerontological and geriatric fields. Its focus is on enhancing practice skills, presenting new knowledge, developing creative program and practice principles, sharing current research findings, and stimulating practice exchange among those who work with the elderly. For more information, or to request products and services, contact the Center at (773) 508-1075.

ACKNOWLEDGMENTS

As with any publication of this magnitude, we owe many thanks to the numerous individuals who helped make this book a reality.

Ron Gould of Ron Gould Studios for his excellent photographs and his skill during the many hours of the photo shoot.

We would like to thank all CJE clients, staff, and volunteers who graciously served as models at the following Council for Jewish Elderly facilities: Joseph and Sylvia Robineau Residence, Herman and Gertrude Klafter Residence, Lieberman Geriatric Health Center, Adult Day Center, Swartzberg House, and the Bernard Horwich Building (part of the Jewish Community Centers of Metropolitan Chicago).

The following chapter authors contributed a vast amount of time and energy to ensure the excellence of this publication by providing the most up-to-date information for each of the units on which they worked:

Michelle Ackerman, B.S. (Jewish Vocational Service)

Sandra Alexander, M.S.W. (Alexander Consulting Services)

Maria Betke, R.N., B.S.N. (Chicago Health Outreach)

Ellen Cervantes, M.S.W. (Bernard Weinger Jewish Community Center)

Anna Fallon, L.C.S.W. (Council for Jewish Elderly)

Kay Francel, R.N. (Council for Jewish Elderly)

Naomi Griffin, L.P.N. (Jewish Vocational Service)

Jo Hammerman, L.C.S.W. (Council for Jewish Elderly)

Carol Harris, B.S.N., R.N. (Council for Jewish Elderly)

Jeanne Heid-Grubman, L.C.S.W. (Catholic Charities)

Amy Keller, M.A. (Center for Applied Gerontology)

Kate Kesteloot Scarborough, B.G.S. (Council for Jewish Elderly)

Barbara Kravitz, M.S., R.N. (Council for Jewish Elderly)

Sherry Lopata, R.N., B.S.N. (Council for Jewish Elderly)

Hedda Lubin, C.P.M., B.A. (Council for Jewish Elderly)

Soli Mostafavipour, R.N., B.S.N. (Council for Jewish Elderly)

Bella Panchmatia, R.N., M.S. (Council for Jewish Elderly)

Dorit Weinberg, M.S., R.D. (Nutrition consultant)

Special thanks go to Sandy Alexander, for her efforts throughout the revision process; Barbara Carter; Lisa Guinta; Amy Keller; Patti Reczek; and Charlotte Schuerman.

The authors and Delmar Publishers wish to thank the following reviewers for helping to shape the final product:

Jody Badgley, R.N., B.A.
Lee County High Tech Center North
Fort Myers, Florida

Carol A. Conti, R.N., M.S. in Nursing Education
Progressive Home Health
Staten Island, New York

Joann Jeannenot, A.A.
Director, Home Care Department
Hampshire County Visting Nurse Association
Northampton, Massachusetts

Mary A. Pasqual
Central County Occupation Center
San Jose, California

Mary Elizabeth Rizzuto, M.S.N., R.N.C.S., C.N.A.A.
Nursing Administrator
Allied Home Health Nursing Services
San Antonio, Texas

Mechelle Sheppard
Home Health Instructor
Sparks State Technical College
Eufaula, Alabama

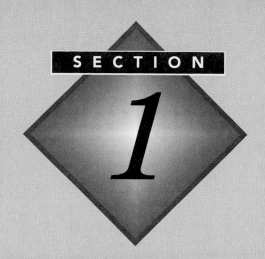

SECTION

1

Becoming a Home Health Aide

Units

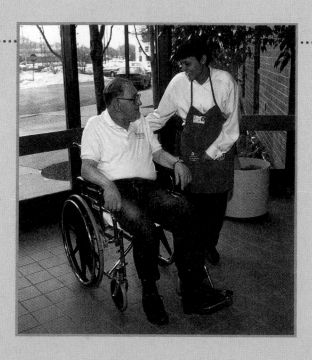

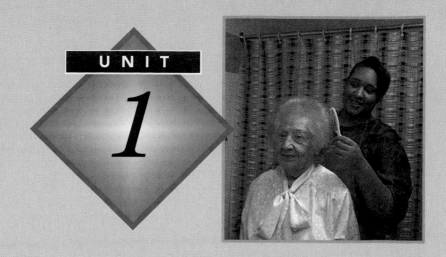

Home Health Services

KEY TERMS

acute illness
case manager (CM)
chronic illness
companion
culture
developmentally disabled
diversity
home care aide
home health aide
home health care agencies
homemaker
homemaker/home health
  aide

homemaker/home care
  agencies
hospice
licensed nurse agencies
licensed practical nurse
  (LPN)
managed care
Medicaid
Medicare
Omnibus Budget Reconcili-
  ation Act (OBRA)
occupational therapist (OT)
personal care worker

physical therapist (PT)
physician (MD)
registered nurse (RN)
social service agencies
social worker (MSW, LCSW,
  LSW)
speech therapist (ST)
terminal illness

LEARNING OBJECTIVES

After studying this unit, you should be able to:

- Name three reasons why the trend toward home care has returned.
- Name two services provided by the home health aide.
- Name members of the health care team.

- Name a type of home care agency.
- Give an example of a managed care organization.
- Describe a hospice.
- Define cultural diversity.

THE DEVELOPMENT OF HOME HEALTH SERVICES

In the early years of our society, a majority of the population lived on farms in rural areas. The family unit was often an extended family, with different generations living together and sharing responsibilities. Family members cared for each other. Women were typically not employed outside of the home. It was their responsibility to care for the children and the frail or disabled members of the family. If the mother could not care for the child, the grandmother or aunt did the caregiving. A member of the community who was trained in medicine or health care may have come to the home for emergencies or, in the case of midwives, for labor and delivery. But, there were few, if any hospitals and nursing homes. Home care agencies did not exist.

The industrial revolution of the 18th and 19th centuries created sweeping economic and social changes in our society. It created jobs in the city and automobiles to get there. Children began to move away from their parents' homes, finding employment in an variety of places. Extended families were replaced by the nuclear family, consisting of the parents and their children. There were more single parents, attempting to raise children on their own.

When the mother became ill or died, the family was thrown into crisis. Often no one else was available to take care of family members. Services were needed to help these families survive.

The first homemaker service was established by a social service agency in the United States in 1903. Its main purpose was to provide child care. In the early 1920s employment agencies advertised for mature, practical women experienced in child care and household management. During the Depression of the 1930s the Work Projects Administration funded a program to train the unemployed as "housekeeping aides." They received formal training and some on-the-job training as well. In 1959, the National Conference on Homemaker Service met in Chicago. It was decided that homemaker service should be given to families with children, chronically ill persons, or aged members. It was advised that these individuals should receive care in the home whenever possible, without regard to family income. In 1960, at another conference, personal care and health care were seen as added duties of a homemaker's job; the term **home health aide** came into use. Home health aides were expected to work only under direct nursing supervision.

In 1976, laws were passed in a few states setting minimum standards for home health aides. In 1987, the **Omnibus Budget Reconciliation Act**, known as **OBRA**, was passed, which mandates national standards for federally funded nursing homes and home health agencies. A variety of topics and issues concerning health care for the elderly and developmentally disabled were covered in this legislation, such as the use of restraints, nursing assistant and home health aide training guidelines, and rights of the clients. The primary goal of OBRA regulations is to improve care both for individuals in long-term care facilities and for those in their own homes.

INCREASE IN NEED FOR HOME CARE SERVICES

Home care is now one of the fastest growing businesses in this country.

There are a number of reasons for the increase in the need for home care. One of the main reasons is that older adults, the main recipients of home care, are the fastest growing population in the country. People are living longer due to advances in health care and modern technology. Approximately 23% of the elderly need assistance with personal care activities and 27% have difficulty in home management activities.

A second reason for the increased need for home care services is the high cost of hospital care and the trend on the part of providers and payers to keep costs down. As a result of this trend, patients are often sent home from the hospital as soon as medically possible. Many of these clients still need follow-up care, which can be provided more economically by a home health agency. This trend has led to the tremendous growth in the field of home health care.

A third reason for the increase in home care is that most individuals prefer to remain in their own homes when they become ill or frail, rather than moving to an unfamiliar setting, such as a nursing home. They wish to sleep in their own beds, eat at their own kitchen tables, and talk on their own telephones. They want to have control over their own life-styles—when they get up in the morning and go to bed at night, what they have for dinner, and who they let into their homes. They want to be near their loved ones, friends, and neighbors.

As a result, there has been a move away from nursing home placement now that more home care services are available. Home care options have increased in response to this desire to remain at home. The goal has been to help seniors "age in place," without having to make a move before necessary.

It is sometimes necessary, however, to make that move to a nursing facility. In many areas of the country, there is a shortage of nursing homes. Those that are available may have long waiting lists. Nursing facilities are being used for individuals who are more frail, ill, or in need of continuous care than was previously the case.

A fourth reason for the steady increase in home care services is the growing acceptance of home as a place to die. **Hospice** services are becoming more available to help a terminally ill patient die with dignity. Although some hospitals offer terminal care facilities, many hospice clients choose to die at home. Doctors, nurses, home health aides, social workers, and volunteers work as a team to make this possible. Bereavement counseling is also offered to family members. The unfortunate and persistent epidemic of acquired immunodeficiency syndrome (AIDS) has resulted in many hospice patients.

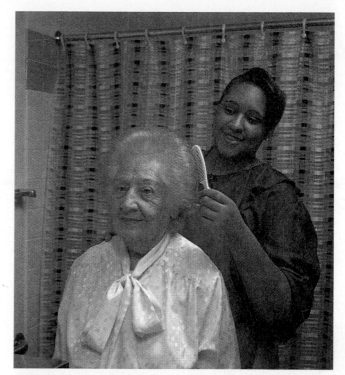

FIGURE 1-1 A home health aide assisting a client with her personal care

TYPES OF HOME CARE WORKERS ·····

Home care workers play key roles in their clients' lives. They perform many of the duties that are necessary for their clients to remain at home. Their duties may fall into two main categories—care of the person and care of the home. Care of the person includes assistance with activities of daily living, such as bathing, dressing, toileting, and simple nursing tasks, such as taking blood pressure or assisting with exercises (Figure 1-1). (See Chapter 2 for more details regarding roles.) Care of the home includes light housekeeping, cooking, shopping, and other homemaking duties (Figure 1-2).

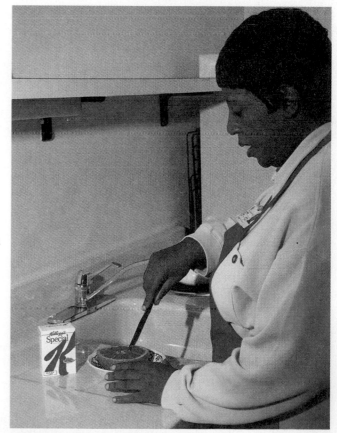

FIGURE 1-2 A home health aide preparing a meal

Care of the person requires more training than care of the home. Some workers do all of the above; others may have more limited roles. The role depends on the amount of training that the worker has had and how the person is classified on the state registry (Figure 1-3). The worker's supervisor designs a separate care plan to be followed for each client. The care plan specifically outlines the home care worker's responsibilities.

FIGURE 1-3 Home health aide functions approved by most states

A. Routine home health aide functions include the following:
 1. With guidance from the nurse or agency supervisor, arranging the schedule so that the client follows the care plan such as increased physical activity and other activities of daily living
 2. Keeping an aide care plan as part of the client record
 3. Taking temperature, pulse, and respiration
 4. Assisting the client on and off the bedpan, commode, or toilet
 5. Assisting with bathing of the client in bed, in the tub, or in the shower as determined by the doctor, nurse, or agency supervisor
 6. Assisting with the care of teeth and mouth
 7. Assisting with grooming—care of hair, including shampooing; shaving; and the ordinary care of the nails
 8. Assisting the client with dressing
 9. Assisting the client with eating
 10. Assisting the client in moving from bed to chair or wheelchair and assisting the client in walking
 11. Accompanying the client to obtain medical care (when practical)
 12. Preparing and serving meals according to instructions
 13. Washing dishes as needed
 14. Making or changing the bed
 15. Reminding clients to take medications on schedule
 16. Doing light housekeeping, i.e., dusting and vacuuming the rooms the clients uses
 17. Listing needed supplies
 18. Shopping for the client if no other arrangement is possible
 19. Doing the client's personal laundry if no family member is available or able; may include necessary ironing and mending
 20. Notifying supervisor or case manager to whom you report of any change in the client's condition
B. Special home health aide functions:
 With permission of the case manager or supervisor, the home health aide may do the following procedures:
 1. Reinforcing dressings and changing simple nonsterile dressings
 2. Applying prescribed ice cap or ice collar
 3. Applying TED hose
 4. Assisting with prescribed skin care
 5. Taking the blood pressure
 6. Assisting with the change of ostomy bags
 7. Measuring intake and output, as ordered
 8. Preparing modified diets, as prescribed by the physician
 9. Assisting the client with prescribed exercises that have been taught by appropriate professional personnel
 10. Helping the client relearn household skills
 11. Assisting with rehabilitation measures

The following are some of the more commonly used titles for home care workers.

Companion—Keeps the client company or maintains safety; usually does not provide personal or homemaking services.

Homemaker—Performs household duties, such as laundry and cooking, as well as light housecleaning.

Personal care worker—Assists with a minimal level of daily living activities, such as meal preparation and companionship, as well as minimal assistance with personal care.

Home health aide—Provides substantial assistance with personal care, such as bathing and dressing, as well as supervised health assistance, such as assistance with rehabilitation activities and self-administered medication.

Homemaker/home health aide—Assists in general household tasks, as well as those listed above for the home health aide.

Home care aide—Works with the client with the goal of assisting the client with independent living under professional supervision (title promoted by the National Association for Home Care).

The Health Care Team

The home health aide is one member of the health care team. Although members may not see each other on a regular basis, the team still exists. Other specially trained health care personnel who are part of the health care team may include:

Physician (MD)—Authorizes home health care treatment; supervises plan of care.

Registered nurse (RN)—Assesses clients' conditions and determines types of personal and nursing care needed; provides direct care to clients, such as treatments and medications; educates clients and families; may supervise home health aide.

Licensed practical nurse (LPN)—Provides direct care to the client, such as treatments and medication; may supervise home care workers.

Case manager (CM)—Assesses overall needs of the client and decides what services should be provided; usually performed by a nurse or social worker; may supervise the home care worker. (Many home care agencies combine the role of the case manager and the registered nurse.)

Social worker (MSW, LCSW, LSW)—Assesses social and emotional aspects of the home situation; assists client and family to cope with problems and to plan for the future; identifies available community resources.

Physical therapist (PT)—Assesses client's ability to stand, walk, climb stairs, transfer, and other activities related to strength and endurance; develops plan of treatment including some exercises done by PT during home visits and others to be assisted by the family and home health aide.

Occupational therapist (OT)—Evaluates client's ability to perform skills necessary for independent daily living, such as bathing, dressing, cooking; works with client to improve abilities; develops plan of care to be assisted by family and home health aide.

Speech therapist (ST)—Assesses client's ability to communicate—hear, speak, understand, and write; works with client to improve abilities. Also assesses swallowing difficulties and works with the client to improve swallowing functions.

TYPES OF HOME CARE AGENCIES .....

Home care agencies differ in many ways: types of services provided, fees for services, policies and procedures, and administrative structure. They are large and small, nonprofit and for profit, Medicare certified and non-Medicare certified. Home care agencies offer a range of services, including short-term medical care, long-term personal care, and housekeeping.

The main categories of home care agencies are:

Homemaker/home care agencies—These agencies provide a variety of nonmedical home support services. They provide homemakers, home health aides, companions, and other home care workers. They usually do not employ nurses. The workers are generally not under medical supervision, and their services are not reimbursed by Medicare.

Home health care agencies—These agencies, some of which are hospital affiliated, focus on the medical aspects of care. Their professionally trained personnel (e.g., registered nurses, licensed practical nurses, physical therapists, etc.) can do dressing changes, monitor vital signs, and perform other tasks as ordered by the physician. Most also offer the services of home health aides who are supervised by professional nurses. Their services may be paid for by Medicare for a period of time if they are ordered by a physician.

Social service agencies—In some communities, home care is available through social service agencies. Most of these organizations are nonprofit; many have a religious affiliation.

Licensed nurse agencies—In addition to private duty registered nurses, licensed practical nurses, or skilled therapists (for physical therapy, occupational therapy, or speech therapy), these agencies often provide home care workers (companions, homemakers, home health aides). Their services are usually not reimbursed by Medicare.

Another option for home care workers is to become self-employed. These workers have the benefits of working independently, but have some challenges as well. They must find their own clients. If their clients are temporarily hospitalized or placed in a nursing facility, they are temporarily without work. These workers are not protected by liability insurance, in case something happens while their clients are under their care. They also are responsible for filing their own income tax and part of their FICA (Social Security contributions).*

REIMBURSEMENT ISSUES INFLUENCING HEALTH CARE

Reimbursement is a rapidly changing area in health care. It is important that the home health aide is aware of these issues and how they af-

fect the worker's agency. The home health aide should always ask a supervisor if there is a question about reimbursement for the services being performed.

Medicare

At the present time, all individuals in the United States who have paid into Social Security are entitled to apply for **Medicare** insurance once they are disabled or become 65 years of age. There are two reimbursement parts to this federally funded program, Part A and Part B. Part A is for hospitalizations, stays in skilled nursing facilities, and home health care. Part B is for physician services, diagnostic tests, and therapies. An additional monthly fee is required to qualify for Part B. Medicare insurance pays for part of the costs of health care, but certainly not all.

To qualify for Medicare reimbursement for home health, an individual must be:

- Confined to home
- Under the care of a doctor who certifies the need for care
- In need of skilled nursing care (as provided by a professional nurse), physical therapy, or speech therapy
- Receiving services from a Medicare-certified agency

Medicaid

Medicaid is a federally and state-funded program that pays for health care services for persons whose income is below a certain amount. The coverage provided to recipients and the minimum income level that makes one eligible varies from state to state. Some states also have programs that allow them to provide services to seniors living in the community whose income is above the Medicaid level. These seniors usually pay according to their incomes. The purpose of these programs is to prevent seniors from moving into nursing homes before it is absolutely necessary. A person can qualify for both Medicare and Medicaid or other community support programs.

Whenever government funding is involved, the federal or state government can regulate the health care industry and demand that certain

*Information in this section was adapted with permission from *Someone Who Cares: A Guide to Hiring an In-Home Caregiver*, Center for Applied Gerontology, 1994.

standards be maintained with regard to health care facilities, health care workers, and educational requirements. The home health aide must be aware of these standards.

Managed Care

Health maintenance organizations (HMOs) are examples of **managed care**. This is a method of health care delivery that attempts to cut costs through providing gatekeepers to control access to and use of physicians, hospitals, nursing facilities, and other forms of care. The goal of this gatekeeper, whether it be a nurse case manager or a physician, is to provide the best quality care for the lowest cost. Home care, for example, may be a less costly and more appealing alternative in certain situations. Managed care companies usually offer their patients fewer choices of physicians, hospitals, nursing homes, and other health providers. The out-of-pocket cost to the patient, however, is usually lower than with traditional insurance.

These companies often apply the same eligibility restrictions as Medicare, although there has been some expansion in recent years. In fact, Medicare has been offering its recipients the choice of taking traditional Medicare coverage or signing up with special Medicare managed care plans. Medicaid also has been developing managed care alternatives.

THE CLIENT

Home care clients are of all ages, from birth to more than 100 years old. They are typically either chronically ill, acutely ill, terminally ill, or developmentally disabled. The majority of the aged individuals are affected by one or more chronic illnesses. A **chronic illness** is a long-term health problem, such as arthritis, diabetes, or Alzheimer's disease, which is not generally expected to be cured. An **acute illness** is one that arises quickly, requires immediate care, and can be expected to go away, such as a common cold, flu, or appendicitis. A **terminal illness** is one that is expected to result in death within a limited period of time. The term **developmentally disabled** means the person has a severe chronic disability, such as cerebral palsy or Down's syndrome.

Home care clients are truly diverse (Figure 1-4). They represent different cultures and ethnic groups—Hispanics, Asians, Eastern Europeans, and so forth. They are different races, including African Americans, Anglo-Americans, and Native Americans. They practice different religions—such as Protestantism, Catholicism, Judaism, Muslim, or Buddhism. Throughout this text, you will find examples of this **diversity** among your clients.

The ethnic makeup of our senior population is rapidly changing. The U.S. Census Bureau expects that by the year 2000 there will be a 57% growth in the Asian American senior population and a 36% increase in the Hispanic senior population. This compares to a 15% growth in senior African Americans and 4% in Anglo-Americans.

Home health workers cannot expect to know everything about every different culture, race, or religion. It is important, however, to realize that there are differences, to be accepting of them and to be willing to learn about them. Home health aides may learn, for example, that Native American medicine and religion cannot be separated and that they will turn to traditional healing practices from time to time. An aide may also learn about the strength of family ties in the Hispanic culture or about the dietary practices of the Orthodox Jewish faith.

Religious practices, traditions, types of food, and the manner in which food is prepared are very often determined by the **culture** and religion of the individual. The home health aide

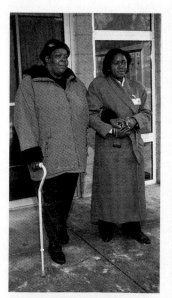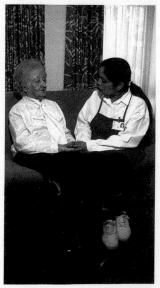

FIGURE 1-4   Home health clients represent many cultures.

must (1) accept the practices of others, (2) be sensitive to the client's needs, and (3) follow the instructions given by the case manager in meeting the needs of the client regardless of religion, color, or belief. An aide must not judge clients, but must allow them the freedom to follow their own practices and beliefs while the aide provides safe and proper care.

In each unit of this text, you will find new words to master and new techniques to learn. As your knowledge grows, so does your confidence as an individual. In becoming a home health aide, you can be proud of your newly acquired skills. Satisfaction comes in being able to serve those who need your skills.

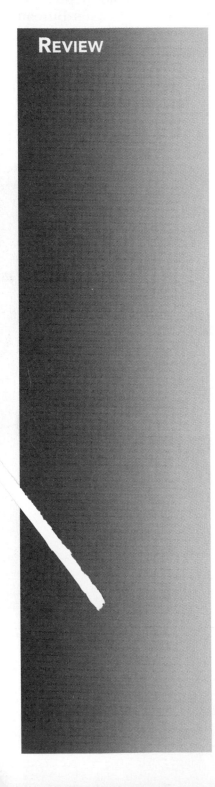

REVIEW

1. List three reasons for the increasing trend toward home care.

2. List two main services provided by the home health aide.

3. Name two differences between Medicare and Medicaid.

4. A _____ helps clients to improve their abilities to perform skills necessary to independent daily living—bathing, dressing, cooking, etc.
   a. Physical therapist
   b. Speech therapist
   c. Physician
   d. Occupational therapist

5. A _____ agency focuses on the medical aspects of home care, many of which are reimbursed by Medicare.
   a. Homemaker/home care agency
   b. Home health care agency
   c. Social service agency
   d. Licensed nurse agency

6. One example of a managed care organization is a:
   a. Nursing home
   b. HMO (health maintenance organization)
   c. Department store
   d. School

7. Payment for the home health aide services is collected by the agency that assumes responsibility for your client. These payments may come from:
   a. Medicare
   b. Medicaid
   c. The client
   d. Any of the above

8. Home health aide care involves:
   a. Client care and housekeeping activities
   b. Supervising client's care
   c. Laundry and wallpapering
   d. Client care and giving injections

9. A hospice cares for clients who are:
   a. Chronically ill
   b. Acutely ill
   c. Terminally ill
   d. Developmentally disabled

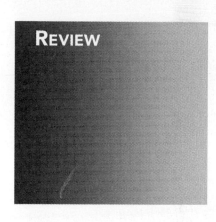

REVIEW

10. A home health aide needs to be aware of the client's:
   a. Cultural differences
   b. Physical needs
   c. Family situations
   d. All of the above

11. (T) F   The U.S. Census Bureau expects there to be a 57% growth in the Asian American population by the year 2000.

12. (T) F   Home health aides should be aware of the reimbursement issues affecting their agencies.

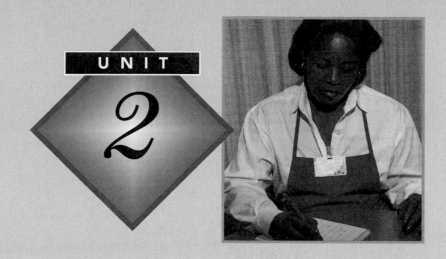

Responsibilities of the Home Health Aide

KEY TERMS

....

abuse	flexible	observation
career	hygiene	oral hygiene
components	interaction	practice
confidentiality	interpersonal	procedure
documentation	relationships	report
ethics	liability	theory
evaluation	negligence	time organization

LEARNING OBJECTIVES

....

After studying this unit, you should be able to:

- List three important qualities of the home health aide.
- Give five examples of actions to avoid that can lead to liability.
- Explain why accurate observation, reporting, and documentation are important tasks.
- Give examples of good personal hygiene.
- Define ethics, and identify two examples of ethical practice.
- List five "rights" of the client.
- List three "rights" of the home health aide.
- Define client abuse.
- List four kinds of abuse.

SKILLS AND QUALITIES OF THE HOME HEALTH AIDE

A **career** is the occupation or profession for which one has been specially educated. Teacher, lawyer, electrician, and home health aide are examples of careers. In addition to the training and education that are required for each career, certain personal qualities or characteristics make people good at what they do. It is important for a teacher to like children, for a lawyer to be a good communicator, and for an electrician to be cautious and not take risks. Likewise, a number of special qualities make for a good home health aide.

If one were to read an ad in the newspaper, it may read something like what is shown in Figure 2-1.

Flexibility

The home health aide will encounter irregular working hours and must be able to adjust to a variety of assignments, settings, and equipment.

Working Hours.   Working hours may be irregular. Primarily the working hours will be during the day, but occasionally a home health aide may be required to work during the night. The aide may be asked to work on varying shifts or on weekends. It is common for a home health aide to be assigned several part-time cases. Three different clients might be visited in one day or on different days of the week. Due to this irregularity of assignments, a home health aide must be **flexible** and have access to transportation. This means being able to quickly adjust from one type of situation to another and being able to feel comfortable meeting new people.

Variety of Assignments.   The aide must adjust to different family situations and varied health care needs of the clients. In one home, the aide might be expected to care for infants, preschool children, and teenagers. In another home, there may be only middle-aged or elderly people. No two family situations are the same. This means the aide will have to establish new interpersonal relationships in each case. The medical conditions can range from ill infants to terminally ill clients. The aide must be prepared to give safe and proper care in each situation.

Variety of Settings and Equipment.   The aide must adapt also to homes that are not as well equipped as others. Some homes have modern equipment and beautiful furnishings. Other homes offer the bare necessities of life. The home health aide must not make judgments about people based on their belongings. Some clients prefer simple living. The aide also should remember that most people who live in poverty do not do so by choice. The home health aide will be expected to treat all clients with dignity regardless of their financial position. Each human being is entitled to respectful and dignified care. That is the only kind of care that a home health aide is trained to perform (Figure 2-2).

Ability to Follow Instructions

The being "able" part is what you are learning in this class. At first glance, the role of the home health aide may appear to be simple. It is made up of everyday tasks: keeping a house in order, preparing and cleaning up after meals, and providing for the comfort and safety of a client. Students may feel that they already know how to take care of a house. Most people have been doing housekeeping tasks since early childhood. They think there is nothing new to learn. The student may ask, "Why don't we get to the important things? I want to take care of the sick. Why should I waste my time relearning homemaking skills?" However, everyone can benefit by learning new ways to do certain jobs. Once the new method is learned, the aide can compare it with the old way and may discover a more efficient technique.

By learning to focus on the components of a task, the aide will find understanding comes

---

WANTED:

Home health aides to care for persons in their own homes. Applicants must have the following qualities:

- Flexible
- Willing and able to follow instructions
- Well-organized

- Good interpersonal skills
- Observant
- Ethical
- Good personal hygiene

FIGURE 2-1   Sample ad in the newspaper

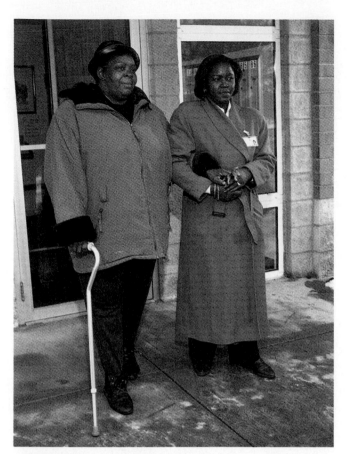

FIGURE 2-2   An aide ambulating a client outside

more easily. **Components** are the separate parts that make up a whole. Learning how to do something, when to do it, and what should be done first will add up to a more complete understanding. Students must learn how and when to do all the tasks that need to be done. They also learn what tasks are most important. In this way, the student completing the course will become a successful home health aide.

There are many ways to do some tasks, for example, preparing a meal. There will be certain essential components of the task that if not completed correctly and in the right order will mean the task has been done wrong. For example, you need to wash your hands first. You need to follow the client's dietary requirements, but you may prepare any of a variety of foods. You can toast the bread before or after you slice a tomato, but you must put ingredients away and clean up after preparing food. Other tasks, however, have rigid procedures and only one way to proceed, such as washing hands and taking an oral temperature. A **procedure** is a list of steps used to complete a task. A procedure can be either a nursing task or a homemaking task.

There are usually two parts to the instruction given to the home health aide. The first is called theory. **Theory** is the information that forms a basis for action. In classroom lectures and in the assigned readings, the student learns theory. The second component is devoted to practice. **Practice** is the actual performance of the procedures. Practice is combined with the theory to enable the student to build skills in both areas at the same time. The home health aide learns client care procedures and homemaking procedures.

The student will need to demonstrate a designated list of procedures satisfactorily in front of an instructor. Each procedure will be demonstrated by the instructor before the student performs the procedure. The instructor will give the student a copy of the procedure with all the required steps listed. Use these procedure guidelines in practicing each procedure in the laboratory. Your instructor will determine if you have learned the procedure correctly by giving you an evaluation. An **evaluation** may consist of written tests or demonstrations where you actually perform the procedure. Evaluation helps the student know which areas require extra study or practice.

Willingness to Follow Instructions

As important as being able to follow the instructions of your supervisor is being willing to follow them. Before taking a case, a home health aide should be sure to ask for all vital information. In addition, the supervisor will provide a home care plan for the client, outlining the specific care to be provided and the aide's responsibilities. This includes duties, client needs, and the name and telephone number of the person to be contacted in emergencies.

Both ability and willingness to follow instructions affect the home health aide's liability when things go wrong.

LIABILITY

Liability refers to the degree to which you are held responsible for something that goes wrong on the job. Probably the most important protection from liability that is available to you is to *do* *only and exactly what your supervisor instructs you to do.* When you follow these instructions, your agency assumes responsibility for your actions. There are some pitfalls that you should recognize and avoid:

1. *Doing more than is assigned.* Practice saying "no" in a nice way, encouraging the client to contact the supervisor if more services are wanted. When you do something that was not assigned, you are assuming responsibility (liability) for these acts, and your agency is no longer responsible.

2. *Doing less than is assigned.* This may put the client in danger and lead to a charge of **negligence,** which means "an action or lack of action that leads to an accident or injury."

3. *Doing hasty, careless, or poor-quality work.* You have received training in the proper way to carry out your work activities. It is your responsibility to work carefully. Sometimes, even with the greatest amount of care being taken, accidents happen: a valuable vase breaks while you are dusting it or a client falls. If you have been carrying out your assigned duties and exercising a normal amount of care, you usually are not held liable for the damage or injury that results; agencies carry liability insurance to cover these kinds of accidents.

4. *Using your car for work activities without notifying your insurance company.* This particularly applies to taking clients out in your car, even to the doctor's office or clinic appointments, without letting your insurance agency know. If an accident occurs, you might be liable for injury. It is also a good idea to be sure the agency approves of your taking clients in the car (Figures 2-3 and 2-4).

5. *Failing to do accurate reporting and documentation.* If you see a client doing something wrong, such as failing to take medicine properly, abusing another family member, or being abused by others, and you do not include that in your report because you tell yourself, "She doesn't like the taste of that medicine and anyway, it's so expensive," or "He's such a nice man, he couldn't possibly have meant to bruise his wife like that," you are leaving yourself open to charges of negligence.

6. *Failing to act in an emergency.* You should know what the emergency plan is for each client you care for, and you should be pre-

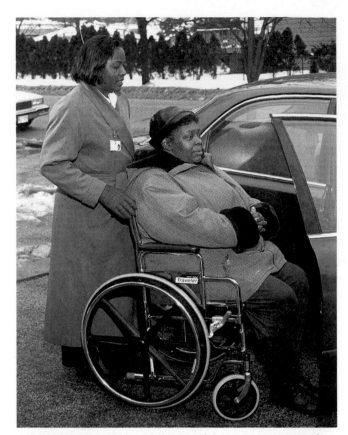

FIGURE 2-3 Always have the permission of your agency before transporting a client in your own car.

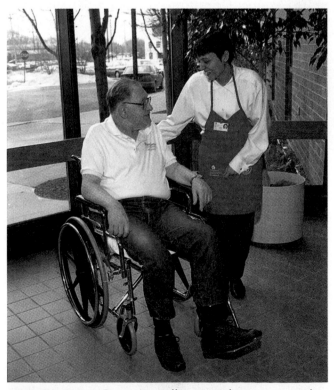

FIGURE 2-4 Occasionally an aide may need to accompany a client to the outpatient department of a hospital for therapy.

pared to follow it. In a life-threatening situation, call for an ambulance before calling the supervisor. Do not try to perform first aid or cardiopulmonary resuscitation (CPR) if you have not been trained to do so.

7. *Attempting to do things that are beyond your abilities.* It is okay to say, "I don't know how to do that. Let's see if we can get someone who does." You are not employed as a nurse, a plumber, an electrician, or a counselor . . . do not try to be one.

8. *Injuring yourself or the client* by doing something you are not assigned or adequately trained to do. If you have been assigned to do something you do not feel comfortable doing, ask for more training. Trying to do something without assignment and adequate training, such as moving a client with a Hoyer lift, can leave you liable for injury that results.

9. *Failing to report* unsafe working conditions that later cause injury to you or another home health aide. Do not take unnecessary risks. Follow the agency procedures for reporting.

Organizational Skills

A successful aide possesses good organizational skills. An aide must manage time well to be able to complete all the tasks required in the allotted time. The instructions may include light housekeeping, laundry and ironing, meal preparation, marketing, and personal care of the client. The aide will have to decide the best way to plan each day's activities. This will require flexibility, practical judgment, and **time organization.** Some pitfalls to avoid are:

- Not replacing or ordering supplies when needed from your case manager
- Gossiping with the client or family member instead of working
- Watching a favorite television show
- Jumping from one task to another and one room to another without organizing priorities
- Putting off unpleasant tasks because they are disagreeable
- Talking to friends on the telephone or doing personal business
- Stopping frequently for a cup of coffee
- Trying to do too much in one day and, thus, doing nothing well

The best way to deal with a new set of circumstances is to look over the situation care-

fully and get organized. On entering a new situation, it is human nature to think about the end result. Often one is tempted to try to do everything in one day. This leads to frustration, and nothing gets done well. Begin by asking where supplies are stored. Communicate with the family and supervisor to find out exactly what is expected. Prepare a written plan each day for the cases assigned (Figures 2-5A and B). At the end of the working day, see what did not get done. Revise the plan for the next day. It is best to select only one big project for each day. After the routine tasks and client care procedures are done for the day, tackle the larger job. These tasks can be planned for periods when the client does not require your full attention. The household often will function better as a result of preplanning and organization.

A home health aide may be assigned to work with several clients each week. The aide should prepare a schedule for each assignment. In this

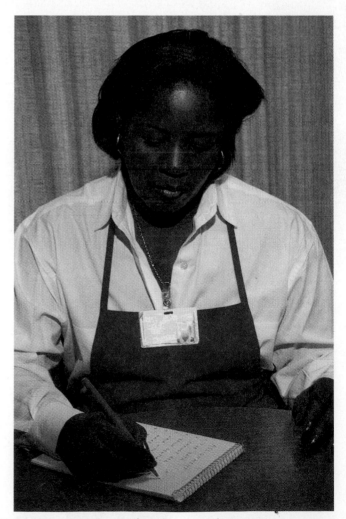

FIGURE 2-5A   Aide planning her assignment before the start of her work day

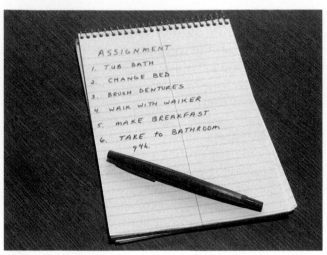

FIGURE 2-5B This is a sample list of tasks to be completed by the aide.

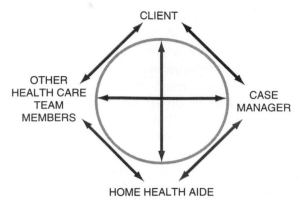

FIGURE 2-6 A home health aide needs to interact with all members of the health care team and is an important member of the team.

way the aide's time can be used most efficiently. Each daily plan should be flexible enough to allow for the unexpected. The supervisor can make suggestions and help define the duties in each case. The aide must perform these duties in the time allotted.

When beginning a new job, the aide must adjust to the client's or family's routine. Aides should not reorganize the entire house or daily schedule to suit themselves. Major changes should be made only with the approval of the client or a responsible family member. An aide's job is to make the family comfortable and to assist them, not to change their life-style. A well-organized home health aide saves time and effort by planning ahead and anticipating possible problems.

INTERPERSONAL SKILLS

When people live, work, or play together, one person acts and the other reacts or responds to the act. This process is called an **interaction.** Figure 2-6 shows that several persons may be involved in a situation—the arrows point to all the possible interactions.

People are expected to handle interactions as a part of everyday life. The feeling and understanding that result from the interactions between two or more persons form what are called **interpersonal relationships.** To the person entering a service occupation, interpersonal relationships can determine success or

failure. Each of the persons involved in these relationships is entitled to be treated with dignity. Everyone should follow the golden rule—treat others as you would like to be treated. This helps to establish good interpersonal relationships.

In Figures 2-6, 2-7, and 2-8, look at the combinations of relationships that may develop for the home health aide. Home health aides must remember that they are entering a home where an illness or problem already exists. An illness or problem may cause the family members to be unhappy or disorganized. Anger, fear, and other emotional reactions may be obvious. The client may be in pain, cranky, sad, or depressed. The home health aide who is aware of the source of the problem often finds it easier to accept the family's behavior. As a result, awkward interpersonal relationships often can be avoided.

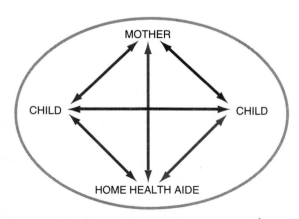

FIGURE 2-7 Many interactions may take place between the home health aide and family members.

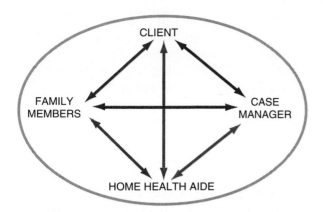

FIGURE 2-8 Learning to handle relationships is part of the home health aide's job.

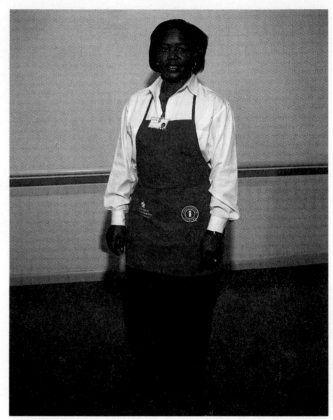

FIGURE 2-9 A well-groomed home health aide. Note the smile on her face and her neat appearance. Also note that aide wears little makeup or jewelry and that she wears a name tag on her uniform.

Clients may ask the aide to perform skills that have not been included in the nurse's instructions or in the aide's training. How can the aide inform the client that what has been requested is not part of the assigned duties? Anger and hostility accomplish nothing. The aide should say, "This procedure was not included in my training. I would have to contact my supervisor." If the request involves a housekeeping task that is not part of the nurse's instruction, the aide might say, "There are many things I can do, and am ready to do. However, I am required to follow the nurse's instruction, and your care plan does not state that particular task."

GOOD PERSONAL HEALTH AND HYGIENE

A home health aide must observe the personal **hygiene** standards expected of any health team member (Figure 2-9). When working in other people's homes, the aide should reflect the highest standards. This means being clean and well groomed each workday. The person who goes on a job unbathed, with dirty hair and nails, and wearing wrinkled, stained clothes makes a bad impression. A sloppy appearance implies that the person also has a poor self-image and sloppy working habits.

An aide should wear a clean uniform, clean undergarments, and comfortable, polished shoes.

An aide who is appropriately dressed or in the proper uniform creates a more professional appearance and makes the client feel more comfortable. Home care agencies vary greatly in their dress codes. A few agencies do require a designated uniform, whereas others may allow the aide to wear comfortable, clean, untattered street clothes. Most agencies do not allow their home health aides to wear blue jeans or shorts. In all situations, the aide must follow the agency's dress code or uniform requirement.

It is also important for the home health aide to wear a name tag at all times. The name tag gives the name of the aide and the proper title.

Bathing, brushing the teeth, and wearing a neat hair style is also part of good grooming. Fingernails should be short, smooth, and clean. Jewelry should be limited. Small post earrings for pierced ears are usually acceptable. Bracelets and dangling necklaces are not worn because they may catch on bedding or furniture. A ring might scratch the client or become lost.

Good grooming is important not only for appearance but also for safety reasons. Jewelry and rough fingernails could cause scratches. The danger of infection is always present if the skin has been scratched. Dirt and germs may easily enter an opening in the skin. Infected wounds heal more slowly among clients who are affected with other serious illnesses. The home health aide must not add pain or discomfort to the client by being careless.

Personal cleanliness is also necessary to prevent and remove body odors. A home health aide is in close contact with clients; odors can be quite offensive. Remember, some clients may be allergic to perfumes. Body odors should be removed with soap and water, not covered up with perfume. A considerate home health aide will check mouth odor as well. Brushing teeth regularly and using mouthwash helps prevent mouth odors. Eating garlic and onions and smoking cigarettes increases the need for oral hygiene. **Oral hygiene** means keeping the mouth clean and healthy. One important way to improve oral hygiene is to have annual dental checkups. It must be emphasized that an aide should not smoke while on duty. Clients with lung disease, allergies, respiratory illness, or personal distaste for the smell of cigarettes may have an adverse reaction to cigarette smoke.

SKILLS OF OBSERVATION

In many cases, the client is with the home health aide more than any other human being. If there is a problem, the aide may be the only, or at least the most likely, person to notice it. The client may be developing a rash, losing weight, or becoming confused—all indications that there may be a problem. If the problem is noticed and professional assistance is obtained, it may be resolved. If not, the situation may be life-threatening. That is why the aide's skills of **observation** are so important.

All five senses (seeing, hearing, touching, smelling, and tasting) should be used in the day-to-day work of the home health aide. Let's consider each sense:

1. Seeing
   Look at the client carefully, watching for any changes since your last visit. Some of the things you might note are facial expression, posture, skin color and cleanliness, rashes, discharges, redness, swelling, evenness of facial features, way of walking (gait), steadiness, stains on clothing.
   Look at the home for safety hazards (frayed electric cords, wet floors, throw rugs, loose steps), cleanliness, medications sitting out, food supply, spots, stains, and spills on clothing, furniture, or floors.

2. Hearing
   Listen to the client. What is being said? How is it being said? Is the client's speech clear or slurred? Is it logical or nonsensical? Are the words sad, angry, friendly, or hostile? Do you hear wheezing, coughing, or gasping for breath?
   Listen to the home. Does the faucet drip? Does the refrigerator vibrate? Is the radio or television volume too loud to permit conversation? Are the telephone and doorbell loud enough for the client to hear?

3. Touching
   Does the client's skin feel hot, cold, or moist? Is it rough, or puffy? What is the pulse rate?
   Are the sheets dry? Is the diaper wet? Is the bread dried out? Are the crackers soggy? Is the bath water too hot?

4. Smelling
   Does the client have bad breath or body odor? Does the odor smell like perspiration, urine, feces, alcohol, or fruit? Is there an odor from a wound or dressing?
   How do the bathroom, bedroom, and kitchen smell? How does the inside of the refrigerator smell? Have items of food spoiled?

5. Tasting
   Is the food too salty or too spicy?

REPORTING

Some important instructions that you need during your orientation to the agency are how to **report** information, who to report it to, and when to report it. You have a right to know these "who, what, when, and how" procedures, and a responsibility to ask if you are not told.

In most agencies, one person will be in charge of the care given to the client. This person may be called the supervisor or case manager. This is the person you probably will be instructed to contact when you have information to share about the client.

You will need to exercise judgment in making these reports. Some things need to be reported immediately, even while you are with the client, such as falls. Some things need to be reported as soon as you leave the home. Other things can wait until a regular conference, staffing, or written report. Anything you learn that puts the client in danger should be reported immediately. Such things usually involve physical problems (e.g., chest pain, falls, or deep cuts). Other observations may leave you unsure, and you would want to talk them over with the supervisor at your first opportunity. Some observations that leave you unsure might be forgetfulness, decreased appetite, or reduced social contacts. Still other things can wait for regular contact times.

Throughout your career as a home health aide, and especially as a beginner, you should remember that it is *always* better to report something even if you are not sure how important it is, rather than to risk endangering the client, the agency, and yourself by not reporting it. Good supervisors can help you learn how to sort out the "crisis" from the "unusual," and develop good judgment in reporting. You should never feel or be made to feel that the supervisor is "too busy" or that your information might be "too unimportant." Your supervisor is employed to help you give good client care, and, as you read earlier, an important part of that care is what you observe and report. When you talk over your observations and your feelings with the supervisor, you can speak freely and voice your opinions and small details. All of these help the supervisor to make decisions; he or she can help you learn to be more concise and accurate in your oral reports as time goes by.

DOCUMENTING

Writing down your observations and actions, or **documentation,** is an important part of your job. Your agency will show you the forms they want you to use and will tell you how often you need to document something in writing, where to do it, and where and when to turn it in.

There is a saying that "The job's not over till the paperwork's done." This certainly holds true in home health care. The information you write, which may be called a "narrative," "observation," "notes," or "charting," becomes part of the client's record, or chart. The information contained in client records is of critical importance for these reasons:

1. It is a lasting record of what was done to, for, and by the client. If it is not charted, it is considered not to have been done.
2. It is a record of what was observed about the client.
3. It is a record of how the client reacted to the care that was given.
4. It contains information that can be used by other team members in evaluating the care that was given and in deciding if changes in the care plan should be made.
5. If the client or family is unhappy with services and decides to complain, or, in the event of legal action, the client record can be used to show that certain things were done on certain dates and times.

When you are writing these reports, it is important that you:

1. *Be factual.* Write only those things that you know to be true, not what someone told you or what you think might be true.
2. *Be objective.* Write what you actually did, saw, heard, smelled, felt, or tasted. Do not try to interpret the cause or the feelings that went along with the observation. If you feel that you really must put something in the record that is your own interpretation, identify it as such.

   Do not diagnose. If the client complains of pains in his chest and arm, do not write, "Mr. Peterson had a heart attack and I called the ambulance." Instead, write, "Mr. Peterson complained of severe pains in his chest and upper left arm. His face was pale and moist. I called the ambulance."

   If you observed a large discolored area on the client's arm, write a description of it. Do not write, "Mrs. Jones has a big bruise on her arm where I think her husband grabbed her when he got mad because she wet the bed." However, if the client told you this was what had happened, you could record it as, "Mrs. Jones told me that her husband was angry because she had wet the bed, and he grabbed her by the arm. There is a two-inch discolored, purple area on her left forearm just below the elbow."

3. *Be concise.* Plan your words before you write them. Use enough words to give clear information, but do not "write a book." The important facts should be obvious to another person reading your notes.

4. *Be neat.* Take care that your handwriting or printing is legible. If your writing is very small or very sprawling, try to improve it. If you make a mistake, cross it out with a single line and initial the mistake; this shows you made and corrected the error.

5. *Be accurate.* Be sure the record shows exactly what you did, and if it is appropriate, what the client's reaction was. If you were not able to carry out some activity that was assigned, give the reason ("I couldn't do the laundry because the washer was broken"). This shows that you did not forget the activity or purposely fail to do it. Be sure measurements (pulse, temperature, intake, and output) are correct.

6. *Sign and date every entry in the record.* Most agencies will want you to sign your name and title (Mary Simmons, HHA) at the end of every entry. It is important to put the date (month, day, and year) and the time the visit began and ended.

7. *Be sure what you write relates to the goals* set for and by the client. Do not let yourself fall in the bad habit of continually writing "No change," "Client was okay today," or other meaningless phrases. If the goal is to have the client learn better housekeeping methods, you might write, "Today, Mrs. Kitt washed the dishes immediately after lunch."

8. *Be descriptive.* "The kitchen was a mess" does not give as much information as "The sink was piled full of dishes coated with dried food. Spilled milk had soured on the floor. Roaches were crawling across the counter."

9. *Use the correct words and abbreviations.* Unit 3 has lists of the proper words and approved abbreviations to use in describing your observations. Try to use these words properly, instead of using slang, and learn their correct spelling. Your reports will be more respected if you learn to use the right words and correct abbreviations. Figures 2-10 A and B show a sample charting form for the home health aide to complete.

ETHICAL BEHAVIOR

Ethics is a standard or code of behavior. It is a code concerned with what is "right" and what is "wrong." Doctors and nurses take an oath when they are licensed in which they promise to help and care for clients without causing unnecessary pain or suffering. Although there is no written code for home health aides, they are expected to uphold a definite set of standards as they practice their profession.

Ethical Standards

- Be honest in your dealings with clients and coworkers. Stealing involves not only the taking of objects or money, it involves falsifying reports of time and activities.
- Never discuss the financial, emotional, family, medical, or other problems of the client with outsiders. **Confidentiality** is a commitment to keep your client's affairs private. The home health aide must not discuss the client's health, family situation, finances, or any other personal matter with anyone except the supervisor. This includes the worker's family and friends.
- Respect the cultural and religious practices of the client and family.
- Never walk out in the middle of an assignment. Some people may be more pleasant to work with than others. If a personality conflict or the work load is impossible to deal with, the aide should try to finish the shift, then call the case manager and explain the problem. If the aide is working a private case or did not get the job through an agency, the problem should be discussed directly with the employer. Having accepted the duties as an employee, a home health aide is ethically bound to give service for the wages paid.
- Refuse tips and gifts.
- Report possible cases of abuse.
- Do not have any sexual contact with a client.
- Safeguard the confidential information you acquired from any source concerning the client.

NURSES NAME: _____

BOSTON REGIONAL MEDICAL CENTER/HEALTH CARE AT HOME
Home Health Aide Worksheet

YEAR: _____

Patient: _____ Employee: _____

	SUN	MON	TUES	WED	THUR	FRI	SAT
REMEMBER: Begin new worksheet each week and turn in to HHA Department. Report any changes or observations to the nurse. — Date:							
Visit Length:							

PERSONAL CARE
Bath - Sponge/Tub/Shower							
Bath - Partial/Complete							
Hair - Shampoo/Grooming							
Shave							
Nails (File Only)							
Mouth Care							
Bed Making							
Help with Dressing							
Help with Toileting							
Transfer to chair/wheelchair							
Positioning Turn q ____ hours							
Foot Care - Lotion/Massage							

NUTRITION
Special Diet
Meal Preparation B L D
Feeding/Serving
Encourage Fluids

HOUSEHOLD
Marketing
Laundry
Light Housework (BR, Kitchen, Bath, Living Room)

SPECIAL SERVICES
Special Skin Care
Weigh Patient
Catheter Care
Empty Drainage Bag
Measure Intake and Output
Check Bowel Elimination
Ostomy Care
Dressing Change/Wound Care
Exercise (instructed by PT/OT/RN)
Ambulation - Walker, etc.
Accompany to M.D.
Temperature - Oral/Axillary
Blood Pressure
Pulse
Respirations
Assist with Medication

Initials	Signature and Title	Initials	Signature and Title

OBSERVATION NOTES: (Continued on back) _____

Worksheet Reviewed By: _____

HCAH 2.089 Oct 93

FIGURE 2-10A The home health aide worksheet. The care given each day is documented by the home health aide. (Courtesy Boston Regional Medical Center/Health Care at Home, Stoneham, MA)

WORKSHEET CONTINUATION

The space below is provided to record special treatments, problems and other "Observation Notes". Make certain that all notes are dated and signed, using both name and title. Record vital signs on page one on this worksheet, using the flow sheet section under Special Services.

NOTE: Any treatments, problems or other observation notes must be communicated verbally to Nurse/Therapist and/or Supervisor.

Initials	Signature and Title	Initials	Signature and Title

2.089

FIGURE 2-10B Treatments, problems, and observations are documented on this side of the worksheet. (Courtesy Boston Regional Medical Center/Health Care at Home, Stoneham, MA)

- Do not adjust the client's care plan without permission of the case manager.

Professional Standards

- Maintain high standards of personal health and appearance.
- Be dependable and reliable. When accepting a job, you must be on time and prepared to fulfill all obligations.
- Carry out the responsibilities of the job in the best way you possibly can. This means being sure you understand the assignment and how to do it and asking questions when you are in doubt.
- Show respect for the client's privacy and modesty.
- Recognize and respect the right of clients to determine their life-style, even if it is not one you would choose.
- Keep your professional life separate from your personal life. Personal problems of the home health aide should not be discussed with the client or the client's family. Working hours should be addressed to the needs of the clients.
- Control any negative reactions to chronic disability or the living conditions of the client.
- Maintain safe conditions in the working environment. An aide needs to follow basic rules of safety in caring for the client and when working with equipment and supplies.
- Do not use client's medications for your own health problems.

CLIENT'S RIGHTS

The home health aide must respect the rights of the clients. The following is a list of common client rights that are mandated by Medicare and Medicaid regulations:

1. Every client shall be treated with consideration, respect, and full recognition of the client's dignity and individuality.
2. Every client shall receive care, treatment, and services that are adequate, appropriate, and in compliance with relevant federal and state law.
3. Every client has the right to be free from mental and physical abuse.
4. Every client shall be informed of these rights in writing.
5. Every client who is responsible for a fee for service shall be given a statement of the services available by the agency and related charges.
6. Every client shall participate in the development of the plan of care and discharge plan and be informed of all treatments, when and how services will be provided, and the name and functions of any person and affiliated agency providing care and services.
7. Every client has the right to refuse treatment after being fully informed of and understanding the consequence of such actions.
8. Every client shall be informed of the procedure for submitting complaints to the agency. If the client is not satisfied by the agency response, the client may complain to the state Department of Health and Social Services.
9. Every client shall have the right to recommend changes in policies and services to agency staff, the area office representatives of the department, or any outside representative of the client's choice free from restraints, interference, coercion, discrimination, or reprisal.
10. Every client shall receive respect and privacy, including confidential treatment of client records, and the right to refuse release of records to any individuals outside the agency.
11. Every client has the right to privacy.
12. Every client has the right to request change of caregiver.
13. Every client has the right to be informed of the state consumer hotline telephone number.

HOME HEALTH AIDE'S RIGHTS

As an employee of an agency or your client, you also have rights. Examples of your rights are:

1. The right to take pride in a job well done
2. The right to make suggestions and complaints within designated channels without fear of retaliation

3. The right not to be abused physically, verbally, or sexually by clients
4. The right to recommend care plan changes designed to facilitate care delivery and reduce caregiver stress
5. The right to be informed when complaints concerning client treatment are alleged against you
6. The right to a fair hearing with your case manager
7. The right to a confidential investigation
8. The right to be informed of the investigation's outcome

CLIENT ABUSE

Client abuse, neglect, or mistreatment will not be tolerated by your employer or your supervisor. All home health aides are expected to use a professional, caring approach with all clients. There are many forms of abuse. **Abuse** is treatment that reasonably could cause physical pain, physical injury, mental anguish, or fear. Abuse may be verbal, sexual, physical, mental, bodily punishment, involuntary seclusion, mistreatment, or neglect.

- *Verbal abuse* is using depreciative terms or remarks either orally, written, or by gestures to describe someone.
- *Sexual abuse* is making sexual advances to someone or fondling another in inappropriate places.
- *Physical abuse* is hitting, slapping, or pinching another person. Another example is forcing a treatment on a person that the person has requested not to be done.
- *Mental abuse* is threatening or humiliating an individual.
- *Involuntary seclusion* is placing the client in his or her room without the person's consent or not allowing the individual to visit with others.
- *Mistreatment* is using profanity or obscene words, shouting, teasing, or any other method to punish or humiliate another person.
- *Negligence* is failing to follow the established procedures for the care of an individual.

If a home health aide knows that a client is being abused by the client's family or by another caregiver, the aide is obligated by law to report it. If the home health aide does not report it, the aide is just as guilty as the person doing the abusing.

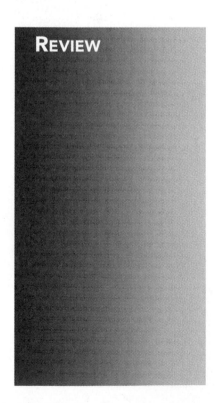

REVIEW

1. The home health aide will be expected to adapt to:
   a. Irregular hours
   b. A variety of assignments and settings
   c. A variety of different types of equipment
   d. All are correct

2. The home health aide should watch for which of the following changes in a client because it may be a sign that there is a problem:
   a. Cuts
   b. Weight loss
   c. Bluish lip color
   d. Increasing "forgetfulness"
   e. All of the above

3. The case manager asks the aide to do something for a client but the aide does not know how to do it. The aide should:
   a. Ask a family member in the home to do it
   b. Call the agency and ask for another worker to help you
   c. Look in her pocket manual and try to find out how to do it
   d. Tell the case manager immediately that she does not know how to do it

4. Ethical conduct for a home health aide involves:
   a. Doing everything the client asks you to do
   b. Discussing your personal problems with the client to relieve the client's boredom
   c. Carrying out the responsibilities of your job in the best way you can
   d. All of the above.

5. Which of the following is a form of abuse?
   a. Refusing to give a diabetic client candy
   b. Forcing a client to be fed through a stomach tube after the client told the doctor "no" for this method of receiving nourishment
   c. Making sexual advancements toward your client
   d. Forgetting to give your client a bath

6. List five actions that could lead to liability and should be avoided.

7. List five rights of clients.

8. List three rights of home health aides.

9. Give four examples of good personal hygiene.

10. T F It is not unethical for a home health aide to discuss a client's health or life-style with friends if they do not know or live near the client.

11. Mrs. Stanley, 85 years old, lives with her 50-year-old son, Harold, who is struggling with an alcohol problem. While bathing her, you observe a number of unexplainable bruises on Mrs. Stanley's arms. You also notice that Harold is short-tempered with his mother. You are suspicious that Harold is abusing Mrs. Stanley. What should you do in this situation? What should you do if Mrs. Stanley admits the abuse but asks you not to tell anyone? What are other possible signs of abuse that a home health aide could observe?

12. Agency Care Well does not provide transportation services for its clients. Mr. Baxter, a 78-year-old client, realizes that this is the case but needs a ride to the grocery store. He asks you to drive him there after your regular work hours. He offers to pay you twice your normal hourly wage. Should you provide the ride for Mr. Baxter? If not, why not? What other solutions might there be to Mr. Baxter's problem?

13. A client of yours is so grateful for your attention that she offers you a gift. You politely decline, but the client insists. What should you do?

14. A new client to which you have been assigned is rude and insulting. You feel so angry that you want to walk off the job. What could you do instead? What factors might be causing your client to be so difficult?

15. You and your client have developed a good relationship with the cashier at the supermarket, where you shop together every

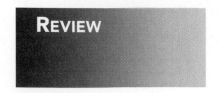

week. One week your client is unable to go shopping with you because of an illness. The cashier is concerned by your client's absence and asks you what is wrong. Give examples of some appropriate responses that would not violate the confidentiality of your client.

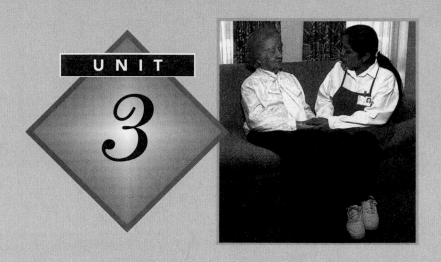

UNIT 3

Developing Effective Communication Skills

KEY TERMS

active listening
body language
communication
invalidate

listening
nonverbal
   communication
nonjudgmental

paraphrase
passive listening
platitude
restate

LEARNING OBJECTIVES

After studying this unit, you should be able to:

- Explain the difference between verbal and nonverbal communication.
- Define the components of basic communication.
- List factors that promote good communication between worker and supervisor.
- Practice active listening.

- Use some of the techniques to improve communication with clients.
- Be more deliberate in communicating with friends, coworkers, and clients.
- Demonstrate the following:
  PROCEDURE 1   Inserting a Hearing Aid

The ability to communicate effectively may be the most important skill that a care provider can learn. **Communication** is the successful transmission of information from one person to another. A care provider's work with people consists primarily of performing tasks, but it also includes establishing positive relationships. The care provider often must communicate why a certain task needs to be done or perhaps coax the person to help with the task. The care provider may also communicate concern—or frustration—in nonverbal ways. Communication with the client's family may involve explaining the reasons why the care provider cannot do certain tasks the family wants, or the need to encourage the family to offer more assistance.

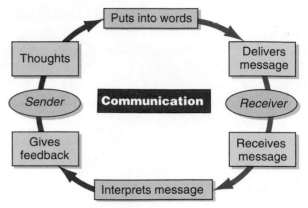

FIGURE 3-1 The communication process. (From Cervantes, Heid-Grubman, Schuerman, The Center for Applied Gerontology, *The Paraprofessional in Home Health and Long-Term Care—Training Modules for Working with Older Adults*, Health Professions Press, P.O. Box 10624, Baltimore, MD 21285-0624 1995. Reprinted with permission.)

COMMUNICATION IN THE WORKPLACE

Good communication is essential in the worker-supervisor relationship. A worker who knows what, how, and to whom she should report is an effective team member. When she hears the respect of her supervisor, she will feel better about the work she is doing.

Communicating, something that we all do every day, sounds easy, but it is actually a complicated process. There are three key aspects of communication: how messages are sent and received, active listening, and nonverbal communication.

SEND A CLEAR MESSAGE

Communication is a two-way process. The sender must send a message and the receiver must receive it for communication to occur. However, the communication is not successful unless the meaning of the message sent and the one received are the same. This is not easy to accomplish. At many points something can go wrong. Figure 3-1 is a graphic description of the communication process.

Problems in communication can begin before words are even spoken. We have all experienced times when our thoughts are unclear. Although we are not sure what we want to say,

we say it anyway. The resulting confusion is no surprise. Taking the time to think through what is really bothering us or what we need from communication will help. In Figure 3-1 we see that "thoughts" are the actual beginning of the communication process. Taking the time to organize our thoughts is the basis for all clear communication.

For example, a care provider may know that she is unhappy with her work, but she cannot explain why she is unhappy because she simply does not know. She could blame her supervisor. She could blame her clients. She could blame herself. In any case, she needs help sorting out her thoughts. Sitting down with a trusted friend or coworker to talk over what she is experiencing will help the worker to organize her thoughts, so that she can communicate clearly the changes she would like to make in her work situation. There are times when we can identify that others are disorganized in their thoughts and not communicating clearly. Our clients may be angry but not know where their anger is coming from. They just know they are angry. They need help sorting things out.

We run into quite a few problems putting our thoughts into words. One major problem is that we often neglect to communicate at all. For many different reasons, we do not talk to each other, and the result is rarely good. When clear communication of expectations has not taken place, mistakes happen that could have been avoided. Care providers often have thoughts, feelings, and information that the supervisor should know about. When the care providers do not communicate with the supervisor, problems can occur. For example, a worker may feel angry because the supervisor has given her a very difficult client when she is feeling work-related stress or "burned out." The supervisor will not know how the worker is feeling unless she mentions it. Only then can she get the support she needs.

Putting the thoughts into words and actually delivering the message are also important steps. Often we have organized our thoughts and rehearsed how we want to say them, but we find it hard to deliver the message. If the worker who is feeling work-related stress is afraid her supervisor will not receive the message well or will "interpret" the message in the wrong way, she will find it very hard to deliver the message.

Good communication involves *two* people. Thinking of our example and looking at Figure 3-1, the worker feels work-related stress and thinks about how to talk to her supervisor ("thoughts"). She tells her supervisor how she is feeling ("puts into words" and "delivers message"). The supervisor listens to the worker ("receives message"), thinks about all of the complex cases the worker is carrying right now ("interprets the message"), and tells the worker that she is carrying a lot of complex cases right now, it is no wonder that the worker is feeling some stress ("gives feedback").

OBSERVATION

The home health aide is in a unique position to observe client needs in the home environment. Through frequent observation and interaction with the client, the aide will see changes in the client's behavior and the environment. In this role the aide has two responsibilities: to orient the client and to provide observations to other members of the care team.

Including orientation to space and time as a part of her routine with the client may be helpful to some clients. "Good morning, Mrs. Jones. It's 9 o'clock, time for your breakfast. You know, this is the coldest January 5th I can remember." For many homebound ill people, one day is sim-

ilar to another. Reminders of the day, the time, the season, and life outside their home are helpful. If a client seems unable to remember even after this orientation, the home health aide will report this to other health care team members or the family.

For the work team to be effective, the home health aide must make sure that she is providing as much detail as possible about the client to other members of the health care team. Observing and reporting are key aspects of the care provider's work. She is the eyes and ears of the family and of the employer. Good case notes can help keep families and other professionals up-to-date and informed about the client. Figure 3-2 includes some commonly used abbreviations that may be encountered and used in writing case notes. Figure 3-3 includes a list of abbreviations used in the diagnosis of a condition or disease of a client. Accurate and clear communication is the goal of these notes. If the notes are generally for family caregivers, these abbreviations will be helpful only if they are understood by everyone who needs to use the notes!

POSITIVE FEEDBACK

For some reason, many of us have difficulty complimenting others and receiving compliments. We may be thinking a kind thought, but we do not put it into words. Unless the other person is a mind reader, it means nothing. In *The One-Minute Manager* (1983), Dr. Ken Blanchard suggests a new supervisory technique. He recommends that, rather than watching to see what people do wrong, supervisors should try to discover them doing something right and then pay them a compliment. This praise reinforces the correct behavior, shows that the supervisor is paying attention to the person, and enhances the worker's self-esteem.

Blanchard's lesson is not just for supervisors. Workers need to learn it as well. Do you know how much a family caregiver or client appreciates a compliment? For example, you might say to your client, "Mr. Jones, you are walking better and better each day! Today you walked 10 feet, twice as far as last week. It won't be long before you are walking without my help. Congratulations!"

FIGURE 3-2 Standard medical abbreviations must be learned to understand medical orders and to chart correctly.

$\bar{a}$ - before
ad lib - as desired
ac - before meals
ADLs - activities of daily living
Amb - ambulatory
bid - twice a day
BM - bowel movement
BP - blood pressure
BRP - bathroom privileges
C - Celsius
$\bar{c}$ - with
CBR - complete bed rest
cc - cubic centimeter
c/o - complains of
CPR - cardiopulmonary resuscitation
dc - discontinue
dsg - dressing
F - Fahrenheit
Fe - iron
HOB - head of bed
HOH - hard of hearing
HS - hour of sleep
Ht - height
I & O - intake and output
K - potassium
Lab - laboratory
lb - pound
mL - milliliter
Na - sodium salt
NPO - nothing by mouth

O_2 - oxygen
od - every day
OT - occupational therapy
oz - ounce
$\bar{p}$ - after
pc - after meals
PO - by mouth
prep - prepare for
prn - when needed or necessary
pt - patient
PT - physiotherapy, physical therapy
q2h - every 2 hours
q3h - every 3 hours
q4h - every 4 hours
qd - every day
qid - four times a day
qod - every other day
ROM - range of motion exercises
$\bar{s}$ - without
SOB - short of breath
Spec - specimen
SSE - soapsuds enema
stat - immediately
Temp - (T) - temperature
tid - three times a day
TLC - tender loving care
TPR - temperature, pulse, respiration
VS - vital signs: TPR and BP
w/c - wheelchair
Wt - weight

FIGURE 3-3 Abbreviations used in the diagnosis of a condition or disease. Many times more than one diagnosis will be listed for a client.

AIDS - Acquired immunodeficiency syndrome
Alz - Alzheimer
ARC - AIDS-related complex
ASHD - Arteriosclerosis (hardening of the
    arteries)
CA - Cancer
CBS - Chronic brain syndrome
CHF - congestive heart failure
COPD - Chronic obstructive pulmonary disease
CVA - Cerebral vascular accident (stroke)
DD - Developmentally disabled
DJD - Degenerative joint disease

DM - Diabetes mellitus
Fx - Fracture
MI - Myocardial infarction (major heart
    condition)
MS - Multiple sclerosis
PID - Pelvic inflammatory disease
TB - Tuberculosis
TIA - Transient ischemic attack (small stroke)
URI - Upper respiratory infection
UTI - Urinary tract infections
VD - Venereal disease

Or you might say to a wife taking care of her husband, "Mrs. Smith, your husband is not easy to take care of. I know he is a very finicky eater. He has gained 2 pounds since last week. You have been working on cooking Mr. Smith's favorite foods. Keep up the good work." Practice positive feedback with clients, friends, and supervisors.

PUTTING THOUGHTS INTO WORDS

The message being sent often has more than one meaning, and the receiver must try to figure out what the sender really means. There are many common phrases and words that have a wide range of meanings. Consider the following words and phrases: often, occasionally, always, almost always, sometimes, seldom, never. Misunderstanding simple words like these can cause problems. A client may want her bathroom cleaned "often." To her this means daily, but to the worker it means once per week. In this example, the client's anger and the worker's frustration may be avoided if the meaning of the word is clarified.

There is not likely to be total agreement on many terms that we commonly use. We must be very careful that the understanding of the sender and the receiver is the same. Communication can be difficult when the message is not clear enough and when the person who receives the message does not ask for clarification. To clarify what is meant, you can ask a series of questions to make sure you understand. This is doubly important to do if your client is from another culture.

MESSAGE DELIVERY

Any message can be delivered in a variety of ways. Comedians say that the success of a joke depends on delivery. Tone of voice, facial expressions, **body language,** and gestures all affect how a message is delivered. For example, tone of voice can make a profound difference in the way a message is sent. **Nonverbal communication** also may include eye contact, posture, and the distance between people. Try repeating the following messages using different tones of voice:

> *"That's OK, I'm not angry."*
> *"I'm glad my mother-in-law is coming to dinner."*
> *"No, I'm not busy."*
> *"You were sick yesterday."*
> *"That is not my job."*

RECEIVING MESSAGES

Many factors can affect how a message is received. Hearing loss, medications, disabilities, and depression can have major effects on how a client receives a communication. Clients with hearing or speech impairments need special attention. Procedure 1 discusses the proper method of inserting a hearing aid.

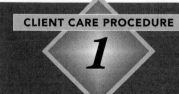

CLIENT CARE PROCEDURE

1

Inserting a Hearing Aid

PURPOSE

- To increase the hearing ability of the client
- To ensure the client's optimal use of the hearing aid

NOTE: Many types of hearing aids are on the market today. They all take special batteries.

The batteries generally do not last a long time, some only 24 hours. Always check to see if your client has an adequate supply of batteries on hand.

(continues)

CLIENT CARE PROCEDURE **Inserting a Hearing Aid** *(continued)*

PROCEDURE

1. Wash your hands.
2. Check hearing aid appliance to see that the batteries are working and tubing is not cracked (Figure 3-4).
3. Tell the client what you plan to do. You may need to use gestures because client may not be able to hear spoken words.
4. Check inside of client's ear for wax buildup or any other abnormalities.
5. Check to make sure the hearing aid is off or the volume is turned to its lowest level.
6. Handle the hearing aid very carefully. Do not drop it or allow it to get wet. Store in a safe area when client is not wearing it. Be sure hearing aid is clean before giving it to client. Follow manufacturer's directions in cleaning your client's hearing aid.

7. Assist the client in inserting the earmold in the ear canal.

Alternate Actions

8. Place the hearing aid over the client's ear, allowing the earmold to hang free.
9. Adjust the hearing aid behind the client's ear.
10. Grasp the earmold and gently insert the tapered end into the ear canal.
11. Gently twist the earmold into the curve of the ear, pushing upward and inward on the bottom of the earmold, while pulling on the ear lobe with the other hand.
12. Let client turn on switch and adjust volume.
13. Wash your hands.

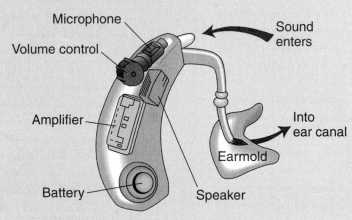

FIGURE 3-4   Parts of a hearing aid

The following list of techniques can be used to improve communication with these clients.

- Be sure you have the person's attention before beginning to speak.
- Face the person and stand reasonably close.
- Lower the pitch of your voice.
- Speak clearly and slowly.
- Use short sentences.
- If the client is speech impaired, speak normally.
- Avoid background noise.
- Encourage the use of nonverbal communication, such as touch, when appropriate.
- Use written communication if you are unable to communicate verbally.

- Do not shout; shouting makes words less clear and may cause pain.
- Do not speak with something in your mouth or with your hands over your lips.
- Give clues about what is being discussed.
- State your name before making a statement or asking a question.
- **Restate** your sentence when you are not understood.
- If you do not understand a part of your client's message, restate the part that you do understand and ask for clarification.
- Talk toward the "better" ear because many people hear better out of one ear.

- Recognize that illness or fatigue reduces the ability of a person with a hearing or speech impairment.
- Do not exhaust the person with irrelevant noise or chatter.
- Visual cues may assist the client; use hand gestures when appropriate; provide the opportunity for lipreading.

Touch is an important form of nonverbal communication. It is helpful for those clients who may need focus to hear the verbal communication. Those who need focusing may be blind, hard of hearing, or confused or they may simply make it clear to the home care worker that they enjoy being touched and respond well to it (Figure 3-5). In some cultures touching is not appropriate, so talk with your supervisor if you are unsure.

Stress and work load are factors that can affect how a worker—or a supervisor—hears messages from coworkers and clients. Also, a limited knowledge of English can be a substantial factor for both clients and care providers in understanding messages.

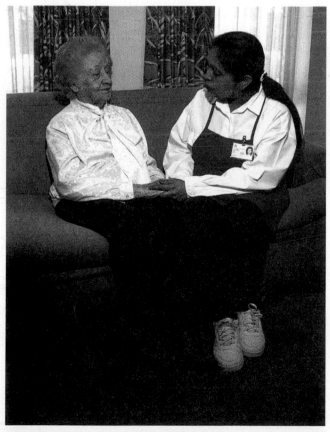

FIGURE 3-5   Encourage the use of nonverbal communication, including touch.

Listening

One reason that a message may not be received correctly is because of poor **listening** skills. It is interesting how little we are taught about how to listen. Yet listening is one of the most important factors in communication. Certain behaviors on the part of the receiver may make it hard to listen. When someone is listening to a message, he or she may be preparing responses instead of listening, thinking of other things, or feeling bored and uninterested with what is being said. Often, people will not completely attend to what is being said because they believe they already know the answer or their biases and stereotypes stand in the way of hearing new information. The frequent distractions in the health care environment make listening difficult, and concentration may be difficult due to fatigue or illness.

A poor listener shows inattention by various means. Some of the behaviors demonstrated by a poor listener are not paying attention to the speaker, listening passively, preparing an answer before the speaker is through talking, rushing the speaker, interrupting the speaker or changing the subject, and becoming emotional. Another common mistake by a listener is to give advice when it is not asked for.

Changing the Subject

It is often tempting to change the subject because the subject is uncomfortable. The client may be depressed and speaking about things that are discouraging to hear. Stay with the client, who may need to talk about something that is deeply troubling. Changing the subject will not take the problem away, but listening may very well ease the load.

Using Platitudes

A **platitude** is a word or a phrase that people use very often for a lot of different situations.

- "Oh, you'll get over it."
- "Just make the most of it."
- "Tomorrow's another day."
- "It's God's will."

You will offer these words of encouragement from time to time, and, at some point in the conversation, these reassurances may be much appreciated. However, when a person comes to you with a problem, platitudes may completely

invalidate her feelings, making her feel that her problems are not important. Platitudes may be useful at a later point in the conversation, after the individual has had the opportunity to express feelings.

Asking Closed-Ended Questions (Yes/No)

Yes/No questions are useful when you want quick answers, but not when you are actually interested in a conversation. Open-ended questions are far more likely to lead to interesting dialogue. Some yes/no questions are: "Do you need help?" or "Would you like to go outside?" Similar questions that are open-ended are: "How may I help you today?" and "Where would you like to go?"

Giving Advice

Do not give your client advice or make recommendations. Just listening to your client will usually help the person to arrive at his or her own decision.

Talking About Yourself

Caregiver-client discussion is not restricted, but the caregiver's role is to listen to the clients, not to air her own problems.

Showing Disapproval and Passing Judgment on the Client

It is extremely important to remain **nonjudgmental** of clients. For example, an elderly client is telling you that her children are so wonderful, but very busy. They really do not have the time to see her. You know the client's son and his wife live only a mile away, yet they visit only once a month, if that often. Even though you may think they are ungrateful children, you would be judgmental if you said what you thought to the client. Your negative comment is based on what you are seeing right now in the client's life. You cannot know all of the details of the relationship of the client with her children. In this case, it would be better to just agree with the client that they are busy or to say that she must miss seeing them more often.

Asking "Why" Questions

Often more information is needed before you can understand what someone means. In that case, a "why" question is often used. Care must be taken when asking "why" questions because they can also send the message that you are judging the other person. Such questions include:

- "Why did you do that?"
- "Why are you thinking that?"

These short, direct questions may suggest that you are disapproving or judging the other person. "Mrs. Jones, I'm not sure why you did that—help me understand so I can do it better next time." Or, "Mr. Smith, why would you think I would do that?" These are softer messages that include the fact that you are inquiring to understand the situation better.

EFFECTIVE LISTENING SKILLS

A person who is an effective listener shows positive behaviors. Paying attention to the speaker, adopting an accepting attitude with a calm, open facial expression and a relaxed, nonthreatening body position, and allowing the speaker plenty of time are just a few ways to be an effective listener. Staying on the subject and being aware of your own emotional reactions to what is being said also help. The following summarizes the ways to listen effectively:

- Pay attention to the speaker.
- Adopt an accepting attitude.
- Allow the speaker plenty of time.
- Be aware of your own emotional responses.
- Use active listening.

As you can see, the process of communication is complicated. At many points the message may be lost. The final factor in good communication is one that is often underestimated. That is when we "interpret the message" that has been sent. At this point, we develop our own understanding of what has been said. **Active listening** is a tool that will allow you to become very involved in the communication process. You can make sure that you understand not only what the speaker has said, but also how the person feels. We do this by giving the speaker feedback about what we have heard. The speaker may then confirm or correct our understanding.

We often assume that we know what a person is saying without checking to make sure that we are correct in those assumptions. When we carefully listen, then check to see if we heard correctly, we are participating in active listening. In **passive listening,** listeners simply sit and hope that they understand what is being said. However, there are many points along the way during which the message may go wrong, so we should work to become active rather than passive listeners. Active listeners become very involved in the process, constantly checking to see if they are on target in what they understand.

There are four active listening behaviors that should be practiced: paraphrasing, reflecting the speaker's feelings, asking for more information, and using nonverbal communication.

Paraphrasing

Paraphrase what has been said. Paraphrasing involves restating, in your own words, what the other person has said; this gives you a chance to check whether your understanding of what has been said is correct. It also gives the speaker a chance to correct you if you have misunderstood. You might say such things as "Do you mean that . . .?" "I understand you are saying . . . ."

Reflecting the Speaker's Feelings

The feelings behind what is being said are often as important as the words, if not more so. Therefore, it is important to try to understand the underlying feelings, attitudes, beliefs, or values. You might make such statements as "That must have made you upset." "I imagine you were thrilled about that." "Does that worry you?"

Asking for More Information

We often need more information to understand what has been said. In most cases, we simply need to ask for clarification. Responses may include: "I'm interested. Tell me more about that." "What happened after that?" "How did you feel when that happened?"

Using Nonverbal Communication

There are many ways through which the speaker can tell whether we are listening. Through our eyes, our posture, and our gestures, we communicate our interest in what is being said.

When an active listener reflects the speaker's feelings, she comments on the feelings behind what is being said, and these feelings can be as important as the words, if not more so. Understanding the underlying feelings, attitudes, beliefs, or values of a statement is useful for a care provider who is creating a successful relationship. Statements such as "That must have made you upset," "I imagine you were thrilled about that," or "Does that worry you?" tell the person you are talking with that you care and that you are paying attention.

We often need more information to understand what has been said. In most cases, we simply need to ask. Your question elicits more information from the speaker and gives him or her the opportunity to expand on the thought. In this way the listener can learn more about the problems, concerns, fear, or joys of the speaker.

REVIEW

Choose the responses that illustrate good listening habits:

1. "My daughter wants me to go into the nursing home."
   a. Well, maybe you should consider it. Things are hard for you here.
   b. How could she say that! After all you've done for her!
   c. How do you feel about that?

2. "I haven't been sleeping well lately."
   a. Try some of these pills. They work great for me.
   b. What's keeping you up?
   c. Don't worry; you'll catch up on your sleep later.

3. "I just can't handle this job anymore."
   a. Is something at work bothering you today?
   b. I know what you mean. I have this client who's driving me crazy!
   c. The pay is terrible, and the hours are long; you should just quit.

4. "My husband and I had a big fight last night."
   a. Again? I don't know why you ever married him.
   b. You're upset about the fight.

5. Mrs. Lindsay is blind. You should:
   a. Touch her to get her attention.
   b. Move furniture and items around to provide for variety.
   c. Provide step-by-step explanation of what you are doing.
   d. Have her walk in front of you as you guide her from behind.

6. You are talking to a client with a hearing loss. You should do all of the following except:
   a. Speak clearly and slowly.
   b. Speak in front of the client so the client can read your lips.
   c. Shout at the client.
   d. Use short sentences and simple words.

7. Body language is:
   a. Use of gestures instead of words.
   b. A form of verbal communication.
   c. Of no concern to the home health aide.
   d. Used only when a client is unable to hear.

8. Match Column I with Column II (abbreviations of diseases).

Column I	Column II
_____ 1. AIDS	a. Alzheimer
_____ 2. CHF	b. acquired immunodeficiency syndrome
_____ 3. DM	c. congestive heart failure
_____ 4. DJD	d. diabetes mellitus
_____ 5. Fx	e. transient ischemic attacks
_____ 6. Alz	f. fracture
_____ 7. TIA	g. degenerative joint disease

9. Match Column I with Column II.

Column I	Column II
_____ 1. ADLs	a. complains of
_____ 2. TLC	b. activities of daily living
_____ 3. qod	c. four times a day
_____ 4. stat	d. tender loving care
_____ 5. HOH	e. immediately
_____ 6. c/o	f. every other day
_____ 7. qid	g. hard of hearing

10. Your client is a 35-year-old woman whose left leg was amputated. She is usually quite sad and lethargic. Today you arrive and she is cheerful. Her hair has been combed and she has cleaned up and gotten dressed. This is all different from the woman you saw just the day before. This change in mood bothers you. Part of you thinks "Oh, well this is good. It makes MY work more pleasant." And part of you is uneasy. You know that when someone has a drastic mood change, something serious can be going on psychologically. What would you do first? What questions would you ask to find out more about her emotional state? Who else needs to know about this sudden mood

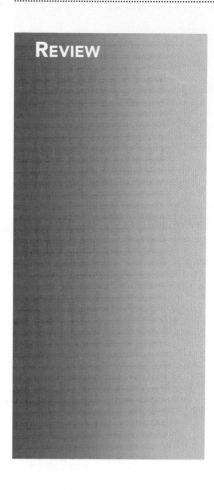

REVIEW

change? What procedures do you follow to communicate your uneasiness?

11. Your older client is a very religious man who uses a wheelchair. He lives with one of his daughters. The other visits regularly. Today you arrive to see that the daughter is visiting and has begun what looks like very heavy cleaning. The client is waiting for his bath and breakfast. You understand from something the daughter says that she thinks the house is dirty and that you have not been doing your job. What would you do first? What is the best attitude to have when approaching the daughter? How do you feel? Can you find out how she feels? Why will it help to know how she feels? What is the main message that you want to get across?

12. You are assigned to work with Mrs. T from 10:00 AM until 12:30 PM on weekdays to prepare a noon meal, with enough planned leftovers for Mrs. T to prepare a light supper for herself. Your supervisor has told you that Mrs. T has very limited money available for food purchases, so you must be careful not to waste food or to plan expensive menus. When you prepare the meal, Mrs. T asks you to share lunch with her. When you say that the extra food is for her leftovers she becomes angry with you and refuses to eat. What are some of the responses you might make that will encourage her to eat, but allow you to refrain from eating her food?

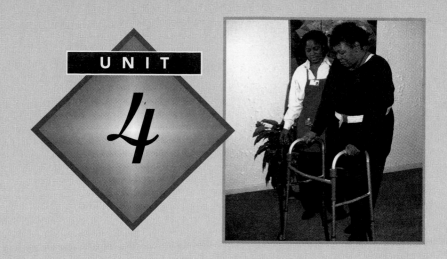

UNIT 4

Safety

KEY TERMS

body mechanics

evacuate

fire extinguisher

gait belt

hazard

peripheral vision

pivot

synchronize

transfer belt

LEARNING OBJECTIVES

After studying this unit, you should be able to:

- Identify the conditions in aging that contribute to the incidence of accidents.
- Identify five causes of accidents around the home.
- List three assistive safety devices used with the frail elderly.

- State the basic rules to follow in the event of a home fire.
- List five safety tips for the home.
- List 10 rules of good body mechanics.

COMMON HAZARDS ····················

According to the National Safety Council, at least 4 million people are injured each year in home accidents. This means that about 1 person in 50 suffers some kind of injury as a result of an accident that occurs in the person's home.

In addition to actual physical **hazards,** human factors are directly related to many home accidents. Statistics show that certain kinds of accidents happen most often in specific age groups (Figure 4-1). Most of these accidents can be prevented.

Young children must be carefully watched at all times. Parents should be aware of the actions of teenagers. Adults should use good judgment and not attempt to do too many things at one time. Carelessness and accidents go hand-in-hand. Because home health aides care for clients in the home, they should be aware of potential hazards in this environment.

An aide should be aware of the effects of medication on the client. Muscle relaxants or tranquilizers can cause clients to become so unsteady that they may fall if they get up from a chair or bed without assistance. If an aide observes that a client becomes disoriented and loses balance easily after taking medication, the aide should inform the supervisor immediately. Sometimes clients have such reactions because of the interactions between several medications or too high a dose of a single medication. It is important that the doctor become aware of these abnormal signs.

Clients who are confused will not remember if they have taken a particular medication. Overmedication can be just as bad as undermedication (Figure 4-2).

Falls and Risks

As the human body ages, the bones become brittle and break easily. Broken hips are a common injury among the elderly.

Many clients may need canes, walkers, or wheelchairs. Before a client uses a cane, walker, crutches, or other device, make certain that each rubber tip is firmly in place and has not worn through.

Some hazards may be avoided by providing a safer environment. Stairways and landings should be kept uncluttered (Figures 4-3 and 4-4). Children's toys, such as skateboards, balls,

blocks, and roller skates, must be put away after use. Waxed and polished floors and stairways can be very dangerous. Scatter rugs in hallways should have a skid-proof backing or be removed completely because they pose a safety hazard in the home. Spills on kitchen and bathroom floors should be wiped up at once so that falls may be avoided.

Do not permit the client to walk about with untied shoelaces. Tripping over the laces can result in serious injury. If the client cannot reach the laces to tie them, even with the use of devices designed for this purpose, the home health aide should tie the laces so they do not present a hazard.

The bathroom is one of the most dangerous rooms in the house for accidents. Bath mats should have a rubber backing so they will not skid. Bathtubs should be equipped with nonskid rubber strips to decrease the danger of slipping when getting in and out of the tub. For older persons, special handrails should be installed to assist them as they use the tub or shower (Figure 4-5). A bath chair should be provided for some elderly clients (Figure 4-6). Faucets for hot water should be clearly marked so that accidental scalding will not occur. Special elevated toilet seats and handrails make it easier for clients to use the toilet safely (Figures 4-7 and 4-8).

When transferring a client from bed to wheelchair, the home health aide must remember to lock the wheels (Figure 4-9). The client is less likely to fall if the chair remains still. If the client is unsteady, it is wise to use a **gait belt** or **transfer belt** while transferring the client. A transfer belt is a wide canvas belt that is placed around the client's waist for the home health aide to hold onto when transferring or walking a client. Be sure to get the proper training before using the gait belt (Figures 4-10 and 4-11).

Another reason clients may fall is due to poor lighting. When elderly clients get up in the middle of the night, it takes their eyes a few more seconds to adjust from the dark to the lightness of the room. Many older adults get up in the middle of the night to use the bathroom; they may not wait a few seconds for their eyes to adjust to the light. It is advisable to keep a night-light on in the bedroom so the adjustment from dark to light is minimal. Another reason for falls by the elderly is due to the loss of

FIGURE 4-1 Age group-related accidents

Age	Accidents
Infants up to 1 year are physically active and willing to touch or taste most anything.	Falls from a bed or table Burns from stoves or heaters Swallowing small objects Small objects stuffed in ears Smothering in bedding/pillows Cuts from sharp, pointed toys Choking on candies or food, toys, or coins
Preschool children are curious and extremely active. They explore most everything by looking, tasting, and touching. They have few fears and no judgment.	Scalding from pulling pot handles on stove Electrocution from playing with electrical cords and outlets Burns from stove or radiators or playing with matches Poisoning from pesticides or cleaning supplies, lead-based paint chips, medicines Falls from chairs, tables, countertops, open windows, or falls into deep holes in ground Drowning in unattended pools Smothering in discarded refrigerators, freezers, and plastic bags Cuts from kitchen knives
Preteen children are adventurous and not aware of dangers. They become involved in play and do not watch for hazards.	Injuries from bicycle and auto accidents. Hit by car when darting into street or between parked cars Poisoning Drowning
Teenagers like to experiment and are influenced by their peers (others in their age groups). They like to show off and are careless.	Injuries from auto, motorbike, or bicycle accidents because of carelessness, drunkenness, or drug abuse Wounds from accidents with guns Burns from careless smoking habits Injuries from carelessness with tools and machinery Drug overdose
Adults have fewer accidents because learning is based on experiences. Self-control and judgment are better developed, but overconfidence, negligence, and carelessness may cause accidents.	Burns from careless use of outside fire, and inside fireplace; from overloading electrical circuits; from smoking in bed Electrical shock from attempting to repair home appliances Using table or chair for climbing instead of sturdy ladder Automobile accidents from carelessness or drunkenness Poisoning or drug abuse from failure to read labels
Old age causes many changes within the body; bones are brittle, eyesight and hearing may fail. Minor accidents may cause great bodily harm.	Falls Burns Cuts and bruises Poisoning because labels cannot be seen due to poor eyesight

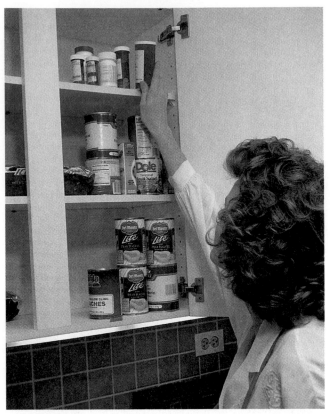

FIGURE 4-2 Keep medication in a safe place if the client is either forgetful or confused.

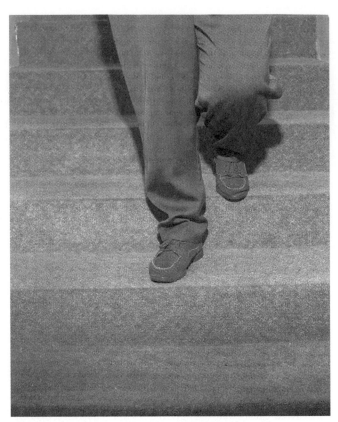

FIGURE 4-4 Uncluttered hallways and stairs can prevent falls and other accidents.

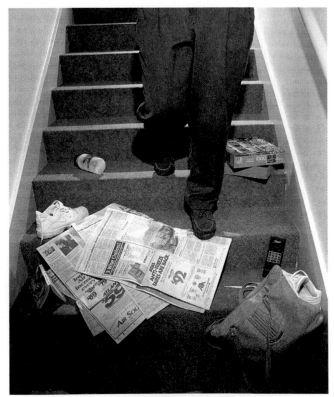

FIGURE 4-3 Cluttered stairways can be hazardous for the elderly client with vision or balance problems.

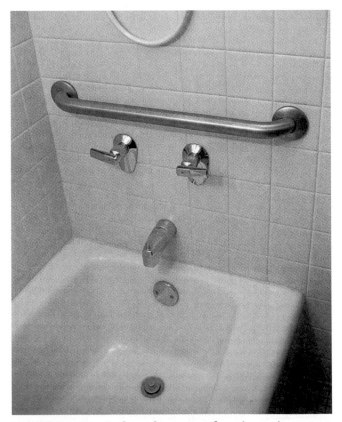

FIGURE 4-5 Safety features for the tub include grab bars and nonskid strips.

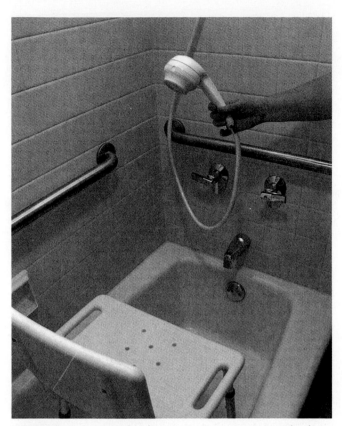

FIGURE 4-6 Bath chairs are recommended for the unsteady client.

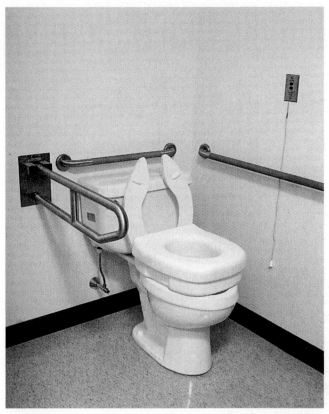

FIGURE 4-8 Seats can be placed easily over toilet.

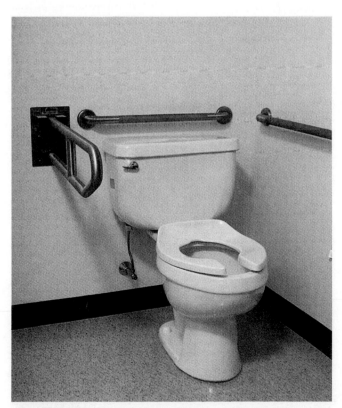

FIGURE 4-7 Raised portable toilet seats allow the client easier transferring onto and off the toilet.

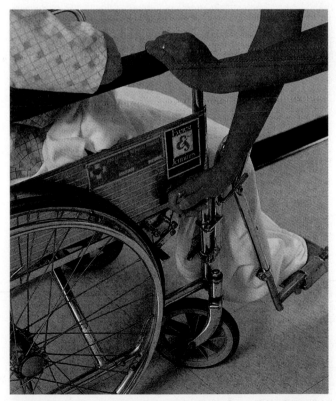

FIGURE 4-9 Lock the wheels of a wheelchair before transferring the client into or out of the chair.

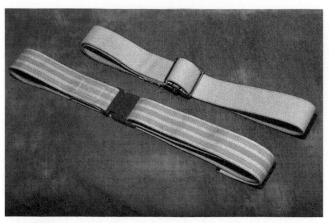

FIGURE 4-10 Gait belts or transfer belts are commonly used to ambulate or transfer a client.

peripheral vision (side vision), which means they can see only things straight ahead and not on the sides.

A care plan for the client will indicate if the use of safety products has been approved. If you recognize any unsafe conditions, or if you have suggestions to make the client's home safer, tell the case manager. Special training

from a nurse or physical therapist is recommended for clients using safety equipment such as walkers and grab bars for the first time. When using a walker, the client's hands must be free to guide the walker. Figure 4-12 shows how the walker can be adapted to carry often-used items. Under no circumstances is the home health aide to initiate the use of canes, walkers, or wheelchairs.

Fire

Few words are more frightening to hear than "Fire, fire!" The smell of smoke or the flash of flames from the kitchen stove can cause panic. Some people are stunned and unable to function. Others rush around wildly trying to save their belongings. The home health aide should advise the client and the client's family whenever a fire safety problem is noticed. If necessary, report your concerns to your supervisor so the family can be notified. All homes should be equipped with ceiling or wall smoke alarms (Figure 4-13). They can run on electricity or batteries. If they run on batteries, the home health aide should check them periodically to see if they need new batteries.

As a home health aide, there are basic rules to follow in case a client's home, or something in it, catches on fire. *Remaining calm* is the

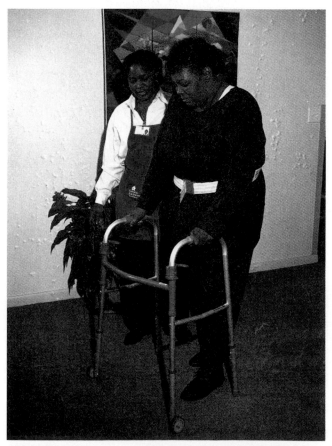

FIGURE 4-11 A gait belt is often used to ambulate a client who is unsteady on her feet.

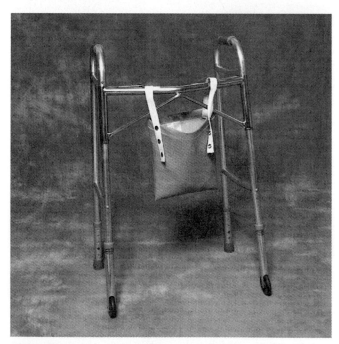

FIGURE 4-12 A walker may have attachments to enable the client to carry often-used items.

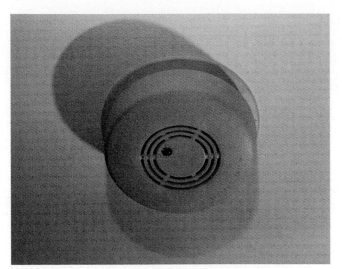

FIGURE 4-13 Smoke alarms should be standard equipment in the client's home.

first and most important rule. Lives can be saved if an emergency plan has been made beforehand. A home health aide, on entering a client's home, should make note of the nearest exit from each room. The telephone number of the fire department should be placed close to the telephone (Figure 4-14).

The aide must consider the client's condition and decide the best way to move the client in case of a fire. At the time of the fire, other decisions also must be made:

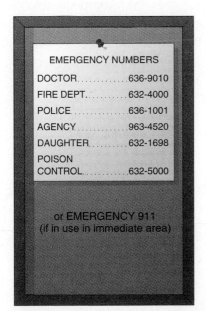

EMERGENCY NUMBERS

DOCTOR............636-9010
FIRE DEPT.........632-4000
POLICE...........636-1001
AGENCY............963-4520
DAUGHTER.........632-1698
POISON
CONTROL...........632-5000

or EMERGENCY 911
(if in use in immediate area)

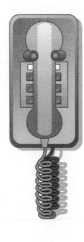

FIGURE 4-14 Important telephone numbers posted next to the telephone may save precious moments at the time of an emergency. Check your local directory for the correct numbers.

1. Determine if the fire is major. If it is minor, put it out at once, following the directions given in Figures 4-15 and 4-16.
2. Decide if there is time to call the fire department before you **evacuate** the client. If there is no time, move the client and call the fire department from a telephone outside the house.
3. If the client or family members are in immediate danger, evacuate them at once.
4. If the client cannot be moved safely, and you are trapped in the client's home, go into a room with a door and window. Close the door and place a rolled blanket, towel, or sheets (wet, if possible) at the bottom of the door to keep the smoke out. Place some signal in any available window that will attract the attention of firefighters.

Waiting for the fire department to arrive is difficult for the home health aide and family members. Under no circumstances should the aide return to the burning building. Family members and neighbors also should be stopped from returning to the building. No personal possession is valuable enough to risk a human life.

Fire Extinguishers. Small fires may be extinguished by using a **fire extinguisher.** There are four main types of fire extinguishers, each of which is used for a specific type of fire.

1. *Class A extinguishers* contain water that is under pressure. They are used to douse fires involving paper, wood, or cloth.
2. *Class B extinguishers* contain carbon dioxide. They are used to put out fires caused by igniting gasoline, oil, paints or other liquids, and cooking fats. These types of fires would spread if water were used to extinguish them. The carbon dioxide smothers the fire, leaving a white powder residue. These extinguishers should be used with caution because the residue they leave may irritate the skin and eyes. Fumes also may be dangerous to inhale.
3. *Class C extinguishers* contain dry chemicals and are used on electrical fires.
4. *Class ABC* or *combination extinguishers* contain a graphite-like chemical. They can be used on any type of fire. The residue that results from their use can cause irritation of the skin and eyes.

If an aide uses a fire extinguisher on a minor fire, the manufacturer's operating instructions

FIGURE 4-15   Basic rules for the home health aide to follow in case of fire in the client's home.

Basic Rules in Case of Fire

1. Know the location of the nearest fire alarm box in the area.
2. Know how to phone for the fire department.
3. Remember the location of the nearest exits.
4. Close any door that will tend to confine the fire.
5. See that everyone is out of danger.
6. Know where a fire extinguisher is located and how to operate it. Check batteries of smoke alarms regularly.
7. Never try to fight a fire in a room filled with smoke; the fumes and lack of air are dangerous.
8. Never try to enter a room where much fire is in evidence.
9. Remember that a woolen blanket or other heavy covering will help to smother a small fire.
10. Keep boxes of inexpensive baking soda handy to extinguish kitchen fires. The boxes can be kept in the refrigerator so you will always be able to find them.
11. Use baking soda instead of water to extinguish small grease, oil, paint, varnish, and similar fires, because water spreads such a fire. Dust the flames with baking soda; this smothers the flames physically and chemically with carbon dioxide gas.
12. Smother small grease fires in cooking utensils by covering them with a lid or long-handled pan, or by throwing baking soda on the blaze.
13. Extinguish small broiling pan fires by first turning off oven and then throwing handfuls of baking soda on the blaze.
14. Throw baking soda on small fires in ashtrays, wastebaskets, or upholstered furniture.
15. Do not try to be a hero. If the small fire does not respond to your efforts to extinguish it immediately, remove the client and yourself from the house as quickly as possible. Call the fire department from a neighbor's house, or flag down passing motorists and ask them to call.

must be followed carefully. Most extinguishers have a lock on the handle that must be unlocked before use (Figures 4-17A and B). The extinguisher should be held firmly and the nozzle aimed at the near edge of the fire. **CAUTION:** Do not aim toward the center of the fire. Discharge the extinguisher, using a slow, side-to-side motion, until the fire has been extinguished. Avoid contact with the chemical residues from the extinguisher. To prevent personal injury, the aide always should stay a safe distance from the fire.

An easy-to-remember method for operating a fire extinguisher is to follow the letters P-A-S-S.

P   Pull the pin at the top of the extinguisher that keeps the handle from being pressed. Break the plastic or thin wire inspection band as the pin is pulled.

A   Aim the nozzle or outlet toward the fire. Some hose assemblies are clipped to the extinguisher body. Release the hose and point.

S   Squeeze the handle above the carrying handle to discharge the contents of the container. The handle can be released to stop the discharge at any time. Before approaching the fire, try a very short test burst to ensure proper operation.

S   Sweep the nozzle back and forth at the base of the flames to disperse the extinguishing agent. After the fire is out, watch for remaining smoldering hot spots or possible reflash of flammable liquids. Make sure that the fire is completely out.

Once an extinguisher has been used in a fire, it must be replaced or recharged. Notify your agency of the need for replacement.

SAFETY TIPS FOR THE HOME

- Free floors of clutter and small objects.
- Wipe dry any spilled water, grease, or food immediately.
- Keep all rugs and carpets in good repair.

FIGURE 4-16 First aid—what to do.

First Aid—What to Do	Home Fire Escape Plan

First Aid—What to Do

If you catch on fire:
DON'T PANIC. DON'T RUN—RUNNING WILL INCREASE THE FLAMES. *Instead:*
1. **Stop.**
2. **Drop** to the ground.
3. **Roll.** Continue to roll until you have completely put out the fire.
4. Remove clothing from the affected area. *Do not* attempt to remove clothing that sticks.
5. Flush area with cool water.
6. Cover with a sterile pad or clean sheet.
7. *Seek immediate medical attention.*

If the burn is from a chemical:
1. Follow steps 4–7 and be sure to flush with cool water for 20–30 minutes.
2. If the eyes are involved, flush the eyes for at least 20 minutes or until medical attention arrives.
3. Remove contact lenses.

If the burn is electrical:
1. Turn off electrical source before touching victim.
2. Check for breathing and pulse. If absent, start Cardiopulmonary Resuscitation (CPR), if qualified.
3. Follow steps 4–7.

Home Fire Escape Plan

- Develop a Family Escape Plan.
- Include 2 exits from each room.
- Plan a meeting place outside the home.
- Practice the plan.

Plan of Escape:
Evacuate!
Do not attempt to fight the fire.
1. If in bed, roll off onto floor.
2. Stay low! Crawl if necessary. Smoke rises, and oxygen will remain near the floor.
3. Cover your mouth and nose with some clothing or material to aid in breathing.
4. Place your hands on any closed door before opening it. If it is hot, *do not open!* Find another exit. If it is not hot, open it slowly, standing to the side. *Do not use elevators.*
5. *If you are trapped in a room:*
   a. Roll a rug or other materials and place across the bottom of the door.
   b. Open a window, both top and bottom, to allow air to enter and smoke to escape.
   c. Telephone for help, if possible.
   d. Attract attention and call for help.

(For further information, call The Burn Center at New York Hospital-Cornell Medical Center, 535 East 68th Street, New York, NY at 212-472-6890.)

- Do not wax the floors; waxed floors are slippery.
- Keep drawers and closet doors closed.
- Install night-lights in the bedroom, hallway, and bathroom.
- Keep a flashlight within easy reach at bedside.

- Do not use small scatter rugs in the bathroom.
- Use plastic or paper cups instead of glass drinking containers in the bathroom.
- Place grab bars in strategic locations around the bathtub, shower, and toilet.
- Never use an electric appliance in the bathtub or shower.

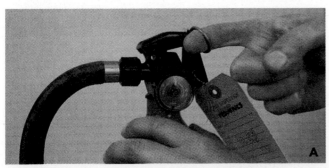 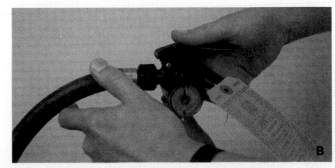

FIGURE 4-17 Use of the fire extinguisher. A. Remove pin. B. Push top handle down.

- Install handrails in stairways.
- Keep stairways and hallways well lit.
- Keep all objects off the stairs.
- Remove scatter rugs, especially at the bottom or the top of stairs. If the client insists on using scatter rugs, place a nonskid backing underneath the rug.
- Arrange the kitchen so heavy cookware and frequently used items are within easy reach.
- Consider using a shower chair if client is unsteady when standing.
- Install smoke alarms and be sure batteries work.
- Store medications in cool, dry area, and out of reach of children and confused adults.

PRINCIPLES OF GOOD BODY MECHANICS

Each year, because of incorrect body and muscle use, millions of dollars are lost in wages and millions of dollars are spent on treatment for unnecessary injuries and disability payments. The most common injuries for the home health aide involve the muscles, ligaments, and joints of the lower back. These injuries are caused by lifting, bending, pulling, twisting, and pushing incorrectly.

Much of your work as a home health aide requires physical effort. To avoid injury to yourself, use good techniques when you lift a client, transfer a client between bed and wheelchair, cook meals, do laundry, or even stand, sit, or walk. All require correct, careful, and efficient use of your muscles to prevent injury and reduce fatigue.

The way in which the body moves and keeps its balance through the use of all its parts is referred to as **body mechanics.** Use of body mechanics means that each part of the body works together. Some muscles are better at pushing than pulling. The body organs are held in their cavities by the muscles surrounding them. When one part of the body is under strain, it may affect other parts of the body.

Your spine is like a flexible, bendable rod with a crossbar near the top where the shoulders and arms are attached. The muscles of the spine are small straps that run up and down the spine. They are designed to hold the spine steady and to bend in different directions. They are not designed to lift heavy loads. The strong muscles of the hips and of the shoulders and arms are there to do the heavy work. When you lift, push, or pull, be aware of the positions of the different parts of your body. Keep your back straight and steady. Bend your knees and use the muscles of the thighs and shoulders to do the work. When you carry an object, hold it close to your body.

Good body mechanics start with proper posture—the way you hold and position each part of your body. Correct posture means that there is a balance between your muscle groups and that the different parts of your body are in good alignment—in the correct position relative to each other (Figures 4-18A and B).

Correct posture makes lifting, pulling, and pushing easier. Correct posture is important at all times—standing, sitting, walking, and lying. A good standing posture begins with having feet flat on the floor, separated by about 12 inches, knees slightly bent, arms at the sides, abdominal muscles tight.

Ten basic rules will help your body and muscles work well for you, prevent injury, and reduce fatigue.

1. Keep your back straight—do not twist or bend.
2. Keep your feet apart, to provide a good base of support (Figure 4-19).
3. Bend from the knees, particularly when lifting—do not bend from the waist or spine (Figure 4-20).
4. Use the weight of your body to help pull or push an object (Figure 4-21).
5. Use the strong muscles of your thighs and shoulders to do the work (Figure 4-22).
6. Hold objects close to your body. This allows your strong shoulder and thigh muscles to work most efficiently (Figure 4-23).
7. Avoid twisting your body as you work and bend. **Pivot** the whole body (Figure 4-24A and B).
8. Push or pull, rather than lift.
9. Always get help if you feel you cannot do the lifting or moving on your own (Figure 4-25).
10. **Synchronize** movements with client or others; count 1 . . . 2 . . . 3 . . . and do the job together.

Remember, it is your body, they are your muscles, and you are responsible for the way you use them.

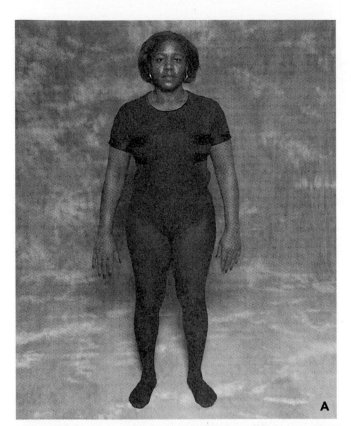

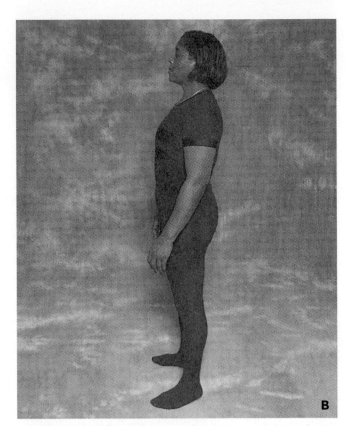

FIGURE 4-18   Correct standing position   A. Front view   B. Side view

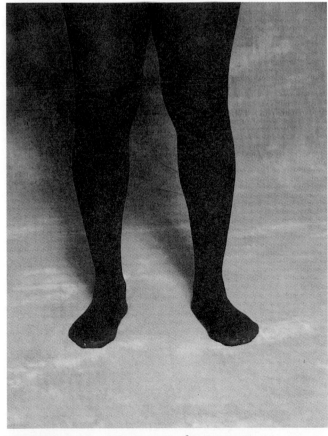

FIGURE 4-19   Keep your feet apart.

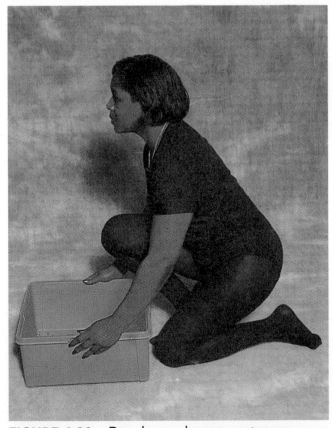

FIGURE 4-20   Bend your knees, not your back.

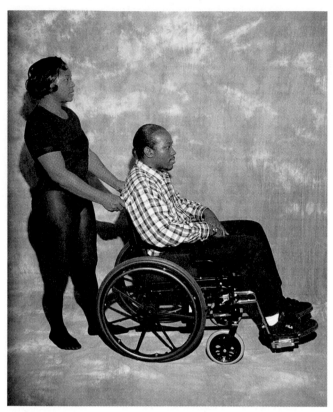

FIGURE 4-21 Push an object rather than lift it.

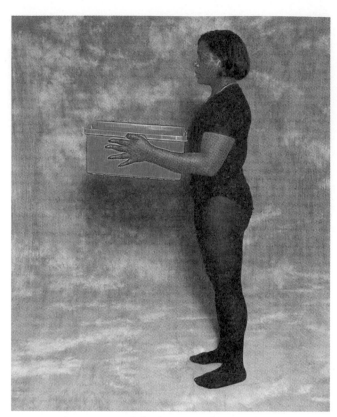

FIGURE 4-23 Hold objects close.

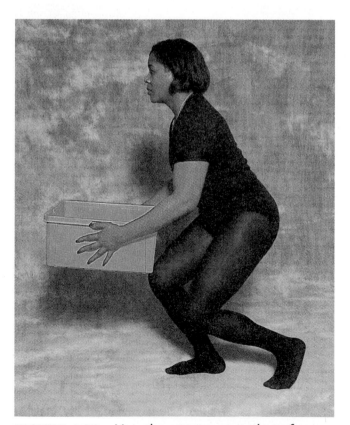

FIGURE 4-22 Use the strong muscles of your thighs and shoulders when lifting.

Applications of Good Body Mechanics to Client Care

Many client care procedures require moving and turning the client. To ensure the safety of the client and to avoid self-injury, the home health aide should apply the techniques of good body mechanics to the work situation. This means that the aide should do the following:

- Stand straight, rather than slouch. Keep the back and shoulder muscles in a straight line.
- Push, pull, slide, or roll the client whenever possible. Try to avoid lifting the client.
- When turning the client, try to make the movement smooth and fluid so that the entire body shifts at the same time.
- When repositioning the client in bed, turn the client toward you rather than away from you. This lessens the danger of the client falling out of bed and keeps your weight more evenly distributed.
- When walking with the client, remain on the client's weak side. Try to stay near chairs or a couch so you can quickly seat the client if the client tires.
- If the client becomes faint while walking, help the client to sit in a chair. If there is no chair

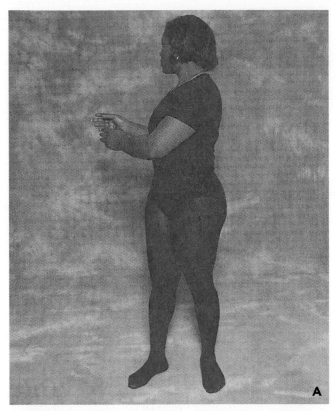

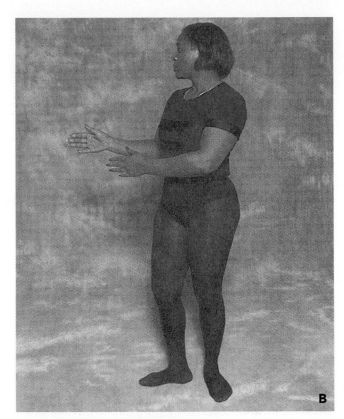

FIGURE 4-24   A. Avoid twisting your body.   B. Pivot instead of twisting.

nearby, help the client slide slowly to the floor. Call for assistance.

• When walking or transferring a client, remember to use a gait or transfer belt (Figure 4-26).

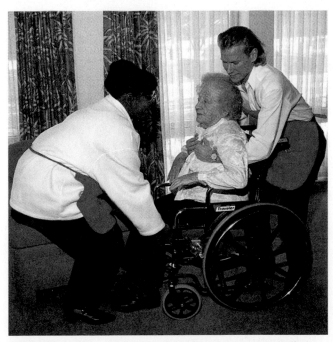

FIGURE 4-25   Determine if you can transfer alone. If not, ask for help.

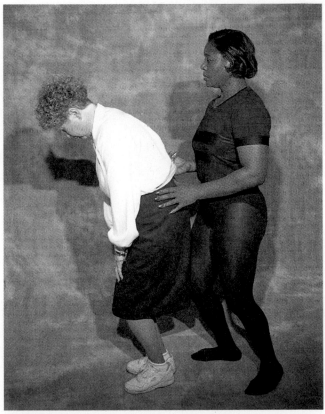

FIGURE 4-26   If an unsteady client starts to fall, slowly lower her to the floor with a transfer belt.

SAFETY OUTSIDE THE CLIENT'S HOME

The home health aide must be aware of safety issues outside the client's home as well as within. The aide must be "streetwise" and safe. To be streetwise each aide must:

1. Be alert.
2. Be observant.
3. Trust own instincts.
4. Know how and when to call 911.

Do's and Don'ts

- Keep your money and identification close to you.
- Wear a fanny pack rather than carry a purse.
- Do not put money or credit cards in shopping bags.
- Do not put your wallet in your back or rear pocket.
- Do not wear flashy jewelry.
- Do not have personal identification on your key chains.

Safety When Walking

- Plan the safest route.
- Choose well-lighted streets, not alleys.

- Avoid vacant lots.
- Take the long way if it is the safest.
- Cross the street and head for a busy, well-lighted area if you are followed.
- Do not hitchhike.

Safety When Driving

- Keep your car in good running condition.
- Plan the safest route.
- Have your keys ready when approaching your car.
- Drive with your doors locked.
- Do not pick up hitchhikers.
- Park in well-lighted areas.
- Stay in your car when you see a street or motorist problem; go to a telephone for help.

Buses and Subways

- Have your money or token ready—do not open your purse.
- Try to sit near driver or conductor.
- Do not stand near edge of subway platform.
- Avoid sitting near the exit doors.
- Do not fall asleep.

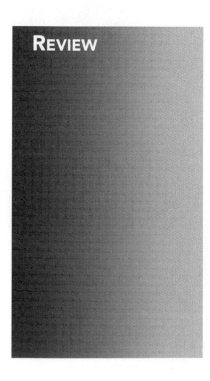

REVIEW

1. T F Bones are more brittle when a person is young.

2. T F Hazards may be avoided by providing a safer environment.

3. T F The most common accidents during old age are falls, burns, cuts and bruises, and poisoning because labels cannot be read due to poor eyesight.

4. T F The bathroom is the most dangerous room in a home.

5. T F Grab bars, nonskid strips, bath chairs, and gait belts are assistive devices that can increase the safety and security of the frail client.

6. You have identified a fire hazard in the client's room. What should you do?
    a. Call 911.
    b. Notify the family.
    c. Notify your case manager.
    d. Evacuate the client if possible.
    e. All of the above.

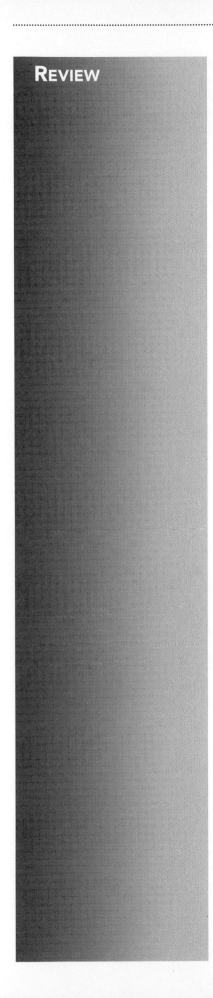

REVIEW

7. The types of fire extinguishers available for home use are:
   a. Class A extinguishers that contain pressurized water; used for paper, wood, cloth fires
   b. Class B extinguishers that contain carbon dioxide; used for gasoline, oil paints, cooking fat fire
   c. Class C extinguishers that contain dry chemicals; used for electrical fires
   d. Class ABC extinguishers that contain graphite-like chemical; used for all fires
   e. All of the above.

8. List five safety tips for the home.

9. What does the term *body mechanics* mean?

10. You are going to pick up the laundry basket from the floor. You should:
    a. Use only one hand for lifting.
    b. Flex your knees.
    c. Bend over at the waist.
    d. Keep your feet close together.

11. When lifting a client, you should keep your _____ straight.
    a. Back
    b. Hips
    c. Knees
    d. Thighs
    e. All of the above

12. Many client care procedures require moving and turning the client. To ensure the safety of the client and to avoid self-injury, the aide should use which of the following good body mechanic techniques:
    a. When turning the client, make smooth fluid movements so that the entire body shifts at the same time.
    b. When repositioning a client in bed, turn the client toward you rather than away from you so the client does not fall and keep your weight evenly distributed.
    c. If a client becomes faint while walking, help the client to sit in a chair; if there is no chair, help the client slide slowly to the floor.
    d. When walking or transferring a client, use a gait belt around the client's waist and hold onto it when transferring or walking the client.
    e. All of the above

13. Your day in the client's home includes a variety of chores and responsibilities including housecleaning, garbage disposal, laundry, transfer of a wheelchair/bed bound client, bathing, meal preparation, and grocery shopping. What actions and procedures will you follow to avoid injury to yourself and your client?

14. You are scheduled to service a client who lives alone in a small house. The client has just had eye surgery and should not bend. The bedrooms and bathroom are on the upper level, the living

room, dining room, and kitchen are on the lower level. Some of the flooring is linoleum, some wood. There are rugs in some of the rooms. The client often leaves things on the stairs so that she will remember to transfer them. There is an overhead light in the bedroom and bathroom and a smoke detector in the hallway near the bedroom. Next to the rear exit the client saves newspapers, glass, plastic, aluminum, and tin containers for recycling. How would you make her environment safer?

15. What actions must the aide take to remain safe when traveling to the client's home?

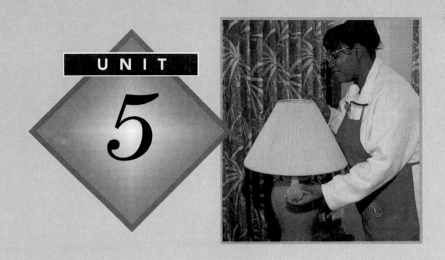

UNIT

5

Homemaking Service

KEY TERMS

bulk	mildew	produce
convenience foods	pathogens	recyclable
delicatessen	perishable	sanitary
fermented	permanent press	staple items
Meals on Wheels	polyester fabrics	

LEARNING OBJECTIVES

After studying this unit, you should be able to:

- List at least four tips used to plan and organize tasks.
- Explain how to care for major home appliances.
- State some ways to combine client care and household tasks.
- Name three factors that determine the home health aide's cleaning plan.
- List five cleaning tasks done daily.
- List five cleaning tasks done only periodically.
- Describe the correct method for separating and disposing of garbage.
- Identify at least four steps used in cleaning a kitchen.

- Identify bathroom tasks the home health aide does daily.
- List four guidelines for planning menus.
- State eight guidelines for buying food.
- List four guidelines for storing food.
- Name five guidelines for preparing meals.
- Identify two ways to sort clothes for washing.
- Identify several methods for removing stains.
- Explain how to wash the clothing and bed linens of a client with an infectious disease.
- Demonstrate the following:
  PROCEDURE 2   Changing an Unoccupied Bed

HOUSEHOLD MANAGEMENT

Managing a household is like operating a daily 24-hour business. Homemakers raise children, manage a budget, provide a clean and livable house, prepare and serve meals, and handle home accidents. It requires intelligence, understanding, and physical labor.

Many home health aides have a basic knowledge for keeping up a house. However, the habits developed in their own homes may not be suitable to all working situations.

The units covering homemaking skills are presented to introduce homemaking techniques to the beginner. However, even the experienced homemaker may learn some helpful new tips.

The home health aide should realize that each home situation may offer different challenges. A professional home health aide must adapt to the physical surroundings of each job. This adjustment requires the use of whatever appliances and supplies the client has available. The home health aide must remember to show as much care for the property of others as is shown for his or her own personal property. The equipment and furnishings used by the home health aide belong to the client. Considerate and cautious care must be used.

The aide should read directions carefully and ask questions before using unfamiliar equipment. If equipment has frayed cords or if appliances do not work, they should be repaired. The aide should notify the case manager or family so that repairs can be made.

When using any cleaning product or appliance, read the labels and directions carefully. This not only makes for proper use, but can limit the number of accidents that might happen. Using rubber gloves helps avoid skin irritation caused by soaps or household chemical products.

When performing regular household duties, the aide should make a list of any items in short supply. Toilet paper, laundry products, food, or other necessities should be purchased before the house supply runs out.

Sometimes a home health aide handles the client's money. Always get a receipt for any purchases you make and place the receipts in a special place. If there is any doubt about what an item costs, or if the client has any questions as to where the money was spent, you can quickly verify your expenditures. Honesty in money matters is an absolute necessity.

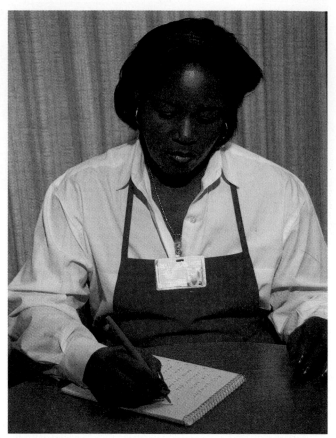

FIGURE 5-1 An aide is planning her work and listing the supplies she needs.

When you are in a client's home and the client requests a cleaning job done a certain way even though you know a better way, you should follow the client's directions.

A few of the homes you will be going to might be very dirty and unkempt; if you are assigned to work at this home for 3 hours, you will not be able to clean it in that short time and get everything spotless. Your client might think differently. If this situation exists, you need to discuss this with your case manager.

Planning and Organization

An important duty of the aide is to plan, organize, and carry out tasks completely. The homemaker who plans the work, organizes the tasks, and starts doing them will find the work load lightened. A home health aide will be given instructions for each assignment. The care of the client is of primary importance, but the household tasks cannot be ignored. The aide should take a few minutes each morning to plan the tasks that should be completed by the day's end (Figure 5-1). This can save time and energy.

- Carry a pad and pencil. Make a note of household supplies that may be needed in each room.
- Post a list of needed supplies on a kitchen bulletin board, or use a small magnet and put the list on the refrigerator door. Remind family members that if they use the last bar of soap or roll of bathroom tissue they should add the item to the list.
- Before starting to clean a room, the home health aide should stop to think which cleaning supplies may be needed. All the supplies needed to complete the work in a particular room should be taken to the room at one time. Carry cleaning supplies from room to room in a plastic container or basket.
- Prevent buildup of dirt by tidying rooms, dusting, wiping surfaces, and sponging up spots as soon as possible.
- Keep a sponge in the kitchen and bathroom for quick wipe-ups.
- Use a tray to carry dishes to and from the table.
- Schedule major jobs for a certain day of the week. For example, vacuum and wash floors on Friday so the house will be ready for weekend use; launder and iron one day; plan weekly marketing on Monday or Wednesday; defrost refrigerator, clean oven, or straighten drawers or cabinets on a day when nothing big is planned.
- Arrange to do two or three tasks at one time. A load of laundry can be put in the machine just before lunchtime. While the machine is running, lunch can be prepared and served to the client. If the laundry has to be done in the laundromat, it can be planned for the same day as the weekly shopping. While hand laundry is soaking, the ironing could be started.
- Learn how to use and care for the equipment in the home (Figure 5-2). Most appliances have an instruction manual. Read it before using the equipment. After using equipment, clean it so it will be ready for the next use. Store small appliances close to where they are used.

COMBINING CLIENT CARE AND HOUSEHOLD TASKS

The order in which tasks are done is not always important. If one knows just what should be completed by the end of the day the work can be arranged around the client's needs. After the client's bath and after the bed linens are changed, the home health aide may decide to

FIGURE 5-2 Proper use and care of household appliances reduce the need for repairs and the risk of personal injury.

Appliance	Purpose and Use	Care and Cleaning
Refrigerator	To retard spoilage of perishable foods. Door should be kept closed when not in use. Temperature control should be set so as to keep foods fresh but not to freeze them. Most refrigerators have zoned cooling. Store foods in a specific area. Meats to be used within 2 or 3 days belong in the meat storage compartment. Fruits and vegetables are kept in the bottom area, milk and dairy products on top shelves. Store leftovers in small airtight containers and use as soon as possible.	Discard leftovers if unused in 3 days. Wipe interior with warm water and baking soda to remove stale odors. At least every 3 or 4 weeks remove shelves and drawers. Wash them in water and detergent. Rinse thoroughly. Place a box of baking soda in refrigerator if odor still present.

(continues)

FIGURE 5-2 *(continued)*

Appliance	Purpose and Use	Care and Cleaning
Freezer compartment of refrigerator	Store frozen foods and weekly meat supply. Mark date of storage and use older products first. Frost-free refrigerators have a tray on the bottom. This tray should be pulled out and cleaned every 2 or 3 months. Persons with lung disorders may be sensitive to the dust and vapors from this area.	To defrost, put pan of hot water in emptied compartment. Turn control knob to defrost. Empty pan under freezer so water does not flood rest of refrigerator or floor. DO NOT USE SHARP KNIFE TO PRY ICE LOOSE. THIS COULD DAMAGE FREEZER COILS. When defrosting is completed, wipe inside with warm water and baking soda. Turn control on and replace foods. If any food has thawed completely, use it at once—do not refreeze foods.
Freezer	Offers large, cold storage area and maintains a constant temperature. Foods may be stored for long periods of time. Some foods cannot be stored longer than 6 months. Instructions on care and wrapping foods for the freezer appear later in the text.	Defrost twice a year. If frost-free model, remove foods and wipe inner surfaces with damp cloth and baking soda.
Stove	Heats food for boiling, broiling, or baking. Uses gas or electricity as a fuel source. Keep pot holders and dish towels away from flame or heat unit. Never use the oven when it is greasy—FIRE HAZARD. Turn off stove when finished cooking. When using gas stoves, be sure the pilot light is burning before turning on gas jet of the burner. When lighting the oven, first light match, then turn on gas jet and put flame to it. Keep body turned away from open oven door for safety. If oven does not light, turn off jet and try again in a few minutes. Make sure gas jet is turned OFF when through using oven.	Wipe up spilled foods at once. Wipe off stove surface once a day. Scour burners and burner pans once a week. When cleaning the oven, follow instructions on cleaner can. Clean as often as needed. When daily spills and grease are cleaned up, a full oven cleaning is not needed as often. Self-cleaning ovens—follow manufacturer's instructions.
Microwave oven	Read instructions before using. Used for rapid food defrosting, quick heating of leftovers, baking, and cooking. Use only the recommended dishes or supplies (paper, plastic) in the microwave. Never use metal containers or dishes with metal trim.	Wipe clean with damp cloth, following instructions in operator's manual. Soap may be used; rinse well and dry interior. If you are unsure about care and cleaning, ask a family member for a demonstration.

(continues)

FIGURE 5-2   *(continued)*

Appliance	Purpose and Use	Care and Cleaning
Dishwasher	Washes dishes at a high water temperature; most dishwashers sterilize dishes. Rinse plates and utensils before placing in dishwasher—or turn on prewash cycle immediately after loading. Use *only* the dishwashing detergent. Wait until there is a full load before putting on wash cycle. (Saves water and electricity.) Do not put plastic, cast iron, or wooden items in dishwasher.	Clean filter once a week and wash interior with water and mild soap, rinse with damp cloth. **CAUTION:** Do not touch coils in dishwasher.
Garbage disposal	Appliance in sink that cuts up discarded food and disposes of it. Follow instructions in manufacturer's guide. Be careful to dispose only the food items listed, not bones or paper. **CAUTION:** Keep hands away from unit while in operation.	**CAUTION:** Do not try to repair; call for plumber if it breaks down. After using, rinse drain with hot water.
Garbage compacter	Crushes garbage to save storage space. Follow instructions in manufacturer's guide. Use it only for those items recommended by manufacturer.	Call professional repairman.
Washing machine	Soaks and agitates clothing. Load as instructed—use correct water temperature for type of clothing. Use soap and bleach as needed according to instructions. Do not overload.	Clean out lint trap. About once a week wipe out inside with soap and water to get rid of grit. Take off agitator and clean carefully. Wipe outer surface after use.
Dryer	Tumbles and heats clothing to dry them. Load according to instructions, using temperature recommended for type of clothes.	Clean lint trap after each use. Wipe outer surface after use. Call repairman if machine works poorly.
Small appliances Automatic blender Mixer Electric fry pan Slicing machine Electric knife Percolator Automatic coffee maker	Follow operating instructions. If you are unsure how to use it, do not use it. Pay special attention to all safety precautions provided by the manufacturer with the appliance.	Wash surface and store conveniently and carefully. Make sure the electric unit does not come in contact with water. Wash coffee maker with soap and water after using. Rinse thoroughly. Once in a while run a cycle of water and baking soda through pot to clean coffee oils away.

clean the client's room. The kitchen could be cleaned after the breakfast meal (Figure 5-3). The client's bathroom cleaning could be done after the bedpan has been used and emptied into the toilet bowl. These examples show how to pair client care procedures with homemaking duties. This technique saves time and energy by avoiding many extra steps a day.

MAINTAINING A CLEAN HOME ENVIRONMENT

The home health aide is normally expected to do general cleaning in the living room, dining room, family room, and bedrooms. Home health aides set up their own routines for completing daily household tasks. Several factors need to be considered:

- Needs of the client
- Size of the home
- Ages of people living in the home
- Number of people living in the home

When you take on the responsibilities for home care, have a master plan. Some tasks must be done several times a day. Some should be done daily or weekly. Others need only be done occasionally (Figure 5-4).

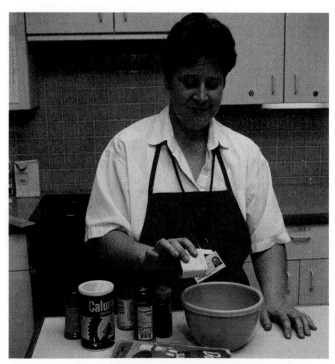

FIGURE 5-3 A clean and uncluttered counter-top makes cooking easier.

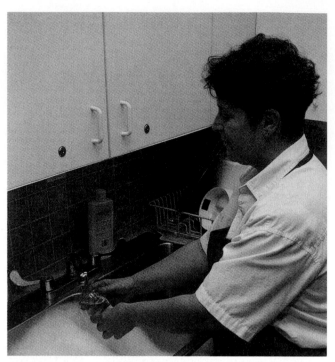

FIGURE 5-4 A client's home needs to be cared for properly. It is a continuous process to keep it clean and orderly.

Daily Cleaning Tasks

Certain tasks should be done every day to keep the house neat and clean. Some daily duties need to be done whether or not they have been assigned. The aide is expected to tidy rooms and clean up spills when they occur. Daily cleaning should not require longer than an hour or an hour and a half. The following duties should be done every day:

- Pick up toys, magazines, newspapers, and clothing. **CAUTION:** Do not discard any of these items without the permission of the client.
- Fluff cushions and pillows, make the beds, or change linens when necessary.
- Dry-dust furniture, lamps, and knickknacks (Figure 5-5).
- Wipe off windowsills and radiators.
- Empty ashtrays and wastebaskets.
- Remove spots and stains using a suitable cleaning product. Test the product first by trying it on a hidden spot. See whether the carpet bleeds or fades. After cleaning a difficult spot, cover it with a clean white cloth until the area dries. Never use soap on carpet stains. Dried soap attracts dirt and can cause permanent damage. To avoid spreading the

stain, work from the outside of the stain toward the center (clean to dirty).

Weekly Cleaning Tasks

Weekly care can be done in more than one way. The aide may want to change the bed linens in every bedroom on the same day or may prefer to completely clean and arrange one bedroom at a time. The aide should always consider the needs of the client before making out a schedule.

Changing Bed Linens. Change bed linens throughout the house. The client's bed may need to be changed more often. Refer to Procedure 2.

Housekeeping Tasks.
* Polish the furniture. Use a flannel cloth, old diaper, or cheesecloth. Use one cloth for dry dusting, another for polishing. Pour polish onto the polishing cloth. **CAUTION:** Do not pour polish directly onto the furniture. Use long strokes along the grain of the wood. Refold cloth and add more polish as needed. Be careful not to spill polish on upholstery or carpets.

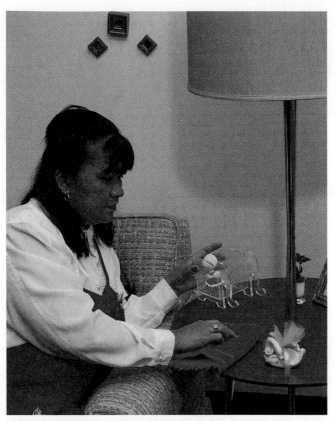

FIGURE 5-5 A home health aide is dusting an end table. Dusting is a task that needs to be done daily.

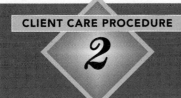

CLIENT CARE PROCEDURE

2

Changing an Unoccupied Bed

PURPOSE

* To apply clean and fresh linens to bed
* To add to the client's comfort by removing wrinkled or soiled sheets

NOTE: Complete one side of the bed entirely before moving to the opposite side. If a fitted sheet for the bottom of bed is not available, and the bed is twin size, it is recommended that a full sheet be used for the bottom. The full sheet, once tucked in, will stay in place longer than a flat twin sheet. Remember to use good body mechanics when making a client's bed.

PROCEDURE

1. Strip bed of dirty linens and place in laundry. Do not rub dirty linens against uniform. Roll linens in and away from aide's body. Wear gloves if linens are soiled.
2. Wash hands.
3. Assemble clean linens: top sheet and fitted bottom sheet (if available), pillow cases, mattress pad, bedspread, and blankets if needed.
4. Place mattress pad on bed and then put clean fitted sheet or flat sheet on bed. If

(continues)

CLIENT CARE PROCEDURE ◆ *2* ◆ **Changing an Unoccupied Bed** *(continued)*

flat sheet is being used, unfold the sheet with the long fold at the center of the bed. Place lower hemline even with the bottom of the mattress (Figure 5-6). If a fitted bottom sheet is used, fit it properly and smoothly around one corner (Figure 5-7).

5. Open sheet gently; do not shake. Starting at the head of the bed, miter the corner and tuck in that side of the sheet (Figures 5-8A–F). A great deal of time is saved by working on only one side of the bed at a time. Sizes of bedrooms differ greatly in clients' homes; you will need to adjust this procedure to your client's bed placement in the room.

6. Place top sheet over the bottom sheet wrong side up. Place hem even with the top edge of the mattress. Place the center fold at the center of the bed. Tuck in top sheet at foot of bed and make a mitered corner (Figures 5-9A–C). **NOTE:** The top sheet, blanket, and spread, if used, may be tucked under the mattress at the same time.

7. Place the blanket back on the bed. Put the top edge 12 inches from the top of the mattress. Place bedspread on the bed.

8. Tuck the blanket and top sheet under the bottom of the mattress at the foot end of the bed. Miter the corner. Fold top sheet over the top edge of the blanket.

9. Walk over to opposite side of bed and make remaining part of the bed.

10. Put pillowcases on pillows. Do not hold the pillow under your chin.

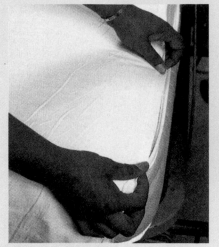

FIGURE 5-6 Place flat bottom sheet even with end of mattress at foot of bed.

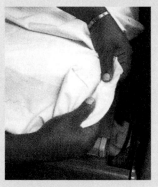

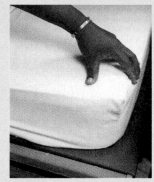

FIGURE 5-7 If a fitted bottom sheet is used, fit it properly and smoothly around one corner.

11. Wash your hands.
12. Document completed task. *(continues)*

- Vacuum floors and carpets, getting under furniture (Figure 5-10). Change or empty the vacuum cleaner bag as required: throw out the dirt in a large paper bag. Avoid bumping the furniture and woodwork with the vacuum cleaner.
- Vacuum upholstery and under seat cushions; vacuum lamp shades and wipe away cobwebs.
- Damp or wet mop floors.

Periodic Cleaning Tasks

Certain areas in the home do not require frequent cleaning. However, the aide should check these areas to be sure that dust and dirt do not collect. The following tasks can be done on an occasional basis.

- Remove cobwebs from the ceilings, walls, curtains, and shades. Use a long-handled dust mop covered with a clean cloth.

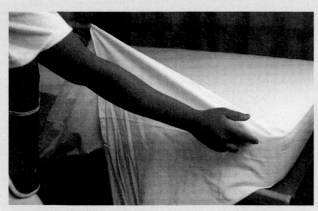

FIGURE 5-8A   To make a mitered corner, pick up sheet hanging at side of bed, about 12 inches from bed, forming a triangle.

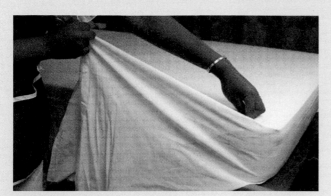

FIGURE 5-8B   Place your finger on bed to form sharp corner.

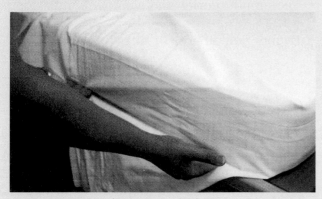

FIGURE 5-8C   Using two hands, tuck sheet well under mattress.

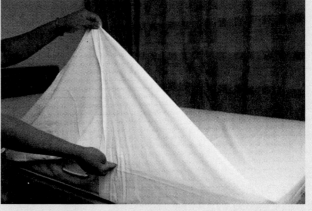

FIGURE 5-8D   Using fingers as a guide, allow sheet to drop straight down. Run fingers along edge of mattress to end forming the mitered triangular corner.

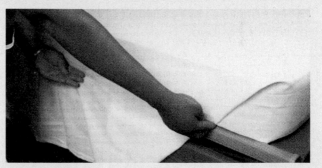

FIGURE 5-8E   Finish tucking in corner and smooth.

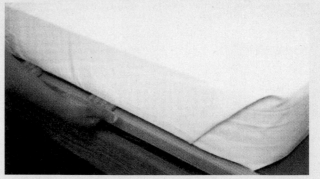

FIGURE 5-8F   The finished mitered corner should look like this.   *(continues)*

- Remove small pictures from the wall and dust behind them. Dust the frames and glass.
- Wipe mirrors or use glass cleaner on them as needed.

- Remove books from shelves and dust both books and shelves.
- Clean lamp bases. Replace burned-out bulbs as needed.

CLIENT CARE PROCEDURE **Changing an Unoccupied Bed** *(continued)*

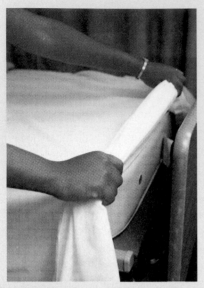

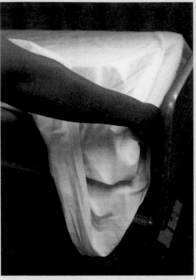

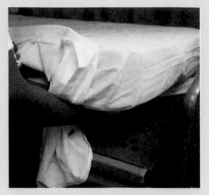

FIGURE 5-9C Bring sheet with opposite hand smoothly over end of mattress.

FIGURE 5-9A Gather about 12 to 18 inches of top sheet at bottom of bed.

FIGURE 5-9B Face foot of bed and lift mattress with near hand.

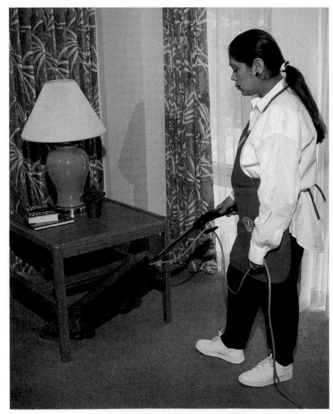

FIGURE 5-10 An aide is vacuuming the living room, a weekly task.

- Damp-wipe lighting fixtures on walls or ceilings (Figure 5-11).
- Hand wash decorative plates and table ornaments in mild soapsuds.
- Vacuum draperies and window blinds (Figure 5-12).
- Launder small area or throw rugs.

Kitchen Maintenance and Cleaning

The client, the family, and the home health aide spend more time in the kitchen than in any other room in the home. Food is prepared, cooked, and consumed in the kitchen. The aide cooks and cleans up after each meal, replaces items used, throws out waste, and stores leftovers. Kitchen work never ends, but it still can be challenging and satisfying when done well. Attractive, nutritious meals can improve the client's physical condition, which is why they must always be made in a clean and healthful environment (Figures 5-13 and 5-14).

Following are some reasons for keeping a kitchen clean and neat:

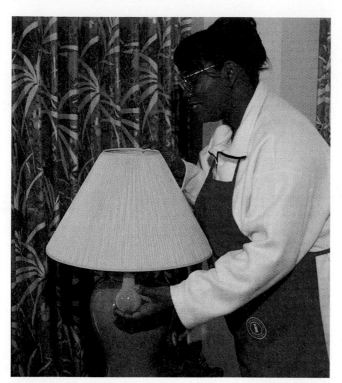

FIGURE 5-11 Minor tasks, such as changing a light bulb, are often part of the home health aide's duties.

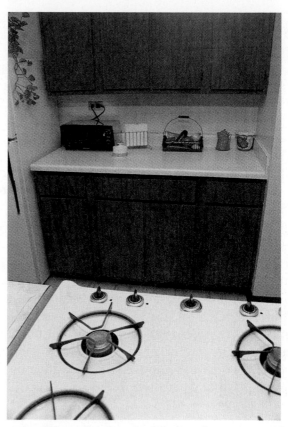

FIGURE 5-13 An example of a neat and orderly kitchen

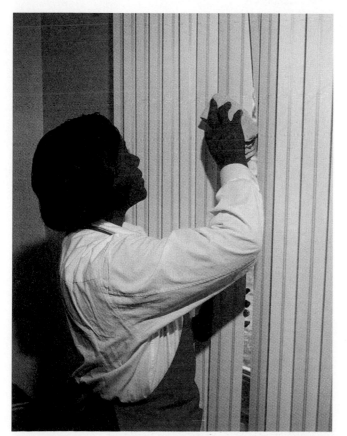

FIGURE 5-12 Cleaning the window blinds is a task that needs to be done on a regular basis.

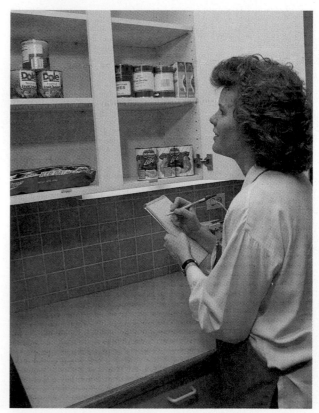

FIGURE 5-14 An aide is checking the cupboards for needed supplies.

- Germs are less likely to grow in a clean kitchen.
- It is easier to prepare meals in a neat area.
- It is quicker to find equipment and supplies that have been properly stored.
- Clean dishes, utensils, and pots are ready for use.
- Accidents are less likely to happen when floors are free of spills.
- Insects (flies, roaches, ants) and rodents (mice or rats) are less likely to appear when food and garbage are properly put away.

Maintaining order is an easier task when the kitchen area is clean. The aide who keeps up with small cleaning tasks will find that it makes work easier (Figures 5-15 and 5-16). Routine cleanup usually takes no more than 15 to 20 minutes after each meal. Major tasks such as cleaning drawers and cabinets require more time. The aide should schedule these to be done at times when routine tasks are light and the client is resting or has visitors.

Disposing of Garbage. Place a heavy plastic bag in a waste container or garbage can. It is required in some cities to separate the glass containers, cans, and other **recyclable** materials (Figure 5-17). You will need to separate the garbage according to local guidelines. In some areas of our country, you will need to place the garbage in specially marked plastic bags. In other states, you may need to save all aluminum cans so that they can be returned to the store for a refund. Empty garbage and trash often to prevent odors that can attract ants, mice, and roaches. Spray the garbage container with a disinfectant.

Dishwashing. If the client has an infectious disease, wash the client's dishes and utensils separately from the other family dishes. Rinse these dishes and utensils in boiling water. This is an aseptic technique used to prevent the spread of germs (**pathogens**) to other members of the family.

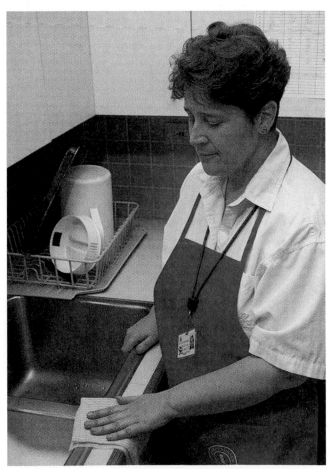

FIGURE 5-15 Keeping the kitchen clean is a continuous daily task.

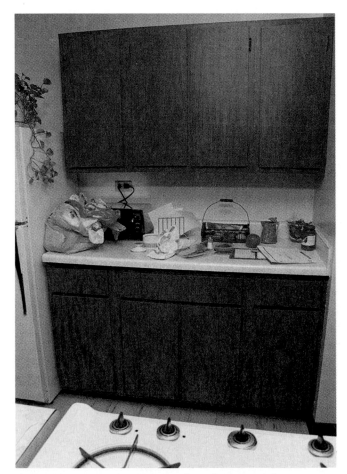

FIGURE 5-16 An example of an untidy kitchen

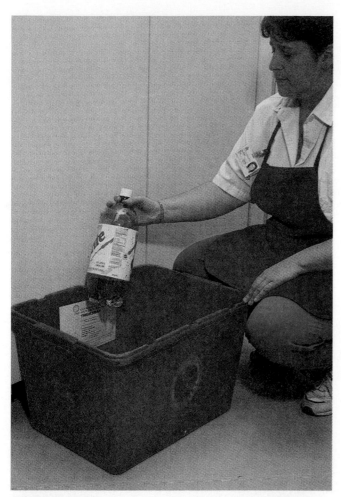

FIGURE 5-17 In many areas, garbage must be separated into recyclable and non-recyclable items.

When washing the family's dishes by hand, use hot water and liquid detergent. Wash the dishes in the following order: cups and glassware, utensils, plates and bowls, pots and pans.

If the water becomes greasy, drain the sink and add fresh water and detergent. After washing them with detergent, rinse the dishes completely with hot water. Place the dishes in a drainer. Air drying is more **sanitary** than drying with a dish towel. Lay a clean dish towel over the dishes as the rest of the kitchen is being cleaned. After the dishes are dry, put them away in cabinets.

Some homes are equipped with automatic dishwashers. Before placing dishes in the dishwasher, scrape and rinse them well. Some machines have a rinse cycle prior to the wash cycle. When using these machines, hand rinsing the dishes may not be necessary before loading. Pour dishwasher detergent into the correct area labeled on the machine. **CAUTION:** Do not use soap powder or liquid detergent. Run the dishwasher only when it is fully loaded. Household kitchen sponges or cleaning cloths can be placed in the top rack of the dishwasher to be disinfected. Pots and pans should be hand washed, rinsed, and stored to dry.

Wiping Surfaces. Use a cloth or sponge, warm water, and detergent to wipe the table, countertops, wall behind the stove, stove top, and outside surfaces of the refrigerator and microwave oven. Be sure to remove grease or splashes caused from cooking foods.

Use a cloth or sponge and vinegar to wipe out the inside of the refrigerator. The inside of the microwave oven should be wiped with warm water and carefully dried.

Wipe the sink; use scouring powder if necessary. Scouring powder helps remove stains and marks left by pans or food wastes. After scouring, be sure to rinse the sink completely. **CAUTION:** Always check with your client before using scouring powder on the sink because many new sinks can be damaged by scouring powder.

Cleaning the Floors. Wipe up any spills with a cloth, sponge, or paper towel as soon as they occur. Do not wipe with a sponge or cloth that is used for other surfaces; keep a separate cloth or sponge for floors only. For general sweeping, use a dust mop or broom. Gather crumbs and dirt on a dustpan and empty the dustpan into a garbage container. Damp mop floors at least once a week. If blood or other body fluids are spilled on a tile floor, you are required to wear gloves and wipe it up with a solution of 10 parts of water to 1 part bleach (Figure 5-18).

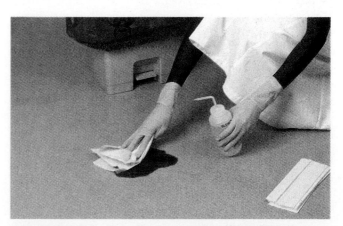

FIGURE 5-18 To clean up blood and body fluid spills, use a solution of bleach and water.

Cleaning Cabinets and Drawers.   Dishes, glassware, and utensils should be stored in clean cabinets and drawers. Water vapor, smoke, and grease from cooking cause a buildup of oily film on kitchen surfaces. The film collects on both the inside and the outside of closed cabinets. The outside of cabinets should be cleaned at least once a week. The inside should be cleaned several times a year. The cleaning product used will depend on the type of cabinet being cleaned. Metal, formica, and wood require different types of cleaning products. Drawers will remain neat if kitchen items are put away in order. Drawers also should be cleaned out several times a year.

Storing Cleaning Supplies.   Cleaning products should be stored in a place that children and confused adults cannot reach. **CAUTION:** Many cleaning products are poisonous. Swallowing even a small amount of a poison can be fatal. In a home where children are living, do not store products under the sink. A high cabinet with a door is the best place to store cleaning products. Brooms, mops, and rags should be put away after use.

Bathroom Maintenance and Cleaning

Bathrooms must be given special care in homes where there is illness. The natural dampness in a bathroom causes the growth of molds and **mildew,** which are unsightly and cause odors. Moisture provides an environment ideally suited for the growth of microorganisms, which may be present in the home. For this reason, the home health aide must be particularly concerned with cleaning techniques (Figure 5-19).

Daily Care.   Bathrooms are used frequently throughout the day and can easily become dirty. The aide should encourage family members to help in keeping the bathroom neat. In addition, a thorough cleaning reduces the risk of spreading disease. The following duties should be done on a daily basis.

- Wash and rinse all surfaces in the bathroom. The outside of the toilet as well as both sides of the toilet seat should be cleaned daily. The shower floor and walls, wall tiles, shower curtain, towel racks, windowsills, and radiator also should be cleaned daily. Use hot water, detergent, and disinfectant.
- Wipe out the tub or shower and sink with cleanser.

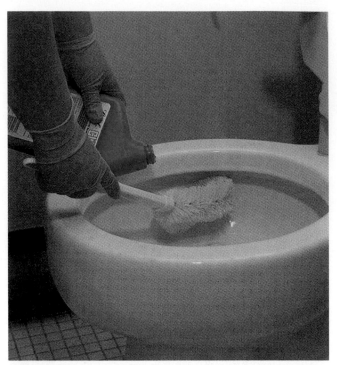

FIGURE 5-19   The client's toilet needs to be cleaned routinely.

- Use a damp cloth to remove water spots from the walls around the sink. Clean the bathroom mirror with a glass cleaner, rinse off the soap dish, and wipe off the toothbrush holder.
- Damp mop bathroom floor.
- Using bathroom cleanser and sponge or cloth, clean and rinse sink and tub.
- Using brush and bowl cleaner, clean the inside of the toilet bowl. Be sure to scrub the area under the top rim of the bowl.
- Bleach in water can be used to remove mildew and mold.
- Empty wastebasket contents into a plastic bag. Line the clean wastebasket with a plastic liner.
- If needed, place a new roll of toilet paper on the roller. If the existing roll is running low, place a fresh roll nearby for easy replacement.
- A laundry hamper kept in the bathroom should be wiped out regularly using hot water and detergent. It is best to wash the client's linens daily. When emptying the family laundry hamper, transfer clothing directly to a laundry basket. Never put soiled clothing on the floor. Germs from the clothing can be transferred to the floor or germs on the floor can be transferred to the clothing. People walking across the floors can transfer these germs to all areas of the home. Hold dirty

laundry away from the body as it is transferred from place to place.

- If possible, open the bathroom window and ventilate the room for a few minutes. Spray around the tub and sink drain with a disinfectant or air freshener.
- Add fresh towels and face cloths to the towel racks. Make a note of any bathroom supplies that need to be purchased, such as shaving cream, toothpaste, soap, tissues, and toilet paper.
- Do not use the same container for both dirty and clean laundry.

Weekly Care.   Some tasks do not need to be done daily. The following tasks can be done weekly or whenever necessary.

- Clean shower stall to remove lime buildup.
- Launder bath mats, small rugs, and throw rugs as needed. **CAUTION:** Do not put rubber-backed mats into the dryer.
- Tidy the linen closet to make it neat.
- Clean the medicine chest. With permission of the family, throw out old medications by flushing them down the toilet. Prescription medicines are normally dated and are marked as to the length of time they may be safely used. All medicines should be labeled. It is unsafe to use medicine from unlabeled bottles.

GENERAL GUIDELINES FOR MEAL PLANNING

There are some general rules to follow when planning nutritious meals for clients. In addition to the general rules listed, the aide should see that an emergency food supply is on hand. The home health aide should take into consideration the ethnic and regional preferences of the client when planning a menu.

Eating Patterns

Generally, people expect to have three meals a day—breakfast, lunch (dinner), dinner (supper) (Figure 5-20). The midday and evening meals are a cultural choice. For example, farmers who work hard during planting and harvesting often expect and need a hot, full meal at noon. They expend so much effort in the morning that they need to replace energy at noon so they can go back to work. Office workers usually do not need nor want more than a light lunch. They

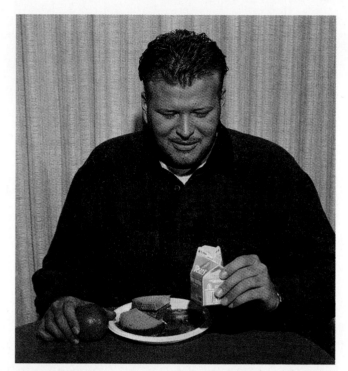

FIGURE 5-20   A man eating a balanced meal

usually prefer to have their main meal in the evening in the comfort of their homes. This gives them a chance to be with their families as they all enjoy a hot meal.

Some older people find that eating the main meal in the evening makes them uncomfortable. They find that they feel better having their main meal at midday and then eating a light meal in the evening. This relieves the feeling of heaviness and discomfort when they go to bed. **Meals on Wheels** (a service that brings hot meals to shut-ins and the elderly) usually provides the food at midday for this reason.

Some elderly who can ambulate prefer the companionship of a meal shared with friends at a local senior citizen center (Figure 5-21).

Some people prefer to have five or six smaller meals that can be divided into a light breakfast, an early light lunch, a midafternoon snack, a small dinner, and a late night snack. Cancer patients are often encouraged to follow this practice. The aide should also remember that persons who are ill may lose their appetites as a result of their condition.

Food Preparation and Appeal

Foods may be prepared in a number of ways. They may be eaten raw. Some can be broiled, baked, fried, boiled, or steamed. Overcooking causes the loss of minerals, vitamins, and other

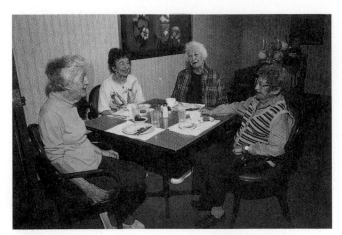

FIGURE 5-21 Many older adults enjoy a daily meal at their local senior citizen center.

nutrients. Some meats, particularly pork and chicken, must be thoroughly cooked.

When planning and preparing food the home health aide must always remember that a menu should provide proper nutrition. This is the most important rule. Foods selected must fall within the limits of those foods allowed by the client's medical condition.

When planning and preparing meals, a home health aide should keep the following in mind:

- Variety
- Appearance
- Flavor and aroma
- Satiety (hunger satisfaction)
- Individual preferences (Figure 5-22)
- Food costs
- Balance

Variety. Variety is necessary to avoid dulling the appetite. People become bored with the same menu day after day. This can cause a loss

FIGURE 5-22 Traditional ethnic, regional, and racial food patterns

Ethnic Group	Bread and Cereal	Eggs, Meat, Fish, Poultry	Dairy Products	Fruits and Vegetables	Seasonings, Etc.
Chinese	Rice, wheat, millet, corn, noodles	Little meat and no beef, fish, including raw fish, eggs of hen, duck, pigeon	Water buffalo milk occasionally, soybean milk, cheese	Soybeans, soybean sprouts, bamboo sprouts, soy curd cooked in lime water, radish leaves, legumes, vegetables, fruits	Sesame seeds, ginger, almonds, soy sauce, sesame, soybean and peanut oils
African American	Hot breads, cookies, pastries, cakes, cereals, white rice, corn breads	Chicken, salt pork, ham, bacon, sausage, salted salmon, salt herring, fish	Milk and milk products, little cheese	Kale, mustard, turnip greens, cabbage, hominy grits, dandelion greens	Molasses, Deep frying
Jewish	Noodles, crusty white seeded rolls, rye bread, pumpernickel bread, chalah, bagels	Koshered meat (from forequarters and organs from beef, lamb, veal), milk not eaten at same meal (not a rule for all Jewish people), fish, chicken	Milk and milk products, cheese	Vegetables (sometimes cooked with meat), fruits, cooked fruits (compote)	Salt, garlic, dill, parsley

(continues)

FIGURE 5-22 *(continued)*

Ethnic Group	Bread and Cereal	Eggs, Meat, Fish, Poultry	Dairy Products	Fruits and Vegetables	Seasonings, Etc.
Italian	Crusty white bread, cornmeal and rice (northern Italy), pasta (southern Italy)	Beef, veal, chicken, eggs, fish	Milk in coffee, cheese (many different kinds)	Broccoli, zucchini, other squash, eggplant, artichokes, string beans, tomatoes, peppers, asparagus, fresh fruit	Olive oil, vinegar, salt, pepper, garlic, basil, wine
Puerto Rican	Rice, beans, noodles, spaghetti, oatmeal, cornmeal	Dry salted codfish, meat, salt pork, sausage, chicken, beef	Coffee with hot milk	Starchy root vegetables, green bananas, plantain, legumes, tomatoes, green pepper, onion, pineapple, papaya, citrus fruits, corn	Lard, herbs, oil, vinegar, hot peppers
Near Eastern	Bulgur (wheat)	Lamb, mutton, chicken, fish, eggs	Fermented milk, sour cream, yogurt, cheese	Nuts, grape leaves	Sheep's butter, olive oil
Greek	Plain wheat bread	Lamb, pork, poultry, eggs, organ meats	Yogurt, cheeses, butter	Onions, tomatoes, legumes, fresh fruit	Olive oil, parsley, lemon, vinegar, olives
Mexican	Lime-treated corn, rice	Little meat (ground beef or pork), poultry, fish	Cheese, evaporated milk as beverage for infants	Pinto beans, tomatoes, potatoes, onions, lettuce	Chili pepper, salt, garlic, herbs

of interest in food. It is important for sick people to receive appealing meals. The same nutrients can usually be obtained from a variety of foods. Variety in the menu helps improve the client's interest in eating.

Appearance. Appearance is the way food looks when it is served. Nicely arranged food adds to the pleasure and enjoyment of eating. When foods are overcooked they become mushy and unappetizing. At the same time overcooking destroys many of the nutrients. Overcooked meats become tough and lose flavor.

Foods that appeal to the eye perk up the appetite. Properly cooked vegetables, for example, retain their natural color. The color enhances the appearance of the vegetables on the plate. The attractiveness of the meal can be illustrated by two examples. Imagine a plate of food consisting of a chicken breast, mashed potatoes, white bread, and cauliflower. This meal would be nutritious but it would look dull and colorless. If the potatoes or cauliflower were replaced by a garden salad and string beans, the meal would look much brighter and more appealing.

Flavor and Aroma. Flavor and aroma set the digestive juices into action. Seasonings most often used are salt, pepper and garlic. However, there are many herbs such as thyme, rosemary, parsley, sage, and basil that can be added to bring out the aroma and sharpen the flavor. Often these herbs and spices can be used when a client is on a salt-free diet. Fresh lemon juice can be squeezed over meat and vegetables also. Because both sight and smell affect the appetite, proper use of seasonings can be of value in planning a menu.

Satiety. Satisfying the pangs of hunger is another reason people eat. Some foods make the stomach feel full but not uncomfortable. This feeling is called satiety. If daily menus are well planned, the satiety value will be provided. Bulk foods such as bread, macaroni, beans, and spaghetti are good fillers.

Individual Preferences. An important factor in meal planning is providing foods that the person likes to eat. There is no logic to explain why some people like certain foods and dislike others. Some individuals want steak served rare; others will only eat it well done. Some people dislike spinach, cabbage, beets, or mushrooms. The home health aide must try to prepare foods the client likes, cooked as the client likes them.

Food Costs. In most homes, it is necessary to work within a budget. Therefore, it is important to check newspaper ads for daily specials, coupons, and seasonal bargains. Fresh fruits and vegetables are lower in price during the summer and fall. At other times it is more economical to purchase frozen, canned, or dried items, such as powdered milk. If money is a consideration, then planning and purchasing must be worked around the prices. Careful planning makes it possible to meet nutritional needs while keeping costs at a minimum.

Balance. All five food groups that appear in the food pyramid should be included daily. Refer to Unit 12, Figure 12-2, for a diagram of the food pyramid.

SHOPPING AND MEAL PREPARATION

Shopping and meal preparation require time and use of special skills. Planning nutritious meals and buying foods the family can afford require knowledge and use of judgment. Storing foods properly is also important. The aide develops these skills with study and practice.

Menus and Shopping Lists

Most meal planning is done for an entire week. Weekly planning saves the home health aide from making frequent trips to the market. The following steps are helpful planning guides.

- Sit down with the client or client's family and ask what foods and menus they want. This could be an important activity for the client because it may foster the client's feelings of being useful and in charge of the care.
- Plan menus for a full week. Make sure that the menu follows any specific guidelines provided by the client's physician.
- Be sure all **staple items,** such as spices and seasonings that are needed for each planned meal, are on hand.
- Make a shopping list and include all items needed in the household (Figure 5-23). Shopping time can be reduced by organizing the shopping list so that all items of one type are under one heading.
- Look in the newspaper and check the prices of products advertised. Cut out any coupons of items on the shopping list.
- Plan to use only the amount of money budgeted for food and supplies.

Purchasing Food

Planning done in the home saves the home health aide time in the store. Shopping should be done at a time when the client can be safely left alone or has a visitor.

Shopping at home is an excellent activity for the housebound client and this is especially true of food shopping. It has several advantages. The client can become involved and interested in choosing foods, planning meals, and, even more importantly, saving money. This activity helps the client remain aware of the "life beyond illness" and can actually make the client feel better and more hopeful about the future. How do you shop at home for food? By reading newspaper and magazine ads and clipping coupons and special company offers. If the client is able to read and has the energy to look through papers and magazines, this might be a challenging and economical way to pass the time.

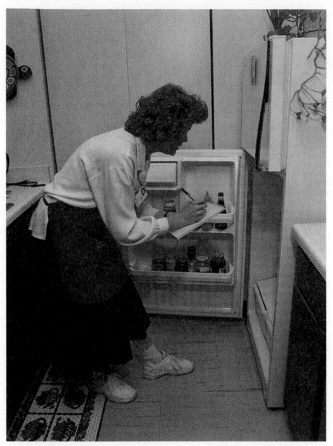

FIGURE 5-23 An aide checking the refrigerator for needed groceries

Check with the client's local grocery store to see if it has special days on which the disabled or elderly can shop and receive extra discounts or assistance. Many large grocery stores have special individual motorized carts to ride while shopping at their stores. Volunteers might be available in your community or through the client's church to assist the client to shop or actually do the shopping for the client. If at all possible, it is beneficial to get your client out of the house and involved in the actual grocery shopping. This gives the client a chance to see other people and also make choices in the grocery shopping. Another benefit is for the client to actually see the "real" cost of food and how expensive certain items are.

A smart shopper plans ahead. If several markets are located within the same general area, it pays to take advantage of money-saving brand or store coupons and buy items at the store where the price is lowest. When prices are particularly low on staple items such as paper and household cleaning supplies or canned goods, then, if money and storage space are available, extra amounts may be purchased. Practical guidelines for shopping are presented in the following list.

1. Avoid going to the grocery store when you are hungry. Sweets and foods not on the shopping list are more likely to be bought when the shopper is hungry.
2. If there is time, walk through the store with the shopping list in hand. Compare prices and decide on the best buys for the budget. If the allowed money will not cover all the items, make substitutions. For example, if beef prices are very high, buy ground beef instead of cube steak. If the quality of fresh **produce** is poor, buy frozen or canned vegetables.
3. Select the needed foods by starting at one side of the store and moving from aisle to aisle. Compare the prices of brand names and store brands. Read labels. Buy the size best suited to the needs of the client or family. Large quantities are not practical if they cannot be stored, handled, or used before the expiration date.
4. Do not buy sale items unless the client normally uses the products and has storage space for them. A bargain the client cannot use is no bargain at all.
5. If the client needs to prepare food when you are not there, you may need to purchase nutritious **convenience foods** that the client can prepare with little assistance. You will need to check food labels if the client has diet restrictions.
6. Be aware of how much area is available for storage of food. Use this space wisely and purchase items that are going to be needed within the month only.
7. If the client just wants a small quantity, it may be wise to purchase a small serving of this in the **delicatessen** rather than preparing a large amount and throwing it away in a few days.
8. If only one person is living in the home, it may be wise to put the bread in the freezer and remove when needed.
9. Powdered or dried milk can be a money saver. Dry milk mixed with water can be added to a quart of skim or whole milk. The flavor may be the same or better and it costs less. The nutritional value is the same as in whole milk.
10. Fresh fruits and vegetables are less expensive during their growing season. Compare

fresh vegetable prices with canned and frozen vegetable prices while vegetables are in season. Out-of-season produce is quite costly.

11. Eggs have the same food value whether they are jumbo, extra large, large, or small. Brown- or white-shelled eggs are equally tasty and nutritious. Large eggs look better when served fried, boiled, or poached. However, for cooking or scrambling, small eggs are the best buy.

12. When buying meat, consider how the meat will be prepared. Most meat cuts have the same food value. Cheaper cuts can be just as tasty when prepared with imagination and care. When comparing the price per pound, consider the waste due to bones and fat. Figure the number of servings needed and the cost per serving.

13. When selecting poultry, buying the whole bird is the best choice. Buying separate parts such as the breast, legs, or thighs is more expensive.

14. If there is enough freezer space in the home, meats can be purchased in **bulk;** there is a considerable saving in the cost per pound. At home, meat can be rewrapped for the freezer in smaller meal-size portions. However, do not buy more than can be used. Waste occurs from overstocking the freezer. Most meats can be safely frozen for up to 6 months. Some meats lose flavor and food value when stored longer. Foods not properly wrapped can be ruined by freezer burn. Be sure to label and date each item put in the freezer.

15. Make sure meats purchased are fresh. If they do not smell, look, or feel right, do not buy them. Fresh meat will regain its shape when poked with a finger. If the meat feels slimy, slick, or soft, do not buy it. If the color is off, the meat may be spoiled already.

16. Do not buy damaged cans, no matter how low the price. Cans with bulging tops, dents, or rust may contain spoiled food.

17. Purchase **perishable** foods last. These include foods that spoil easily, such as milk, meats, and frozen foods.

Storing Food

After returning from the store, the aide should put foods and supplies away. This should be done before any other major task is begun.

- Always refrigerate perishable foods immediately. Lettuce can wilt and milk will spoil if not refrigerated.
- Frozen fruits and vegetables should be placed in the freezer as soon as possible. Do not overstock on frozen foods.
- Wash and clean poultry before refrigerating. If poultry is not planned for a meal within 2 days, wrap, date, label, and freeze it.
- Dried and packaged foods should be stored in airtight containers. Examples of airtight containers are canisters, glass jars with lids, or plastic bags. Many containers of food can be refrigerated if there is room. Otherwise they should be stored so that roaches, ants, or rodents cannot get to them. If safe storage space is limited, buy only small amounts of these foods.
- Canned goods store easily and keep very well. They should not be stored near hot water pipes or near any other source of heat.
- Paper goods and other supplies should be stored nearest the place where they will be used. Toilet paper should be stored near the bathroom and laundry supplies near the washing machine. Cleaning products always should be stored in a closet or cabinet out of the reach of children. Childproof locks may be used if there are small children or confused adults in the home.

Meal Preparation

When preparing meals, the home health aide must check to see if the client has a special diet ordered or if the client has allergies to any foods. Refer to Unit 12 for a discussion on food allergies. Occasionally the client may be taking medications that cannot be taken with certain types of foods. The aide should use the following guidelines when preparing meals:

1. Use sparingly—salad oils, cream, butter, sugar, soft drinks, sweet desserts.
2. Prepare any special diet the dietitian has ordered for the client.
3. Serve skim or 2% milk to limit fat intake.
4. Cook vegetables in a microwave to preserve the nutritional value of the vegetables.
5. Prepare amounts that will be eaten in one or two meals only. Serving the same foods can decrease the client's appetite.

6. Have low-calorie nutritious snacks available so client does not eat high-calorie snacks.
7. Be sure the meal being prepared has adequate fiber foods. Clients who are inactive may develop constipation, which can be prevented with a diet high in fiber.
8. Encourage intake of water or other fluids throughout the day.
9. If client is taking a diuretic, the diet will need to be high in foods that contain potassium, such as bananas, dates, raisins, and orange juice. Be sure to follow the nurse's instructions.
10. If the client is on a low-calorie diet, sugar substitutes should be used as often as possible.
11. Store food at a height convenient for the client to reach.
12. Avoid fried foods as much as possible. Fried foods add more fat to the diet than is necessary.
13. People should limit the number of eggs per week (*not* including eggs used in preparing a dish such as custard).
14. When opening cans, wash the top of the can before piercing with a can opener; this will keep dirt and germs from entering the food. If the contents spew out or are foamy or appear to have bubbles they may have spoiled and must be discarded. After a can has been opened, unused portions should be transferred to a refrigerator container and covered tightly before refrigerating.
15. Check food for spoiling: sour milk, rancid butter, moldy bread, **fermented** fruits, spoiled meats.
16. Throughout the week serve different vegetables, meats, poultry, fish, and meat substitutes. Different spices and herbs also may be used to add variety to meals (Figures 5-24 and 5-25).

FIGURE 5-24 Seasonings and spices add variety and taste to meals.

Seasonings and Spices*	Uses
Allspice	Particularly good with pot roast, in puddings and cereals (tastes like cinnamon, clove, and nutmeg)
Anise	In tossed green salad and other vegetable salads; can be used with pot cheese
Caraway Seeds	Give flavor to bread, pot cheese, cabbage, cauliflower, cereals, and cookies
Cardamom Seeds	Good with curries, soups, and meats
Cayenne	Few grains will be enough to season vegetables, meats, fish, poultry, soups; vegetable, meat, fish, poultry, or egg salads
Chili Peppers	Seasoning soups, rice, dried peas or beans, meat, fish, pot cheese
Cinnamon	Flavors cereals, bread, pot cheese, vegetables such as beans, cabbage, cauliflower, carrots, cucumbers, eggplant, lentils, onions, and peas
Cloves	Can be used in much the same way as cinnamon; particularly nice for flavoring tea
Coriander Seeds	For seasoning stews, curries, soups, and fish
Curry Powder	To season soups, stews, rice, chicken, eggs, meat, fish, and vegetables
Garlic	Flavors soups, sauces, salads and salad dressings, meat, fish, poultry, pot cheese, dried peas or beans
Ginger	Used in much the same way as cinnamon

*Spices and many seasonings are highly perishable unless kept in tightly closed containers. They should be bought in small quantities and renewed at least once a year.

(continues)

FIGURE 5-24   *(continued)*

Seasonings and Spices*	Uses
Mace	Flavors meats, fish, poultry, soup, sauces, stews, potatoes, carrots, snap beans, peas, cabbage, and cauliflower
Dry Mustard	Seasons meats, fish, salad dressings, vegetables, eggs, pot cheese, fish, poultry, and all salads
Nutmeg	Used the same way as mace
Paprika	Gives a bright garnish to vegetables, meats, eggs, pot cheese, fish, poultry, and all salads
Pepper	Adds flavor to meats, fish, poultry, eggs, and vegetables
Poppy Seeds	Used as toppings for bread, rolls, cookies, and cakes; good with pot cheese and in salad dressings
Sesame Seeds	Used on rolls, buns, and bread
Turmeric	Seasons meats, fish, and poultry

17. Most fresh fruit and vegetables should be served raw if possible because of greater nutritional value. They should be cooked unpeeled to give the most food value. Steaming instead of boiling preserves both flavor and food value. The water from fresh vegetables is high in vitamins. This water may be added to meat stock and used for making tasty soups.

18. Save whole milk for drinking. Use dry milk in preparing sauces and gravies. The food value and flavor of dry milk is equal to whole milk.

19. Use leftover meats in a creative way. Add fresh mushrooms to leftover beef and make a brown sauce. Turkey hash, creamed turkey, chicken salad, or sandwiches all can be made with leftovers.

20. Foods not in season may not be the best buy. However, if the client likes a certain food it is well worth the extra cost and may make a pleasant change in the diet. Fresh vegetables should be purchased in the exact amount needed to prevent spoilage.

21. Practice cooking and serving meals. A good cook uses clean, unspoiled raw meats and vegetables and follows recipes. Food should be attractive and served on an attractive table or tray.

Cooking in a Microwave.   Microwave ovens have been in general use for a few years, but they are not a standard appliance in all homes. If one has not had occasion to use a microwave oven, here are a few simple rules.

Never place anything metal (including twist ties, labels with metal content, or dishes with metal trim) in the microwave. It will ruin the oven and probably the metal also. Special microwave utensils, plates, and dishes can be used, as well as glass, china, and paperware. Most microwave owners will have a simple manual with instructions for proper use. Here are a few examples of ways to make use of a microwave.

- Baked potato: Wash and dry thoroughly, then prick the skin with a fork so the steam can escape. Place the potato on a paper towel or paper plate and put in the oven, following instructions for timing. It can take 3 to 5 minutes to have a perfectly baked potato.
- Leftovers: Place in microwave plate or dish, cover with paper towel or wax paper as recommended, and heat at the recommended setting and time. It can take as little as 2 or 3 minutes to heat up leftovers.
- Frozen vegetables: Follow instructions on package. This is an excellent way to prepare frozen vegetables so they remain crisp and taste fresh. Seasoning is done after the food is

FIGURE 5-25 Herbs also may be used to enhance the taste and appeal of many foods.

Herb and Part Used	Uses in Cooking
Basil—leaves	Italian tomato dishes, soups, ragouts, salads, meats, sauces, fruit drinks
Bay—leaves	For flavoring soups, stews, sauces
Chervil—leaves and sometimes fleshy roots	In place of parsley, in fine herbs, salads, sauces, soups, omelettes
Chives—leaves	In fine herbs, salads, omelettes, or anything for which a delicate onion flavor is desired
Dill—seed and young tips	Added to melted sweet butter or salt-free margarine, it makes a fine sauce for fish. In mashed potato, in tossed green, potato, fish, or vegetable salads. Sprinkled on broiled chops
Sweet Marjoram—leaves	Sprinkled over beef, lamb, or pork. Used in veal stew, chopped meat, meat balls. In fine herbs, salads, and fish dishes. Cooked with zucchini
Mint—leaves	Flavors sauces, vegetables, jellies, fruit drinks, vegetable and fruit salads, custards, puddings
Oregano	Can be rubbed over meat before roasting or broiling, or it can be put in the water during the cooking of meat and fish. Used with veal, pork, soups, potatoes, vegetables and fresh salads. (Closely related to marjoram and has a similar flavor)
Parsley—leaves	In fine herbs, for soups, sauces. Popular with boiled potato and many other vegetables. With meat, fish, eggs and with vegetable, meat, or fish salads
Rosemary—leaves	To flavor roast lamb and veal, meat stews, poultry sauces, stuffings
Sage—leaves	In stuffing for meat, poultry, fish, fish chowder
Savory—leaves	Excellent with snap beans, dried peas, lentils. Also good in chopped beef, gravy, meat stew, and croquettes. Can be sprinkled over fish before baking or broiling
Tarragon—leaves	Flavoring for vinegar, sauces, and salad dressings, chicken and other meats; for egg and tomato dishes, sandwiches; in fine herbs
Thyme—leaves	In fine herbs, in stews, soups, sauces, salads. With meat, poultry, fish, tomato dishes. Can be combined with melted butter and served over carrots, onions, and peas

cooked so that vegetables prepared in the microwave can be appropriately seasoned to fit the needs of any diet.

- Defrost: The microwave also may be used to defrost frozen foods quickly so that they can be chosen and prepared at the last minute.
- Meats seem to taste better when cooked by traditional methods—on top of the stove or in the oven or broiler. However, the microwave manual has recipes for cooking all sorts of food.
- Reheat: If for some reason a client's food has become cold (a telephone call interrupting the meal or an emergency of some sort), a microwave-proof dinner plate can be placed directly in the microwave and in just a

minute, the meal will be heated thoroughly without loss of flavor or appetite appeal.

LAUNDRY

Clothes and household linens are expensive. The home aide must be responsible for giving suitable care to these items. Correctly sorting, washing, and ironing clothes requires careful attention.

Sorting Clothes and Linens

Most clothing can be machine washed. However, some articles of clothing must be dry cleaned; others must be hand washed. Most of today's clothes have labels with instructions for proper care. If an item is not labeled, the aide must be able to judge from its appearance. If there is any doubt, the aide should ask a family member which washing method is best.

In general, cotton fabrics can be washed in hot water. Blends of cotton and polyester and cottons of light color should be washed in warm water. Chlorine bleaches are only used for white cottons. There are special bleaches for nylon and **polyester fabrics.** Be careful to follow instructions when using bleaches. Dark fabrics are washed separately from light fabrics (Figure 5-26). Many homemakers wash dark clothes in cold water with cold water detergent. When sorting clothes for the laundry, use the following tips:

- Sort the clothes according to color. Do not wash white clothes with dark items. If possible wash towels separately. You may use a separate load for lingerie and other fabrics needing a gentle cycle.
- Make a separate pile of clothes that must be hand washed or dry cleaned.
- As each item is sorted, check it for spots that might require special care. Collars of shirts and dresses and spots from food or other stains may need special care (Figure 5-27).
- Turn pockets inside out. Be sure to remove pens, pencils, paper, coins, or other items in the pockets.
- Shake dirt, sand, or grass out of clothing before placing it with the other clothes.
- Remove belt buckles or ornaments that might be ruined in the washer.
- Hand wash separately those fabrics in which the colors run or bleed.

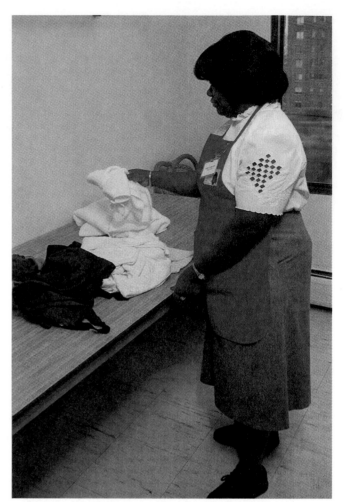

FIGURE 5-26 Dirty laundry is separated according to white and dark colors before the clothes are placed in the washing machine.

- Make sure dark socks do not get mixed with the light or white loads.

Loading the Washing Machine

Loading differs depending on whether the family has a top- or front-loading machine. Before operating the washing machine, the aide should read the directions. If the aide is still in doubt, a family member should be asked to assist. Improper use of a machine could cause personal injury or damage to the clothing or the machine.

- Most top-loading machines will allow you to add the clothes first before the machine fills with water. Pour in correct amount of detergent (Figure 5-28). If bleach is necessary, make sure the bleach mixes well with the water before adding the white clothes. Add softener if necessary. Close the machine and set dial at correct setting. Modern detergents recommend washing clothes for no longer than 12 minutes in the wash cycle.

FIGURE 5-27 Guidelines for removing stains

Stain	How to Remove
Blood	Presoak in cold water; if stain is stubborn rub in detergent, then launder using safe bleach.
Butter, oils	Rub cornstarch on spot or use powdered cleaning product or cleaning fluid according to instructions.
Chocolate	Soak in cold water, and rub detergent directly on stain. Launder in water as warm as the fabric allows.
Coffee, tea	Pour hot water directly on spot, then wash as usual. Use water as hot as the fabric allows.
Cosmetics	Presoak in detergent and water, then launder.
Crayon and candle wax	Scrape off as much as possible. (Crayons have a wax base.) Place blotting paper under spot and on top of spot. Rub hot iron over blotter. The wax should melt into the blotter. Launder, using safe bleach and detergent.
Deodorants	Presoak area with white vinegar, rinse, and launder.
Fruits	Rinse in cold water. If stain is stubborn, put 1 tablespoon of baking soda in a quart of water to neutralize the acid. Rinse and launder.
Grass	Rub detergent into the spot. Launder with safe bleach and detergent.
Ink, magic marker, felt tip pens	Remove washable ink by rubbing cold water and detergent into the spot. Ballpoint pens make a stain that can be removed with dry cleaning fluid. Permament or unwashable inks must be removed by a professional dry cleaner.
Lipstick	Remove with cleaning fluid. Make sure the fluid will not ruin fabric by testing on an inside seam area.
Meat juice, eggs	Scrape off, then sponge area with cold water. Rub in detergent and launder.
Rust	Use dry cleaning fluid, then wash as usual.
Scorch (mark from hot iron)	Dampen a white cotton cloth in cold water to which a small amount of bleach has been added. Quickly rub over the scorched spot. Turn the iron to a cooler setting—wait until the spot has dried, then proceed with ironing. Deeply scorched items may need to be patched.

- For front-loading machines, add detergent and softener as indicated. Put in the clothing and close the door tightly. Set dial for correct setting.
- Unload clean, wet laundry into clean container or basket. Hang outside if allowed, or place in dryer. Figure 5-29 shows a typical laundry room.
- Be sure you do not overload the washing machine.

Pathogens such as human immunodeficiency virus, which causes acquired immunodeficiency syndrome, are not airborne.

However, when handling bed linens and clothing of an infected client, wear gloves and separate the items from other laundry. Bed linens of clients with infectious or contagious diseases should be washed with detergent in the hottest water possible (at least 160°F), using the longest washing cycle. If water temperature is less than 160°F, bleach germicide should be added to the water. Ask the case manager to provide clear instructions so that laundry can be done correctly and safely.

Some clients will not have washing machines and dryers. In that case, you may have to take

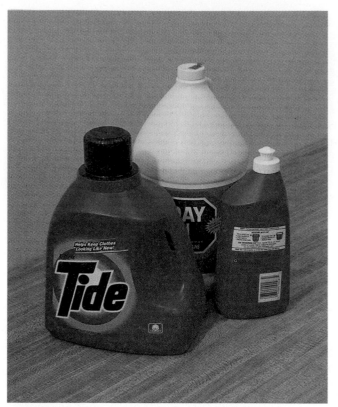

FIGURE 5-28 Common household products used in doing the client's laundry

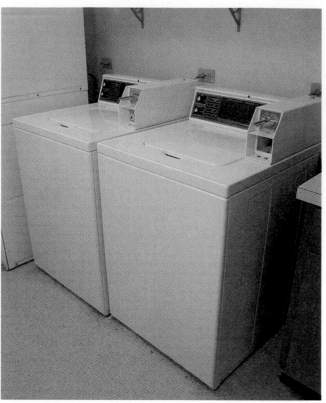

FIGURE 5-29 Laundry rooms with a washer and a dryer are popular today.

the dirty linens and clothing to a laundromat. Some apartments do have laundry rooms that are used by the tenants. If it is necessary to use laundromats or laundry rooms, the home health aide should schedule laundry time when it is safe and convenient to be away from the client and, when using an apartment laundry room, at a time when the machines are available.

When using laundromats and laundry rooms, the aide will need quarters or other small change and should make certain that there is plenty of change on hand. Usually, it is best to take the soap, bleach, and other necessary supplies from the client's home. If you purchase them from vending machines, the cost is much higher. A good idea when using "community" machines (ones that are used by many people) is to wipe them on the inside with a damp cloth before starting to do the wash.

Drying, Ironing, and Mending

Not all clothing requires high heat or long drying cycles. Towels, heavy pants, and sweatshirts usually take the longest time to dry. Nylon, polyester, or any **permanent press** fabrics can be dried quickly. Permanent press clothing should be removed from the dryer as soon as the tumbler has stopped. If clothes are hung or folded at once, few wrinkles will form in them.

Large items such as sheets and blankets should be placed in the dryer separately or no more than two at a time. Folding sheets and blankets as soon as the drying process is finished helps to prevent wrinkling. Some clothing items may need to be drip-dried or laid flat to dry, blocking to shape (such as sweaters). These items usually are not to be wrung out because this twists the fabric fibers.

Cotton clothing that needs to be ironed should be folded neatly. Folding clothing before ironing keeps out unwanted creases and makes ironing easier (Figure 5-30).

- Set up the ironing board and set heat to correct temperature for steam or dry ironing.
- Gather hangers to be used for those items that will need to be hung.

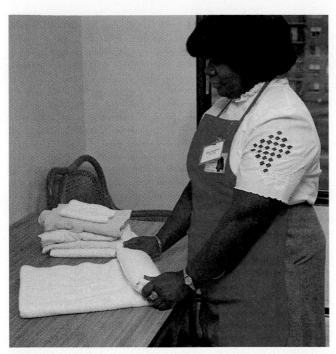

FIGURE 5-30 An aide folding clean laundry before putting it away

- Prepare needles and thread of various colors. Stick the needles at the broad end of the ironing board ready to be used to replace buttons or mend small tears or split seams. Just a few extra minutes spent while handling the ironing to make these small repairs will save time and trouble later. The clothes will be ready for use or storage at once.
- While the ironing is being done, other loads can be put through the wash and dry cycles. Clean the lint traps in the washer and dryer after use. Wipe the inside and outside of machines so they will be ready to use the next time.
- Take the clean and ironed items and store them properly.

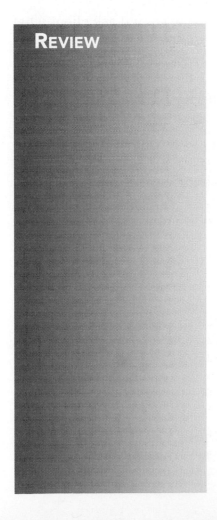

REVIEW

1. Circle the letter that is not a tip for planning and organizing.
   a. Carry a pad and pencil.
   b. Post a list on bulletin board or refrigerator.
   c. Keep all cleaning supplies in the kitchen.
   d. Sponge up spots as soon as possible.
   e. Schedule major jobs for certain days of the week.

2. Circle the letter that is not a tip for appliance care.
   a. Defrost a freezer once a year.
   b. Do not use a sharp knife to pry ice loose from freezer walls.
   c. Store leftovers in airtight containers.
   d. Clean dishwasher filter once a week.
   e. Never use metal containers in a microwave oven.

3. Which are ways to combine client care and household tasks?
   a. The order in which things are done is not always important.
   b. Cleaning the kitchen after the breakfast meal
   c. Cleaning the bathroom after the bedpan has been emptied into the toilet
   d. Cleaning the client's room after the client's bath and the bed linens are changed
   e. All of the above

4. When deciding on a cleaning plan, you should consider:
   a. The needs of the client
   b. The size of the home
   c. The ages of the people living in the home

REVIEW

    d. The number of people living in the home

    e. All of the above

5. List five cleaning tasks done daily.

6. List five cleaning tasks done weekly.

7. List the twelve steps involved in changing a bed.

8. List five cleaning tasks done only periodically.

9. Name five guidelines for preparing meals.

10. Identify two ways to sort clothes for washing.

11. Identify several methods for removing stains.

12. Explain how to wash clothing and bed linens from a client with an infectious disease.

13. T F Some communities require that garbage be separated before disposal.

14. T F Steps in cleaning a kitchen include disposing of garbage, washing dishes, wiping surfaces, cleaning the floors, cleaning cabinets and drawers, and storing cleaning supplies.

15. T F The aide using brush and bowl cleaners, cleans the inside of the toilet bowl daily.

16. T F When planning menus, the aide should ask client what foods the client wants and plan for a full week using only the amount of money budgeted for food and supplies when shopping.

17. T F The following are guidelines for buying foods:

    Avoid going to the grocery store when you are hungry.

    Do not buy sale items unless the client normally uses them.

    Fresh vegetables are less expensive during their growing season.

    When buying meat, consider how the meat will be prepared.

18. T F Wash and clean poultry before refrigerating. If poultry is not planned for a meal within 2 days, wrap and freeze it.

19. You are scheduled to service an incontinent client. When you arrive you encounter piles of laundry, dirty floors, cluttered rooms, soiled bed linens, dirty dishes in the sink, and no food in the refrigerator. The client needs a bath and is hungry but wants to go for a walk to the park. How would you respond to the client's request? How would you organize the other chores on your care plan?

20. You are assigned to do the following tasks in the home for Mr. Tan, a 95-year-old man who is paralyzed on his right side: shower, oral care of dentures, shave, apply topical ointment to

[]

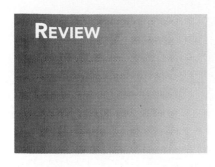

REVIEW

both legs, change his bedding, walk outside for at least two blocks, cook two balanced meals, do his laundry for the week. You are allowed 4 hours to do the tasks. How would you plan your work?

21. Your client is a homebound 72-year-old woman who needs groceries. What factors should you keep in mind in helping her to plan meals? Why is it important to include her in the process of planning meals and developing a shopping list?

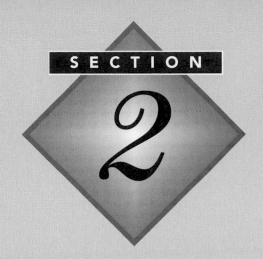

SECTION

2

Stages of Human Development

Units

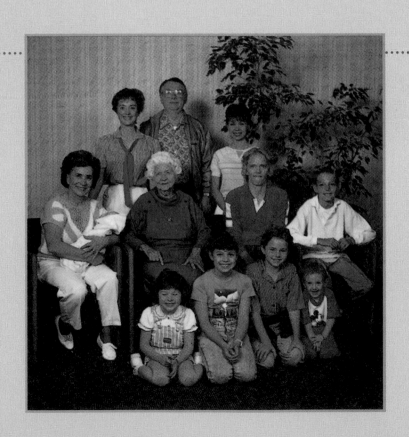

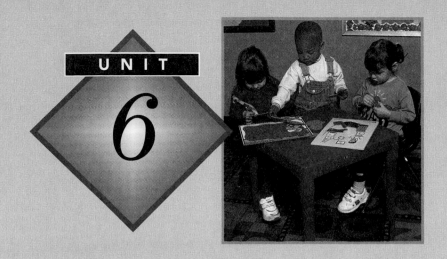

UNIT
6

Infancy to Adolescence

LEARNING OBJECTIVES

After studying this unit, you should be able to:

- Name the five basic human needs.
- Identify three immunizations necessary for infants.
- List six disorders of the newborn.
- List four behavioral patterns associated with abused children.
- Know where and how to report cases of suspected child abuse.
- List four conditions that can occur in an infant if the mother drinks alcohol during pregnancy.

- Describe three characteristics of toddlers.
- Identify three developmental tasks of a preschool-aged child.
- Name two health problems that may affect adolescents.
- Identify changes that occur at puberty.

BECOMING A FAMILY

An aide who is assigned to care for a newborn infant and the mother is usually going into a happy environment. If it is a first child, both parents may be very attentive toward the baby and watch its every move. Of course, the newness wears off, and suddenly they are faced with a demanding, helpless human being for whom they are entirely responsible. Even so, this is usually a positive assignment.

Pregnancy

Conception is the fertilization of the female egg by male sperm. This union forms the **fetus.** The time from conception to birth is called the **gestation period.** When a woman is pregnant, it is essential that she receive prenatal care either from a physician or a midwife. Many complications of pregnancy and birth disorders may be prevented by good prenatal care. It is an important duty as a home health aide to encourage your client to seek prenatal care. If the client is pregnant, the aide should encourage the client to eat a balanced diet. Unit 25 covers pregnancy and maternal care in greater depth.

Labor and Delivery

Infants are most often delivered by a doctor in the hospital. However, in some areas, this situation is changing. There has been increasing use of midwives and home births as alternatives to doctor-attended hospital births. Normally, a woman goes into labor and delivers the baby with the assistance of an obstetrician. The baby moves from the uterus into the vagina and passes out of the body. This normal process can be eased, however, by use of medications, health facilities, and trained personnel.

In some cases it may be necessary to deliver the baby by **cesarean section.** This is a surgical technique in which an abdominal incision is made into the uterus and the infant is lifted out. After a cesarean section, the mother needs extra time to recover. The incision area must be kept clean to prevent infection. The aide may be instructed to assist the mother to clean the incision and apply clean dressings.

Bonding is a process of attachment of mother, father, and infant happening sometime after birth. It is important to remember that each family member bonds differently and at different rates. The newborn infant is placed on the mother's abdomen skin-to-skin so that both parents can make eye contact with the child and feel and cuddle the infant. This initial contact is important because it assists in creating positive emotional ties between the parents and child and the child and the parents. Cuddling and fondling are important in the first few months of the newborn's life. The home health aide needs to encourage a new mother and father to hold, talk, and play with the baby often. The newborn needs to develop a sense of trust and security to develop into a trusting and secure adult.

NORMAL INFANT GROWTH AND DEVELOPMENT

As an infant grows, both physical and mental abilities develop. In the first month, infants are quite helpless. They totally depend on others to meet their basic needs (Figure 6-1). According to American psychologist, Abraham Maslow, all human beings have a hierarchy of five basic needs. He suggests that higher types of needs can only be gratified after a person's basic needs have been met. Maslow's hierarchy is best understood by imagining a triangle shape. At the base of the triangle would be the first basic human need, which is physiologic in nature, that is, food and shelter. After the physiologic needs are met, the second basic need is for safety. Moving up the hierarchy triangle is the third basic need, the need for love and belonging. The fourth basic need is for esteem, which refers to achievement and recognition. The fifth basic need, at the tip of the triangle, is for self-actualization, the highest human need, which is the desire to reach one's fullest potential.

Maslow's hierarchy of needs shows the importance of meeting basic human needs beginning in infancy and moving throughout the life cycle. For instance, the newborn must be fed, changed, cleaned, kept warm and clothed properly, and be kept safe and secure. Infants also need to be held and cuddled. Giving love to the

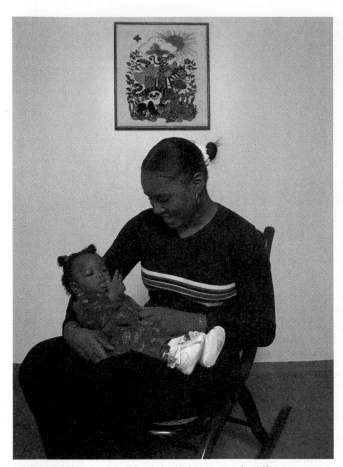

FIGURE 6-1 Mother holding and talking to her baby

infant fulfills a basic need. When these needs are met, the child should have every chance to grow up to be a happy, confident, and fulfilled person.

By age 2 months, babies can raise their heads and may cry when they want to be picked up. Crying is the infant's way of communicating that he or she needs something. Through trial and error parents gradually come to understand the needs of their infants. As infants develop, they notice lights and sounds and begin to babble. They get used to certain patterns, especially the time to eat and time to sleep. Usually by the fourth month an infant sleeps 8 to 12 hours at night and naps during the day. Regular schedules of meals, activities, and sleep are needed and should continue through the first year.

Normal Weight Gain

Normally, infants weigh between 5 and 8 lb (2.3 to 3.6 kg) at birth. During the first 5 days, a weight loss of several ounces is expected. Until birth, all the baby's needs are supplied within the uterus through the umbilical cord. Birth is a shock to the baby's system and it takes a few days for the infant's body to adjust. When the body starts to function, a weight gain of 6 to 8 oz (0.17 to 0.23 kg) a week is normal. Birthweight is usually tripled by age 1. In the second year, the weight increases at a rate of 0.5 lb (0.23 kg) per month.

Nutritionists believe that it is important for children to eat a well-balanced diet. The formation of too many fat cells in childhood can lead to obesity in adulthood. All of the body's systems need the right foods so that they will develop in a strong and healthy way.

Immunizations

Babies are born with a natural **immunity.** This means that they have some built-in resistance to germs for 1 to 3 months. However, once born, a child's body is exposed to many germs. To protect infants from common childhood diseases they are given vaccines (Figure 6-2). At 2, 4, and 6 months, an infant should be given vaccines against diphtheria, pertussis (whooping cough), and tetanus. These three vaccines are combined and given in one injection called a DPT shot. An oral vaccine for poliomyelitis is also given at 2, 4, and 15 months. Vaccines for measles, mumps, and rubella are given after a child is 1 year old. HbCV, a new vaccine for meningitis caused by Hib, is now recommended to be given at 2, 4, 6, and 15 months. A test for tuberculosis is given at 1 year in addition to the vaccines. Boosters of DPT and polio vaccines are given two more times before the child enters school. The American Academy of Pediatrics recommends that children also be protected from the hepatitis B virus (HBV). To be fully protected, children need three doses of the HBV vaccine, which is ordinarily given at birth. However, older children, adolescents, and others living with an infected household member should also receive the three-dose series to be protected from this disease.

Many states do not permit children to begin school until they are properly immunized. Parents should keep records of their children's immunizations. They should also record the diseases contracted by their children and the child's age when the illnesses occurred.

	FIGURE 6-3 *(continued)*	
Condition	**Description**	**Treatment**
Cystic fibrosis	Inherited malfunction of the pancreas, intestine, and sweat glands, and the respiratory system.	No cure; special diet and respiratory care prolong life.
Cleft lip/ cleft palate	Fetal growth incomplete. Infant may have problems feeding. Cleft palate may alter tooth formation and cause speech problems.	Surgical repair; special feeding nipples and special therapy.
Fetal alcohol syndrome	Set of signs and symptoms and problems that newborn babies have if the mother drinks during pregnancy: (1) smaller baby, (2) small head, (3) weak heart or kidney problems, (4) failure to thrive, (5) peculiar-appearing flat face with narrow eyes and drooping lips.	No cure—supportive care. The child may experience some degree of mental retardation for the rest of his/her life.
Sudden infant death syndrome (SIDS)	Baby stopped breathing while asleep.	Place monitor on babies with suspected breathing problems.

premature. Some also judge prematurity by low birthweight. A newborn weighing less than 5 lb may be premature. However, some babies are full term yet weigh less than 5 lb. A newborn in this condition is called a **low birthweight** baby.

Another condition of infancy is sudden infant death syndrome (SIDS) where a baby will stop breathing while asleep. This condition occasionally occurs in infants under 1 year of age. Doctors now recommend that babies be placed on their backs, rather than their stomachs, when sleeping. If breathing disorders are suspected in infants, a monitor may be placed on babies so that an alarm is sounded if the baby stops breathing.

RESPONSIBILITIES OF THE HOME HEALTH AIDE

Often a mother must leave one or more children at home while she is at the hospital. The aide may be assigned to attend to the children then, or after the mother has returned home with the newborn. The children are likely to want to be near the mother and may want to play with the baby. Sometimes older children are too rough with the baby even though they do not intend to be. The children also may be jealous of the new member of the family. This jealousy is called **sibling rivalry.** At these times, the home health aide should give the children extra attention. The aide can make the children feel important by giving them chores to do for the baby or mother. They should be praised for being helpful. Children may need help adjusting to the role of being a big brother or sister. The aide should be sure that the older children wash their hands before touching the baby to prevent the spread of germs and infections. If they have colds they should be kept away from the baby until they are no longer contagious.

Besides the older children, the aide cares for the mother and the newborn. These duties include:

- Bathing the infant
- Diapering
- Feeding the infant
- Preparing the formula
- Doing added laundry such as diapers and crib sheets

- Caring for the mother
- Assisting the mother if she is breast-feeding
- Preventing accidents

See Unit 26 for detailed procedures on assisting with breast-feeding and breast care, bottle-feeding the infant, and giving the infant a sponge bath.

Handling Visitors

Many visitors likely will come to see a newborn infant. One of the aide's duties is to make sure that the mother does not get overtired. A new mother should rest for a period in the morning and afternoon. Most mothers are happy to show off their newborn. However, it is a good idea to plan ahead with the mother as to how to handle visitors. Visitors should not stay too long and should not come in great numbers. The home health aide must encourage the mother to set the standards as to who can and cannot hold the baby. Visitors who have colds or similar infections should be discouraged from going near the baby. The mother and home health aide should wear a disposable mask if they are coughing or have a cold. Although babies are born with some natural immunity to germs, they should not be exposed to disease when it can be avoided.

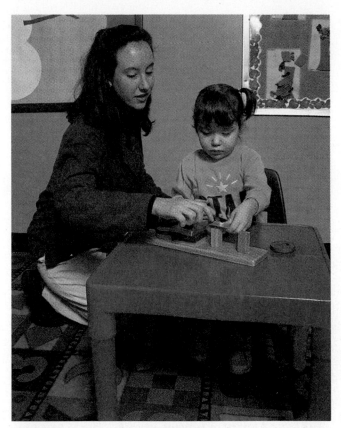

FIGURE 6-4A The toddler begins to develop gross manual skills.

TODDLERS AND PRESCHOOLERS ·········

Ages 1 and 2 are known as the toddler stage. The toddler approaches life with a great deal of interest (Figures 6-4A and B). A favorite activity is exploring the immediate environment, creating a need for safety precautions. Toddlers want to be more independent and experiment with control—testing their parents' limits and discovering their own. This is a time when children start to show possessiveness with belongings and people close to them. At about age 18 months, their favorite word will often be "No!" As infants grow into toddlers, muscle coordination increases, and physical skills expand and improve greatly. Toddlers learn to walk and to feed themselves. Social skills and language become more meaningful.

The period of time between 3 and 5 years is known as the preschool years. Although physical growth and motor development slow down

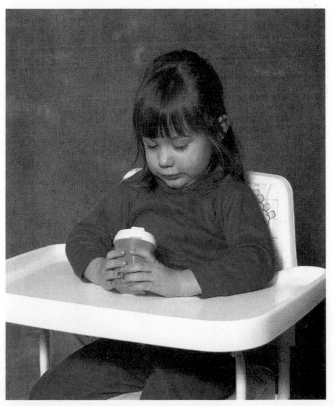

FIGURE 6-4B The toddler begins to use a plastic drinking cup.

a bit, there are many advances in intellectual, social, and emotional growth. By age 3 the child plays alongside other children of the same age (Figure 6-5). The child should be able to start developing some self-control in response to societal rules during this time. The preschooler is learning to be less dependent. This period may seem like a tug of war between the child's reliance on the parent and the need to assert independence. Toilet training is usually mastered by the time the child is 5 and ready to start school.

Safety

Keeping a child physically safe is an ongoing responsibility. Accidents are the primary cause of death in children under 5 years of age. Each year 1 million children are brought for medical care due to accidents; 40,000 to 50,000 children suffer permanent damage and 4,000 die. We know that most accidents can be prevented and all accidents can be minimized.

Childhood injury involves three elements: the child, the object that causes injury, and the environment in which it occurs. Here are several safety checks to ensure a safe environment for young children:

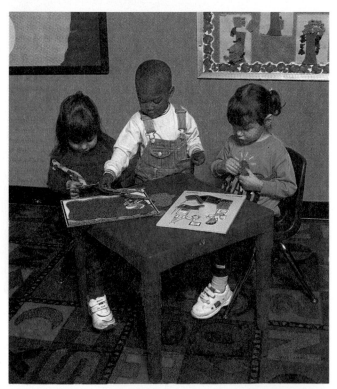

FIGURE 6-5 Learning to play with peers is important for preschoolers.

1. Car seats—The car seat should be federally approved and properly installed. A car seat must be used every time the child is in the car. Car seats should never be placed in the front passenger seat. Inflating air bags can seriously injure and/or suffocate the child. The safest place for a child in a passenger vehicle is in the middle of the back seat, properly buckled in a car seat. If a child weighs less than 20 pounds, the car seat must face the rear of the seat. Be sure you know whether any special attachments are necessary to secure a car seat or a child in the vehicle you are using.

2. Fire prevention—Clothes, especially sleepwear, should be flame-retardant. (Check the clothing label to find out.) Install smoke detectors.

3. Choking—Do not put a pacifier or any object on a string around the baby's neck. Check toys for sharp edges or small parts. Check that all foods for an infant be mashed, ground, or soft enough to swallow without chewing.

4. Poisoning—Keep all medications and household cleaning products out of reach. Use safety latches on cupboards or drawers that contain items that might be dangerous.

5. Burns—Always check the water temperature before placing the baby in the bath. Never hold the baby while cooking at the stove or oven, drinking a hot liquid, or smoking.

6. Falls—Use gates at the bottom of stairways. Supervise the baby at all times on the changing table. Never leave a baby unattended on any surface above floor level. Safety gates should not be placed at the top of stairways because the child could push against them or crawl over them.

7. Drowning—Never leave a small child alone in the bath or around any container with water in it, no matter how little. This includes buckets, wading pools, and the toilet.

8. Strangulation—Keep strings from venetian blinds up and out of the way of a crawling or toddling baby. Do not place the baby's crib near window blinds, where the baby can reach the cords. Remove the drawstrings from parkas and jackets that could catch on playground equipment, causing the child to be strangled.

SCHOOL-AGED CHILDREN ·················

A child beginning school often needs time to adjust to the new situation. The child may one day seem confident and secure and the next day be clingy and dependent. Some children find it difficult to leave the familiarity of home. However, most children enjoy school and being with other children. A school-aged child generally can follow simple instructions and be fairly independent. It is important that children be given small jobs so that they feel a sense of responsibility. Praise for achievements is better than punishments for mistakes. The school-aged child enjoys activities at home and away from home.

ADOLESCENCE ································

Adolescence often refers to the years between the ages of 13 and 19, during which broad developmental changes occur, including intellectual, emotional, social, and physical changes. **Puberty**, on the other hand, is the physical process of growing up, which includes the growth spurts, changing body shape, and maturation of the reproductive system. Pubertal changes occur gradually; they may start as early as age 9 or 10 and not be completed until about age 20 or even a little older in some people.

Physical Changes in Puberty

Puberty begins sometime between the ages of 10 and 15 when the endocrine system releases hormones in both boys and girls. At this time, the secondary sexual characteristics begin to mature. In boys, the beard, underarm, and pubic hair starts to grow and the voice deepens. There is usually a marked growth in both height and weight. At puberty, the testes, scrotum, and penis enlarge and the youth is able to produce sperm.

In young girls, the breasts develop and pubic and underarm hair grows. About every 28 to 35 days the mature female reproductive system releases one or more eggs (ova), and the menstrual cycle begins.

The Teen Years

The teenage years are profoundly influenced by both the physical and mental changes of adolescence. Adolescents begin to take responsibility for their own lives and continually struggle to coordinate the many changes they are experiencing. Many of the concerns at this stage of the life cycle surround the child's dependence on parents, and the youngster's growing independence from them. During adolescence the relationship between parents and children may be challenged, stressed, and gradually redefined. As a home health aide, you rarely will be assigned to care for an adolescent unless there is a physical problem with the youth's health, such as an accident (body in a cast) or childhood cancer.

Open communication between parents and children is healthy and important. If teenagers have a previous history of good communication with their parents, they will be willing to share their concerns and feelings with them. An adolescent wants to feel independent, but needs to know that the family can be depended on (Figure 6-6). This is a time when parental guidance and love are extremely important. During adolescence, children are strongly influenced by their peer group (those of the same age) (Figure 6-7). Showing support, reassurance, and concern for the teenager's well-being is essential.

Common Health Problems in Adolescence

Adolescents are at an age of experimentation. They often express their independence by trying new things. For some adolescents, this experimentation leads to smoking, abuse of drugs

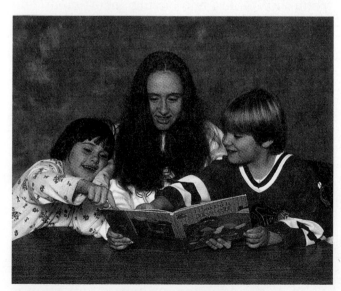

FIGURE 6-6 Adolescent playing with younger members of her family

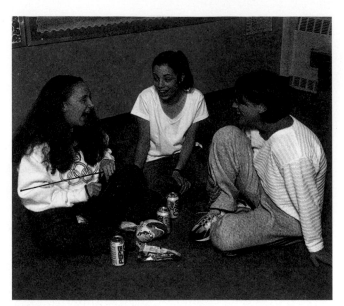

FIGURE 6-7 Peer relationships are important to adolescents who are developing awareness of themselves.

or alcohol, gang involvement, or sexual experimentation.

Sex-related health problems are especially common with adolescents. An active sex life may pose health and emotional problems. **Sexually transmitted diseases (STDs)**, including the human immunodeficiency virus (HIV) and acquired immunodeficiency syndrome (AIDS), may bring about additional very serious problems. (For more information about HIV and AIDS see Unit 24.) In addition, teenage girls must consider the possibility of becoming pregnant. Sex-related health problems often result from the adolescent having insufficient and inaccurate information.

Teenage Pregnancy. In addition to an increase in STDs among adolescents, an increase in teenage pregnancies also has occurred. It currently is estimated that two of every five girls now 14 years old will become pregnant before they are 20 and that one of those five will bear a child. It is now estimated that 42% of teenagers are sexually active. Many teenagers have sex without contraceptives, and when they do go to family planning services, it often is too late.

Few teenagers are ready to handle the responsibilities that accompany pregnancy and parenthood. The decision to raise a child, place the child for adoption, or have an abortion is usually a difficult decision for a teenage girl.

Teenage girls are still growing themselves, both emotionally and physically. Even a healthy, well-adjusted teenager will feel the stress that pregnancy puts on her body. A teenage father may feel emotional stress. The financial and practical aspects of parenthood are usually too much for a teenager to handle.

Pregnancy can be prevented through use of planned birth control methods as well as abstinence from sexual intercourse. Teenagers who are sexually active should be made aware of the methods available. Common birth control methods are the oral contraceptive pill, the diaphragm, the condom, and foam spermaticides. The rhythm method also is practiced by some, but it is not very reliable. Condoms are recommended for the male to use to prevent unwanted pregnancy, and the transmission of STDs.

Religious practices may determine the type of birth control used. In any case, it is wise for the teenager to consult a medical doctor, family planning clinic, or school nurse. The only advice a home health aide should offer is to mention that one of these professionals should be consulted.

Substance Abuse. **Substance abuse** is the use of alcohol or drugs that results in poor treatment of the body. Drug use among adolescents has been on the increase over the past 20 years. Smoking has increased, particularly among Caucasian teenage girls, who often use it as a device to lose weight. It is recognized that "pot" smoking, "pill popping," and the use of hard drugs have increased the crime rate and caused serious physical and mental health problems. Many families have been destroyed because of the aftermath of drug abuse by its members. Drug awareness programs are provided in schools to alert young people to the dangers involved. Legislation has been passed in an effort to stop drug abuse. Television and radio programs continue to tell of the harmful effects of drug abuse.

Parents should see that their children are well informed about the dangers and effects of drug abuse. A loving home environment where the child feels accepted and is able to talk about concerns and feelings helps to deter drug abuse. If a parent sees physical or emotional signs— extreme mood swings, lethargy, overactivity, nervousness, red eyes, sniffling, needle marks, or other unaccountable signals—professional help should be sought.

Alcohol abuse has also become a major problem. Children as young as 6 and 7 years of age are abusing alcohol. One recent report indicated that among youth, the average drinking age nationwide is 11.5 years. Parents often are not as concerned about drinking as they are about other drugs. They seem to think that alcohol is less harmful than drug abuse In fact, youthful drinking is a serious and dangerous problem. Drinking can lead to cirrhosis of the liver, which is irreversible. It also can lead to permanent brain damage. Moreover, drinking is a major cause of death on the highway due to driving while intoxicated (DWI). Although it is illegal to drink under the age of 21, the consumption of alcohol by minors is still a problem. Alcohol is an accepted part of our adult society, but all too often its negative influence reaches the younger generation. Organizations such as Al-Anon and Alateen are educating drinkers and helping them to stop drinking for at least "one day at a time." DARE, or Drug Awareness Resistance Education, is a group organized to prevent young people from getting started on illegal drugs and alcohol.

CHILD ABUSE, MALTREATMENT, AND NEGLECT

According to Social Services Law, Section 412, an abused child is one who is under 18 years of age whose parent, or other legally responsible person, or any person in a caregiver situation:

- Inflicts or allows to be inflicted on such child physical injury by other than accidental means
- Creates or allows to be created a risk of physical injury to such a child by other than accidental means that might cause death or serious disfigurement, impairment of function of any bodily organ
- Commits or allows to be committed, a sex offense against such a child
- Allows, permits, or encourages such a child to engage in prostitution
- Allows such a child to engage in acts or conduct of a sexual nature, such as videotaping sexual acts

Examples of maltreatment and neglect of children include cases in which children are:

- Improperly fed, clothed, or deprived of any emotional support
- Allowed to drink alcohol or given illegal drugs
- Chained or locked in a closet
- Kept in an environment where mice, rats, cockroaches, or other pests can harm the child
- Left alone in an apartment or house or locked in a room while the legally responsible adult is away
- Exposed to lead poison from painted walls or furniture

The "legally responsible person" would include a parent, guardian, or custodian. A home health aide working in the household where such conduct as **child abuse**, neglect, or maltreatment occurs is considered a "legally responsible person." Such behavior is not acceptable on the part of an aide or any other legally responsible person.

Abusive parents or caretakers may have been raised in abusive families themselves. The husband or wife may abuse the spouse. Life crises such as loss of job, debt, or housing problems, and substance abuse of alcohol or drugs or gambling losses can lead to abusive behavior; physical or mental health problems may cause a parent to become abusive; or parents who are too young themselves may lack self-discipline to deal with their own children. Many of these parents are not aware of the damage they are doing to their children and may need help themselves to develop better parenting skills. Parents of mentally or developmentally disabled children may be unable to cope with their children's problems. These parents should be encouraged to join support groups with parents with similar problems.

If an aide becomes aware of abusive treatment, it immediately should be reported to their supervisor or to the state child abuse hotline. In fact, it is mandated by law that any person who suspects that child abuse or neglect is occurring, must report it. The person reporting abuse is not required to investigate or prove the abuse, but rather, just to report even a suspicion of abuse. The person reporting abuse is immune from prosecution and is protected under the law. A report can be made anonymously. Within a certain period of time, an investigation of the abuse will be made by the state.

Abuse comes in many forms. It may be categorized as physical, sexual, emotional, or even neglect. Figure 6-8 lists typical behavior for abused/mistreated children. Child abuse may take place in the homes of any group of people, regardless of income, ethnic origin, or religion. It is most important to remember that if you suspect it, you must report it. Tell your supervisor immediately!

FIGURE 6-8 Observable behavior patterns of abused or mistreated children

Avoid contact with parents or other adults
Become upset when other children cry
Be extremely aggressive
Be extremely withdrawn
Suffer mood swings
Fear going into home—run away from home
Be overly demonstrative and loving to abusive parent
Blame themselves for being "clumsy" or "bad"
Wear long sleeves to conceal injuries
Appear to have low self-esteem
Attempt suicide
Grades go down in school

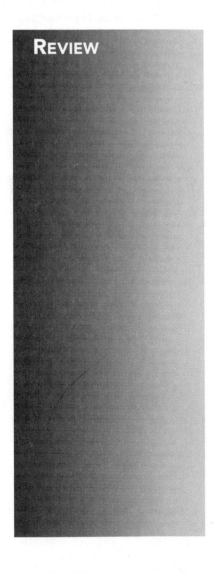

REVIEW

1. What are the five basic needs of a newborn?

2. List three immunizations recommended for infants.

3. Name three developmental tasks of the preschool-aged child.

4. Name two health problems that affect adolescents.

5. What physical changes occur at puberty?

6. Identify four behavior patterns of abused/mistreated children.

7. Give three examples of child abuse.

8. What is an aide's responsibility if child abuse is suspected?

9. Why is it important for the aide to allow the mother to assume as much care of the newborn baby as possible? What would you look for and document relating to the mother's "bonding" with her infant?

10. What kind of observations would you be likely to make in caring for a newborn infant? An older baby? A toddler?

11. An infant needs to be:
    a. Toilet trained immediately
    b. Weaned to a cup by 6 months
    c. Kept awake during the day so it will sleep at night
    d. Loved, held, and fed regularly

12. Typical characteristics of adolescence are:
    a. Strongly influenced by peers
    b. Growing desire for independence from parents
    c. Possible problem with substance abuse
    d. All of the above

13. Match Column I with Column II (childhood conditions).

Column I	Column II
_C_ 1. PKU	a. inherited malfunction of the pancreas
_D_ 2. hydrocephalus	b. chromosome abnormality
_B_ 3. Down's syndrome	c. unable to break down a certain amino acid
_A_ 4. cystic fibrosis	d. defect in the absorption of brain fluid and head is enlarged
_E_ 5. sickle cell anemia	e. abnormal sickle-shaped red blood cells that are very fragile

14. Signs and symptoms of fetal alcohol syndrome are:
    a. Small head
    b. Weak heart
    c. Flat face with drooping lips
    d. All of the above

15. As you go into a home to help a new mother with her newborn, you see two other preschoolers who are dirty and improperly clothed for the weather. You see evidence of roaches, rats, and peeling paint. What signs would you look for in the children's behavior patterns that might indicate an abusive situation in the home? What should you do? Why? What are the consequences?

16. You are helping a 16-year-old new mom who does not know much about babies. She appears uncomfortable and awkward holding her baby, and does not want to cuddle the baby. Why might she be behaving this way? What would you do? Why?

17. You are making your first visit to a new client, who is a young mother with two children, ages 18 months and 3 years. What observations could you make to assess whether the mother is attending to basic safety issues for her young children? What recommendations would you make to the mother to improve the safety of her home for her children?

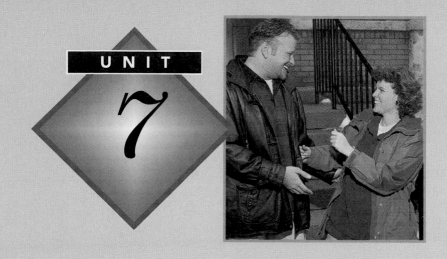

UNIT 7

Early and Middle Adulthood

KEY TERMS

early adulthood
empty nest syndrome
mammogram
menopause

middle adulthood
multiple sclerosis
Pap smear
preventive health measure

prognosis
rheumatoid arthritis
self-esteem
sigmoidoscopy

LEARNING OBJECTIVES

After studying this unit, you should be able to:

- List the causes of health problems in the early adult years.
- Describe the adjustments that often must be dealt with in the middle adult years.
- State why preventive health measures are important.
- Describe the changes that occur during the early and middle adult years in terms of family relationships.

- List two reasons a home health aide should encourage the client to exercise.
- List two activities a disabled client can become involved in outside of the home.

EARLY ADULTHOOD

Early adulthood generally refers to the ages of 20 to 39 years. This is the time of life when formal education is usually completed. Most young adults enter the labor force and begin to assume increased responsibilities.

During early adulthood, most individuals are concerned with improving themselves. They may change jobs often. Many look forward to better jobs, higher wages, and greater opportunities. As young people make these changes, they must constantly make personal adjustments.

During early adulthood, close personal relationships take on greater significance. Some young adults choose to marry; some also choose to start a family. If both partners are working, they need to arrange their personal lives around their jobs. This effort helps produce harmonious relationships with each other. They must learn to share duties and work together as a team.

Early Adulthood Adjustments

During early adulthood, the body normally works efficiently. It remains at a high level of health for about 30 or 40 years (Figures 7-1A and B). The body heals quickly through childhood, adolescence, and early and middle adulthood.

Health problems in early adulthood often accompany parenthood. Normal pregnancy, pregnancy with complications, and reproductive system disorders can occur in the adult woman. If an infant is born with birth defects or serious medical problems, parents may experience considerable stress and financial burdens. Other health problems can result from conditions related to automobile accidents and job-related injuries.

Many health professionals recommend taking certain **preventive health measures** to maintain a person's health and well-being and to prevent the development of health problems. For example, all persons should have a physical examination at least every 3 years. The early detection of diseases such as cancer, heart disease, diabetes, and emotional stress often leads to a better **prognosis** (outcome). Also, women should do a breast self-examination every month. They should have a vaginal examination that includes a **Pap smear** every year. The American Cancer Society recommends that

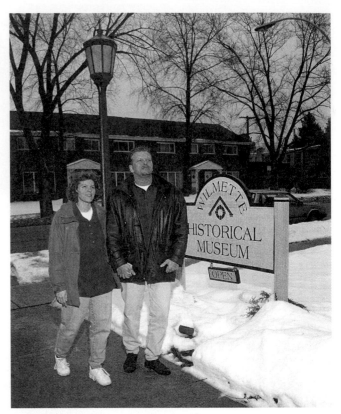

FIGURE 7-1A Young couple enjoying an outdoor activity

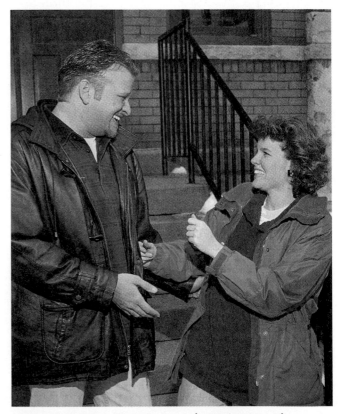

FIGURE 7-1B Young couple enjoying the company of one another

women receive a **mammogram** (x-ray of breasts) between the ages of 35 and 39, every 1 or 2 years from ages 40 to 49, and yearly for women over age 50. It also is recommended that both men and women have a **sigmoidoscopy** (rectal examination with a special tube) every 3 to 5 years after the age of 50.

MIDDLE ADULTHOOD

Society places great demands on a person in **middle adulthood** from 40 to 65 years of age. It is during this period that people are expected to be highly successful and productive as well as financially secure (Figure 7-2). If a woman has chosen to remain at home with her children, this may be the time when she decides to re-enter the work force.

During the middle adult years, people often assess their accomplishments. Some may question how worthwhile their work or other achievements have been and seek a change. This change may take the form of a different life-style—a separation from their marriage partner, or a change in career or place of residence. Often during this stage of life, individuals are asked to take responsibility for care of their aging parents. The roles of parent and child often reverse once the parent is unable to manage all of his or her care. The phenomenon of daughters caring for their aging parents and their own children is so common that Dr. Elaine Brody has dubbed this middle generation the "Sandwich Generation." At times this can be a difficult and stressful period in both the parent's and child's lives.

Physically, those in their middle adult years will notice some changes. Their hair may turn gray or recede, and their eyesight may diminish. Weight gain may occur as a result of a general slowing of their metabolism and inactivity. Hormonal changes that occur during **menopause,** when a woman's periods stop, may result in mood swings, changes in sleeping patterns, increased anxiety, or other physical symptoms.

Middle Adulthood Adjustments

People in the middle adult years may have to make several major adjustments. These adjustments are in response to a change in some area of their lives.

Family Relationships. The middle years are generally the time when grown children leave the home. Parents who have been very involved in their children's lives may feel at a loss when this occurs (**empty nest syndrome**). As the children mature and gain independence, their own roles and responsibilities may become first priorities, and their ties with their family may become more remote. However, this can be a time when parents and children form close, adult relationships with each other. This also can be a time of freedom and creativity for the parents as they find they have more time to spend with each other and more time to develop their own mutual interests.

Effects of Exercise. It is important during the early and middle years of adulthood to become involved in a regular exercise program. At any age, the unexercised body—though free of symptoms of illness—will rust out long before it ever will wear out. Inactivity can make people old before their time. Just as inactivity accelerates aging, activity slows down the aging process. One of the best exercises is walking. Some other alternatives to walking are swimming, riding a stationary or moving bicycle, and dancing. If you are working in a home with a young or middle-aged adult, you should try to encourage the client to do some type of

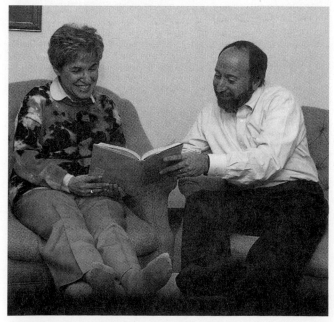

FIGURE 7-2 Middle-aged couple enjoying a leisurely day together

exercise within his or her limits. Adults should always have a medical checkup before beginning an exercise program.

Retirement. Retirement is a major adjustment for most individuals. Often, an individual's identity and sense of **self-esteem** are closely linked with one's job. Retirement from gainful employment may erode one's self-esteem. It also may remove a person from close relationships formed in the workplace. Retirement for some people is very enjoyable; they have more time for hobbies and travel. Individuals who have not planned for retirement can find it difficult, especially if they have not planned financially for it or have no hobbies. One must remain mentally and physically active to keep the body at its peak. Remember the old saying, "If you don't use it, you'll lose it."

COMMON HEALTH PROBLEMS

Multiple sclerosis, a nervous system disorder, is the major crippler of young and middle-aged adults. The range of activity that these clients can do varies greatly. As a home health aide, you will need to use your creativity and ingenuity to encourage this client to do as much exercise as possible.

Rheumatoid arthritis is also a disease that can afflict individuals in this age group. When working with these individuals, it is better to do exercises with them later in the day. In the morning the client has more pain in movement, but as the day progresses, the pain will diminish. This client benefits greatly from swimming in warm water pools. In certain situations, arthritic clients will benefit from taking a pain pill before starting an exercise routine.

Acceptance of Illness or Disability

It is often difficult for individuals to accept the fact that they need assistance from others to do their activities of daily living (ADLs). At times, the client might express anger at the home health aide because of the disability. The client may be frustrated and not know how to cope with these frustrations. Every person differs. With the assistance of your case manager or supervisor, you will be given special instructions to follow on how to handle these clients.

Emotional Needs

Two of the most important aspects of care of clients with disabilities or disabling conditions are to keep them physically and mentally active and to try to meet some of their emotional needs. These individuals have the same basic needs as a healthy individual of the same age (Figure 7-3). It is a little easier for a disabled person to remain physically active than it was years ago. With modern technology, a client can be transported even if confined to a wheelchair. Special vans are available to help transport disabled clients (Figure 7-4). Many restaurants and public places have wheelchair access and also special accommodations for toileting.

Shopping malls and grocery stores sometimes have designated times for the disabled to shop and designated parking. Occasionally stores will have extra help available to assist clients in their shopping needs. Many churches

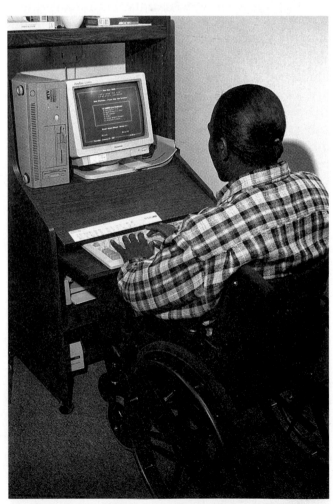

FIGURE 7-3 Adults confined to wheelchairs have the same basic needs as other adults the same age.

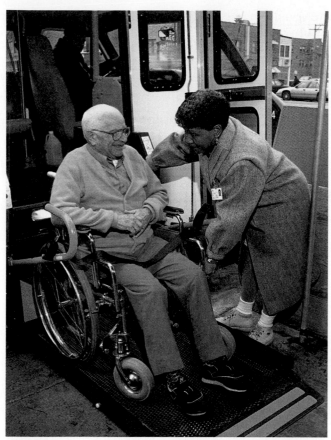

FIGURE 7-4 An aide assisting a client into a van

have special activities for individuals to attend, depending on their interest. In some areas of the country, there are activities for the developmentally disabled, such as the Special Olympics, in which your client may want to become involved. Your role is to encourage your client to participate and attend such functions. In most scenarios, the case manager initially will arrange for transportation and coordination of these activities. Your role will be to assist the client in getting ready to attend, including having the client dressed properly and having all the supplies needed with the client, such as medications, money, and toileting supplies. If the client plans to attend a special family event, you will need to see that the client's hair is clean and stylish and that the client is dressed appropriately for the event. Usually a member of the family will transport the client to the event. Always check to see if the client has all supplies necessary for the time he or she will be gone. Your goal is to make it as pleasant as possible for the client and also the family members. Be sure the family members know how to operate any special equipment and are instructed on any special care that the client may require.

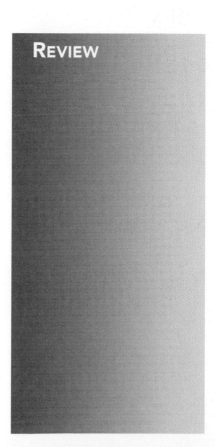

REVIEW

1. Name three causes of health problems in the early adult years.

2. List three adjustments that may need to be made during the middle adult years.

3. During what period of life does society expect the most from an individual?

4. Why are preventive health measures important?

5. List two activities a home health aide can involve a disabled client in outside of the client's home.

6. List two benefits of regular exercise.

7. The developmental tasks of early adulthood include:
   a. Focusing on improving themselves
   b. Developing close personal relationships
   c. Making career choices
   d. All of the above

8. Middle adult years are a time when adjustments are made due to:
   a. Grown children leaving home
   b. Aging parents who may be brought into the home
   c. Chronic illness that may begin
   d. All of the above

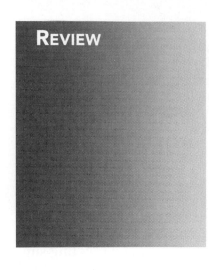

REVIEW

9. T F Multiple sclerosis, a nervous system disorder, is a major crippler of young adults.

10. T F Women over 50 years of age should have a Pap smear and mammogram every year as a preventive health measure.

12. You have been helping a 24-year-old paraplegic man who stays at home and says he's bored and depressed. What can you offer this man? List reasons why outside activities are important.

13. Your client, a 59-year-old woman, just had surgery and has received a diagnosis of cancer. She speaks of feeling listless and depressed. What might this woman be going through? What might you do?

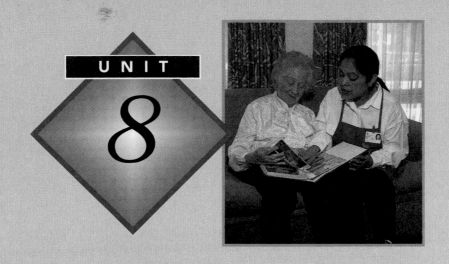

Older Adulthood

KEY TERMS

acuity
aged
carbohydrates
cataracts

dementia
depression
glaucoma
incontinence

osteoporosis
over the counter
reminiscence
somaticize

LEARNING OBJECTIVES

After studying this unit, you should be able to:

- Name some of the normal age-related changes.
- Describe common changes to hearing and how to help older clients cope.
- Describe common changes to vision and how to help the older person.

- Describe reminiscence and how it can be helpful to an older person with depression or dementia.
- Describe dementia.
- Describe depression.

No on Test on →

Older adulthood is generally regarded as the period of time beginning at age 65. However, it cannot be definitely stated at what time in life people become old, for age is more a matter of physical and mental aging than it is of chronological processes. Tremendous variations exist. Some people are physically and mentally old at 45, others seem young even at the age of 75.

The terms aging and aged also must be clarified. Aging is a process that begins with conception and ends with death. The term **aged** means old or mature. Because of an increasing life expectancy, our perceptions of the age at which an individual is old may not be entirely accurate. Approximately one in eight people is over age 65. Today, if a person lives to be 65 and is in reasonably good health, that person can expect to live 14 to 20 more years. In fact, the fastest growing age group of the population in the United States is those over 85. The largest proportion of the aged population are healthy, alert, able, working and contributing members of society. The losses associated with aging years ago are now generally thought to be attributed to disuse.

There is some natural decrease in function or speed of functioning as people age; however, most older people are able to care for themselves. Some choose to have others help them with certain tasks. These people may have had help all their lives and continue to want that help. Others may choose to conserve their energies for tasks they enjoy. Home health aides are an important part of care provided to older, less able people. Although many elderly people live alone, most are not alone. Families and friends remain important supports for people throughout their lives.

NORMAL AGE-RELATED PHYSICAL CHANGES

There are common age-related changes and losses that older people face (Figure 8-1). Remember that common does not mean that all older people are experiencing each of these changes. Not only must a home health aide be sensitive to the conditions the older person may be coping with, he or she also must be careful not to assume that all older people experience them or experience them the same way.

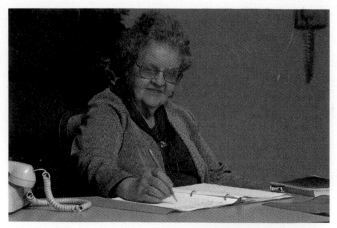

FIGURE 8-1 There are common age-related changes and losses that older people face.

Hearing Loss

Decreasing hearing **acuity**, or sensitivity, is a common problem for many older people, especially men. Because hearing loss is so commonly associated with being "old," many people deny or play down their loss so as not to appear old. Figure 8-2 identifies some common hearing changes and ways the home health aide can help older adults with these losses.

Vision Loss

A moderate degree of failing eyesight is normal to aging, is not serious, and can usually be corrected with special eyeglasses. As people age, they will need more light whether they have visual problems or not. Also, many low-vision aids are available, including magnifiers, telescopes, and large print materials.

However, cataracts and diseases of the eyes are serious because they can lead to loss of vision. Both **cataracts** (clouding of the lens) and **glaucoma** (build-up of fluid within the eyeball) can usually be treated. These illnesses can affect one or both eyes. Because they tend to come on gradually and are often painless, they are often mistaken by older adults as being normal signs of aging. It is important for older adults to see an ophthamologist promptly if a vision problem occurs.

Helping an older person with these kinds of losses can present a special challenge for the home health aide (Figure 8-3). In America's increasingly visual society—television, movies, computers—vision loss can be very isolating. Aware home health aides can make every day easier for the older adults they assist.

FIGURE 8-2   Hearing changes and ways to help. (Courtesy of Glantz-Richman Rehabilitation Associates, Ltd.)

Hearing changes	Ways to help
• There is a decline in auditory acuity with age called presbycusis. This age-related hearing loss is usually greater for men than for women. The reason for this decline is not known, but it is suspected that men are exposed to more damaging noise during their lifetimes, possibly resulting from being in the military service or due to the nature of their jobs.	• Any older person may need your help in compensating for hearing loss. While people with visual impairments can compensate by bringing things closer, those with hearing loss cannot similarly compensate. • Speak slowly and clearly, and do not change the topic abruptly. Be sure to face the person at eye level and have light on your face so lipreading is possible. Ask the person what you can do to make hearing easier.
• Hearing loss is worse at high frequencies, meaning that some sounds are heard while others are not. Sounds may be distorted, or heard incorrectly, and thus misinterpreted.	• Try to lower your voice rather than allowing your voice to become high or shrill. Women should be especially careful about this. • A sound system used for music, entertainment, or oral presentations should be adjusted so that the bass and lower tones are predominant.
• People with normal hearing have a wide range between the quietest sound they hear and the loudest, which is painful or irritating. For people with hearing loss, this range may be much narrower. Sounds may have to be quite loud to be heard, and sensitivity is increased. If sounds are even a little louder, they may be too loud to be understood or may even be painful.	• Talk to those people with hearing impairments to find out the optimum tone to use. Do not assume that simply making things louder will solve the problem. • Be aware of the fact that noise or music may be irritating and may cause anxiety for persons with hearing loss, even if it has no effect on you. Be especially aware of this situation when you are working with people who are unable to communicate their needs to you. Note signs of anxiety, and try changing noise levels.
• Hearing loss is greater for consonants than for vowels. S, Z, T, F, and G sounds are particularly difficult to discriminate, which causes difficulty in hearing words correctly. Words that are similar can be particularly difficult to discriminate.	• People should be aware of the fact that even if sounds can be heard, they may not always be heard correctly. The suggestions previously mentioned can be followed; in addition, it is helpful to limit the competing stimuli of background noise. Choose a quiet, private place for talking.
• Some hearing deficits can be helped by the use of hearing aids, but these must be worn and adjusted correctly to help. They also regularly require new batteries. Some people never learn to use their hearing aids correctly, or they do not get new batteries often enough.	• Older persons can purchase hearing aids from reputable firms and should learn their proper use. Family members or caregivers serving older persons also should learn how to help adjust or insert the aid or how to change batteries when it is necessary. *(continues)*

FIGURE 8-2   *(continued)*

Hearing changes	Ways to help
• Some hearing deficits cannot be helped by hearing aids, and the person's hearing is so poor that verbal communication is difficult.	• Encourage the use of nonverbal communication such as big smiles, waving, pointing, or demonstrating. Offer opportunities for activity and social interaction that require no spoken communication. For example, cooking and cleaning up can be done in complete silence by two or more people who have good understanding and cooperation. Also, use writing as a form of communication. Those who appear to be very impaired can understand written statements and questions.
• Hearing and following a conversation can take tremendous amounts of effort and energy for someone with hearing loss. Motivation, the context of the environment and general feelings of well-being and energy can make a difference in the ability to understand verbal communication. Lack of any or all of these may result in apparent "selective hearing."	• We should try to be more tolerant of "selective hearing." This syndrome is often annoying for those who interact with people with hearing loss, but in some cases there may be some legitimate reasons for it to occur. • Provide opportunities for people to participate in activities that are enjoyable but require little conversation—for example, playing cards, doing puzzles, preparing food, and taking walks.
• Depression and paranoid reactions are common among older persons with hearing loss. When they cannot hear what is being said, they may begin to think that people are talking about them and saying negative things.	• Do everything possible to compensate hearing loss and to ensure that people know what is going on and what the conversation is about. If the conversation does not concern them, tell them what the topic is so that they will not feel left out or talked about.
• Hearing is important to more than communication. It is a way of getting signals from the environment, so it also relates to safety.	• People who work or live with a person with hearing loss should keep this in mind. People in the community also should realize that when an older person crosses the street, he or she may not hear a car horn.

Urination

As part of normal aging, bladder and kidney size decrease and urination becomes more frequent. Although more and more advertisements are appearing for "adult diapers" or "protective undergarments," urinary **incontinence** is not a normal part of aging; it affects only 10% to 15% of the aging population. Incontinence is more often a symptom of some other illness or problem. The inability to hold urine can be profoundly embarrassing for an older person. Often an older person will decrease the amount of fluids they take in each day or per-

haps not take their "water" pill as the doctor instructs. Both of these solutions can have serious consequences for the older person's health. More effective is to encourage the older person to drink at least six 8-oz glasses of fluids each day—ideally, water or fruit juice—and to plan for the client to use the toilet every 2 to 3 hours to "train" the bladder, not allowing it to become distended. Suggest a decrease in the amount of caffeine because it can irritate the bladder. Finally, encourage the older person to talk with his or her doctor. Exercise, medication, or changes in medication all can help the older person maintain continence.

FIGURE 8-3   Vision changes and ways to help. (Courtesy of Glantz-Richman Rehabilitation Associates, Ltd.)

Vision changes	Ways to help
• As a person ages, the lens in the eye yellows and thickens. The muscles that control pupil size also weaken. As a result, the older eye requires more light than the younger eye. To see clearly, a 65-year-old eye needs more than twice as much light as a 20-year-old eye.	• Provide adequate lighting. Be aware of poor lighting and that the older person may be unable to see obstacles, read signs, or recognize familiar people when the lighting is poor.
• The lens grows unevenly and becomes striated. The lens tends to refract the light that passes through it, causing glare problems. A small amount of glare that may hardly bother a younger person may cause great difficulties for the older person. Glare also may cause anxiety and inability to concentrate.	• Carefully adjust shades or drapes throughout the day to avoid glare from windows. Avoid shiny surfaces that reflect light. Tabletops, waxed floors, vinyl upholstery, and mirrors may create glare. • Sunglasses, big-brimmed hats, or sunshades may help when clients are outdoors or riding in a car. When clients cannot express themselves, caregivers must watch for signs of anxiety due to glare.
• Changes in the lens make color perception more difficult. Pastel colors (pink, yellow, pale blue) may all look alike. Brown, dark blue, and black may be difficult to identify correctly.	• Do not interpret inability to identify colors as a sign of confusion. • Do not expect older people to use pastels and very dark colors in a color-coding system. Clients should not depend upon color to help them take the correct pill.
• The older eye does not adapt quickly to changes in light levels. Abrupt changes can be hazardous and may cause falls and other accidents.	• Place lights strategically and keep some lights on so that changes in lighting will be more gradual. For example, nightlights in bedrooms will help. • When there is an abrupt change in the light level, an older person should wait until the eyes have adapted before continuing to walk. • Be careful when placing furniture just inside an entryway. An older person who enters a building may bump into things that are just inside the door if his or her eyes have not yet adjusted to the change in lighting.
• Conditions of the eye that cause vision loss are very common among older people. However, most older people are not totally blind and can be taught to use their residual vision. More than half of the severe visual impairments occur in people 65 and over. Legal blindness is most common in this age group. The changes in vision occur slowly, and older people are often unaware of them.	• Older people should have their eyes examined by an ophthamologist regularly. • Moving closer to things is one of the best ways to see them better. • Extra-large things are easier to see. These include large-print dials, controls, and buttons.

(continues)

FIGURE 8-3 *(continued)*

Vision changes	Ways to help
	• Contrasting colors make things easier to see. For example, doorways can contrast with the wall, wall sides can contrast with the tablecloth, the chair seat can contrast with the floor, and personal items can contrast with a covering on the dresser top. • Avoid clutter. It is difficult to distinguish crowded items. • Don't change the furniture arrangement unless it is necessary; if you do, ensure that older people become familiar with the new layout.
• Glaucoma is an insidious eye disease that has no noticeable symptoms until irreversible damage is done. It involves a loss of vision due to raised intraocular pressure, which damages the optic nerve. Glaucoma can be controlled and vision loss prevented if it is detected in time.	• There is currently a simple and painless test for glaucoma that older adults should be made aware of. They also should realize the importance of having the test.
• At this time there is no known prevention for cataracts, but they can be successfully treated by the surgical removal of the lens that has become cloudy and opaque. The surgery is usually performed when the vision loss has become severe. The lack of a natural lens in the eye is compensated for by special optical lenses that can be recognized by their thickness and the magnification of the person's eyes behind them.	• If a person has had cataract surgery and wears the special glasses, he or she may still experience some difficulty seeing. The person may need help reading, crossing the street, and doing other things that we assume should be easy. Those wearing the special lenses also may be unsure of themselves and want extra reassurance or assistance. However, people who are very proud may need extra assistance but may refuse to ask for it. Ask people how they might be assisted.
• Cataract glasses make objects seem larger. It is sometimes difficult for an older person to adjust to these distortions. A person wearing cataract glasses also has a blind spot at each side where the glasses cannot provide correction. This situation causes things to appear suddenly—to pop into a person's visual field. There is a new technique of implanting a lens in the eye at the time of surgery that has proven very successful. With implanted lenses, some of the problems of visual field change and size distortions are solved.	• Some people are self-conscious about the fact that the lenses make their eyes appear large and may need reassurance. • To avoid startling someone who wears cataract glasses, approach slowly from the front, rather than from the side.

(continues)

FIGURE 8-3 *(continued)*

Vision changes	Ways to help
• Macular degeneration is a condition that causes loss of central vision as the macula, the area of the retina responsible for central vision, deteriorates. This condition is neither preventable nor curable. It will not, however, cause total blindness because peripheral vision is not affected. A current method being tested to slow the advance of macular degeneration uses a laser to cauterize the hemorrhaging blood vessels in the retina.	• It may be reassuring to tell the person that he or she will not be totally blind from the disease but will retain peripheral vision. • Low-vision aids such as magnifying glasses can be of some help to those in the less-advanced stages of macular degeneration. • Persons with macular degeneration may seem not to have a severe vision problem. Due to their peripheral vision, they can move around independently without bumping into things and may appear to see quite well. When they talk about their vision problems, other people may not believe them and think they are looking for unnecessary extra help or attention.
• There is some indication that a relationship exists between visual loss and mental function.	• Compensation and correction for vision problems may possibly lead to better mental functioning. It is worth a try.
• Persons who have visual deficits are unable to benefit from the nonverbal feedback important to communication. They cannot see the smiles, frowns, or other facial expressions that are an important part of conversation.	• When conversing with persons who have vision problems, use touch to compensate. For example, holding, squeezing, or patting someone's hand lets the person know where you are and assures the person that you have not walked away.
• Dining can present special problems for people with visual impairments. These people may have difficulty eating independently or be afraid to dine socially because they might spill or make mistakes. Food that is difficult to see is not appealing.	• For those with low vision, place settings should be uncluttered, colors should contrast, and glare should be limited. A tablecloth or place mat can lessen glare. Someone should name the foods and tell where each is located. Finger foods and snack time should be provided regularly to allow people to feel more comfortable about their ability to eat appropriately.
• Those who have vision problems may be unsure of themselves in social situations and may even be fearful if they are in unfamiliar surroundings and situations.	• Help people with vision problems to look attractive, and reassure them honestly about their appearance. Always explain the layout of a room and describe the people who are present and those who will accompany them to social activities. Do not leave them alone until they have someone they can talk with or until they are touching a table, chair, or wall that will help with their orientation.

Taste and Smell

Much of what we believe to be the taste of food is really smell. The senses of taste and smell decline significantly with age. Consequently, eating and cooking can become much more difficult. A cook who uses "a little of this and a pinch of that" relies on both smell and taste to know when it is right. Appetite, too, is affected by smell. How many times have you walked by a bakery and wanted "just a bite"? A home health aide can compensate for these losses by taking extra care to ensure that food looks appealing. Including a variety of textures (smooth or crunchy) and temperatures (hot or cold) can help make food more appealing. Consider other things that make mealtime more appealing: music, conversation, or pretty dishes. Additionally, check the contents of the refrigerator to verify that the food is fresh. Again, if the older person's sense of smell or taste is less acute, he or she may not notice that food has spoiled.

Nutritional Concerns

American society often is said to be obsessed with food. Every day newspaper articles discuss decreasing fat, increasing fiber, using vitamin supplements, and being within ideal weight ranges. An older person may need to consider all these things and more. Many older people suffer, to varying degrees, from one or more chronic health conditions. Further, many take one or more medications daily. These facts, coupled with the natural changes due to aging, getting the right food, and maintaining good nutrition, can be a great challenge for some older people. They may be less physically active than they were earlier in their lives, and they may be living alone or with one other person. As noted earlier, their sense of smell and taste may be less acute than in times past. It is important, too, to be aware of any dietary restrictions due to the older person's medical condition, for example, diabetes or heart disease. It often is easy to turn to packaged foods or "tea and toast."

A home health aide can assist the older person by offering a variety of foods, focusing on fruits and vegetables, and on **carbohydrates**. Carbohydrates include breads, cereals, and starches. Preparing a number of smaller meals or snacks, especially earlier in the day, may make it easier for the older person to get the needed nutrition without feeling too full. Food may need to be sweeter or saltier to taste "right" to the older person. Salt or sweetener added after food is cooked provides a great taste punch. If the older person has been placed on a salt-restricted diet, encourage the use of salt substitutes, if you have the doctor's approval, or add spice mixtures or lemon to give food the "kick" that salt can provide. Tomato products have a fairly high natural sodium content; pairing them with blander foods can be tastier without increasing sodium.

Exercise, Bone Density, and Osteoporosis

Exercise and aging are not words we normally put together, but we should. If an older person has always exercised or is just now beginning, there are health benefits. Even mild exercise, done regularly, can improve digestion, increase muscle mass, improve sleep, and elevate mood. If the older person has a chronic health condition, he or she should first consult the doctor before beginning an exercise plan. The home health aide can accompany the older person on a walk, encourage or assist with exercises recommended by a physical therapist, or suggest stretching exercises (Figure 8-4). All these things will help the older person to "use it, not lose it!"

Osteoporosis is a thinning of the bone density caused by loss of bone mass and bone strength. It is most common in women, affecting about 25% of those over age 60. There has been a great deal of focus in the media about calcium and osteoporosis, but weight-bearing exercise also is helpful. Weight-bearing exercise could be walking or aerobic dance or Tai Chi. Community centers often offer low-cost classes during the day.

Sleep

Generally, as we age, sleep is of shorter duration, but the same amount. That is to say, we often sleep as many hours as we did when we were younger, but each period of sleep lasts a shorter length of time. It is not uncommon for people to be less physically active as they grow older. Additionally, the bladder gets smaller so the need to urinate becomes more frequent. These three factors often can leave the older person feeling as if he or she never gets a good night's sleep. A home health aide knows these

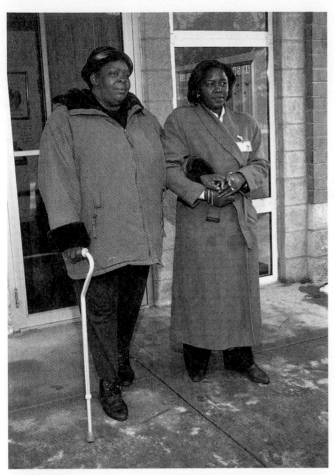

FIGURE 8-4 The home health aide can encourage or assist the older adult with exercises.

changes are normal, but listens and observes carefully because the aide also knows that disrupted or poor sleep patterns can be symptoms of drug interactions or, possibly, depression. Reassurance to the older person about the amount of sleep he or she is getting may help. It also may help to ask the older person why he or she is concerned. This can be the opening to a new kind of conversation, where the older person can confide worries or frustrations he or she has not been willing to share before.

Medication

Because many older people suffer, to some extent, from one or more chronic health conditions, it stands to reason they also may take a number of medications. In fact, the elderly take more than 25% of all drugs prescribed in the United States. This can present special concerns for which the home health aide should be alert.

If the older person is taking more than one medication, whether it is prescription or **over**

the counter (nonprescription) these drugs can interact and produce side effects or complications. The home health aide should be especially alert when there is a change in medication or a change in the way medication is taken.

Decreased kidney function means drugs pass through the system of an older person more slowly. A medication and dosage that works well for someone at 65 may not be right for that same person when he or she is 75. The home health aide is often the person who sees the client most frequently and over the longest period of time. Awareness of subtle changes can be, literally, a real lifesaver to the older person.

AGE-RELATED MENTAL CHANGES······

Although a common pattern of physical changes occurs as people age, mental changes are more unique to the individual. For example, there is not an aged personality. Most older people's personalities or natures remain as they were when they were younger.

Change is a constant in life and if one lives long enough, there is a lot of it! Think about the number of changes an older person may experience: retirement, relocation, grandchildren and great-grandchildren, physical changes, and technological changes. There are at least two common threads in most older people's lives: change and loss.

Depression

Physical changes that occur naturally as we age can make keeping up with change difficult. Change is not always neutral. Sometimes change is loss: death of a family member or friend, or loss of vision or illness, for example. For a person of any age, these kinds of losses can be serious blows. For some older people they can be overwhelming. It can feel as if losses are coming faster than they can handle. The older person grieves for each loss. **Depression** may describe the kinds of emotions a person feels after a loss or multiple losses. Depression is more than just feeling "blue" or "down" one day. Depression is a persistent sadness that makes it difficult to do day-to-day tasks. Clinical depression is a medical illness that is discussed in more detail in Unit 11.

Physical and Visual Clues. Depression interferes with an older person's daily functioning and activities. Often a depressed person is not concerned about personal appearance, and neglects hair, teeth, and skin care. A depressed person may look sad without complaining about being sad. Depression also may cause a person to want to stay in bed more than is normal.

Home health aides may be the only people who see these older persons regularly. They have the opportunity to observe clients closely over time. This activity is an important part of their job. Being able to identify signs of depression and knowing when to report changes in behavior to a supervisor are crucial skills. Many symptoms of depression are the same as symptoms of other serious problems: dementia, malnourishment, medication misuse, or alcoholism. A trained, skilled home health aide will know what is normal for the older person and can identify changes.

Untreated Depression in Older People. Although depression in older people responds well to treatment, it often goes untreated. Depression goes undiagnosed in older people for a variety of reasons. Some people, including older people themselves, believe that sadness and depression are a natural part of aging. Home health aides should know that sadness and depression are not natural parts of aging. Clinical depression is not the result of growing old. It does not happen to all older people. Even people with chronic illness, financial problems, or other difficulties should not suffer from depression.

Another reason that depression is often misdiagnosed is that many people, including older people themselves, are not able to recognize the signs and symptoms of the disease. Physical illness can mask depression, and depression, in turn, can look like a physical illness.

Older people also may deny being depressed because they feel that admitting to the feelings of depression is a sign of weakness. They may fear being labeled as weak or even crazy. Many older people were raised during a time in which it was not socially acceptable to be depressed. Old attitudes hang on and can prevent many older people from coming to terms with the fact that they have a debilitating and even life-threatening illness.

Some clients find it normal to talk about physical illness and express physical pain, but not to express emotional pain. They may **somaticize,** or give physical symptoms, to their depression. For example, headaches and stomachaches will be treated instead of the depression that brings on these symptoms.

Depressed people may drink heavily in an attempt to relieve their feelings of sadness, but heavy drinking can make things worse. The use of drugs also can cause depression. Some people abuse drugs to try to relieve their symptoms.

Dementia

Dementia or confusion is not part of the common age-related changes that older people experience. Dementia is a persistent mental deterioration that can involve memory, problem solving, learning, and other mental functions. These problems are severe enough to interfere with daily living activities. Many conditions can cause or mimic dementia. Many are completely reversible. Others, sadly, are not. Some common causes of reversible dementia are: urinary tract infections, nutritional imbalance, dehydration, medication reactions or medication interactions, and depression. Some causes that are not reversible are: vascular dementia (stroke), Parkinson's disease, and Alzheimer's disease (discussed in detail in Unit 22).

Many older people fear "losing their minds" most of all. This fear can be double-edged. The older person may want reassurance that it is normal to forget where their keys are, for example. They also may go to great lengths to cover up such lapses, hoping that if no one notices, it did not really happen. Knowing how worrisome this topic can be, a home health aide who notices confusion or memory loss must be diplomatic in raising her concerns with both client and family. Be alert to changes in a client's behavior and aware of other symptoms as well. Many times the home health aide sees problems first, when they are easiest to correct. Trust your observation skills and talk with others involved in the client's care.

REMINISCENCE

Reminiscence, or remembering, can be a helpful and enjoyable pastime for some older people. For clients with memory loss, older memories from childhood or early adulthood often remain clear while yesterday or early this morning are hazy. For people suffering from grief or depression, reminiscence can remind them of happier times and successes in their lives. A home health aide can prompt the older person by asking questions to spark a memory (Figure 8-5). For example, the aide can ask the following questions:

1. How did your family prepare for important holidays (Christmas, Passover, Ramadan) when you were a child? When you first had children of your own?
2. What is your favorite birthday memory? What was your best birthday gift?
3. Who is the member of your family (past or present) who is most like you? Why? Tell me about this person.
4. What is your favorite song? What were you doing when you heard it?
5. Did you have a nickname? Who gave you the name and why?
6. What was your home like when you were a child? Who lived there?

In addition, the home health aide can use props to stimulate reminiscence, such as family photographs, music, holiday decorations, postcards, travel books, or baby things. Reminiscence is an important tool for the home health aide who is working with an older adult with depression or dementia.

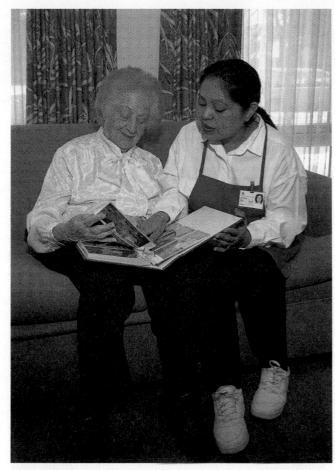

FIGURE 8-5   Reminiscence can be a helpful and enjoyable pastime for older adults with depression or dementia.

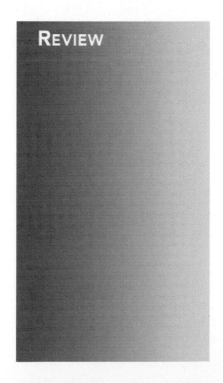

REVIEW

1. Which of the following can cause dementia or dementia-like symptoms?
   a. Stroke
   b. Stress
   c. Aging
   d. Urinary tract infection
   e. All of the above

2. Which of the following would not be helpful to someone with vision problems?
   a. Providing adequate lighting
   b. Speaking louder
   c. Providing finger foods as snacks

3. Which of the following are helpful when working with an older person with hearing loss?
   a. Speaking slowly and clearly
   b. Pitching your voice lower
   c. Avoiding background noise or music
   d. Suggesting activities that do not require conversation
   e. All of the above

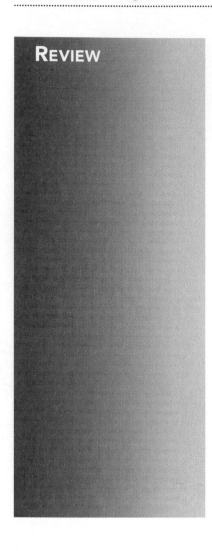

REVIEW

4. T   F   Most older people have no one to help them with their activities of daily living.

5. T   F   Urinary incontinence is a common problem for older women.

6. T   F   Older people sleep fewer hours than younger people.

7. List the ways reminiscence can help a depressed or demented older person.

8. List two ways to prevent incontinence.

9. List three factors that affect the sleeping patterns of older adults.

10. Name three reasons depression can go undiagnosed or untreated in older people.

11. On Thursday you arrive at the home of a longtime client. The client is surprised to see you, saying, "Why are you working on Sunday?" You realize that this client has not been herself lately. What do you do?

12. Your client, an 85-year-old diabetic, has a significant vision loss and as a result is inactive. Although you know your client is on a restricted diet, she continues to ask you to provide her with high-calorie sweet snacks. What steps could you take to help your client, while being mindful of her diet restrictions? What factors might be contributing to her wanting snacks all the time? What alternatives could you suggest that would take her mind off the snacks, but encourage a healthier life-style?

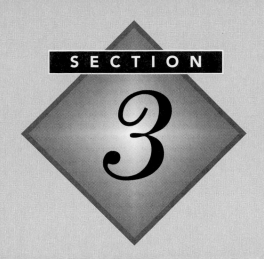
Preventing the Spread
of Infectious Disease

Unit

9 Principles of Infection Control

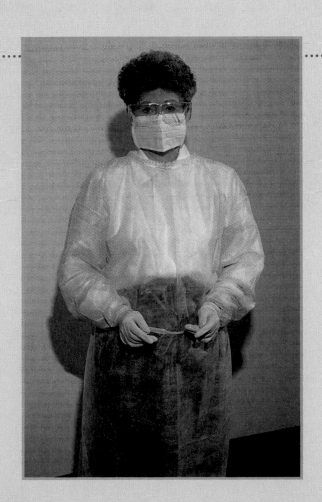

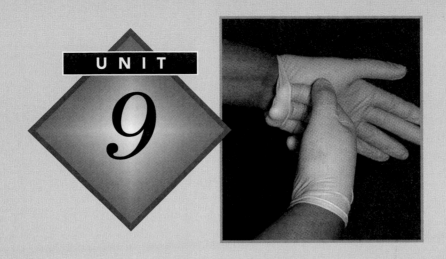

UNIT 9

Principles of Infection Control

KEY TERMS

aseptic techniques
bacteria
contaminated
disinfection
fungi
germs
hepatitis B
incubation period

infection
infection control
infectious disease
isolation
jaundice
microorganisms
pathogens
protozoa

rickettsiae
standard precautions
sterile
transmission-based
    precautions
tuberculosis
virus

LEARNING OBJECTIVES

After studying this unit, you should be able to:

- Name three different types of microorganisms.
- Describe standard precautions.
- List three modes of transmission (the ways germs can spread from one person to another).
- List two contagious/infectious diseases.
- Explain signs and symptoms and nursing care for a client with tuberculosis.
- List six rules to follow when caring for a client with an infectious disease.
- Give examples of situations requiring standard precautions.
- Name the single most effective precaution to prevent the spread of infections.

- List five examples of when aides must wash their hands.
- Explain the purpose of each procedure.
- Demonstrate the following:
  PROCEDURE 3 Handwashing
  PROCEDURE 4 Gloving
  PROCEDURE 5 Putting On and Removing Personal Protective Equipment
  PROCEDURE 6 Collecting Specimen from Client on Transmission-Based Precautions

INFECTIOUS DISEASE ·······················

An **infection** is the invasion of body tissue by disease-producing organisms. An **infectious disease** is one that is readily communicable or easily passed on to others (contagious).

CAUSES OF PHYSICAL ILLNESSES ·········

Microorganisms are so small that they can be seen only under a high-powered microscope. There are good microorganisms and microorganisms that can cause disease. The microorganisms that are capable of causing disease are called **germs** or **pathogens.** The time between the entry of germs into the body and the appearance of the first sign of disease is called the **incubation period.** Strong, healthy people are more able to fight off pathogens than weak or unhealthy people.

There are many different types of microorganisms (Figures 9-1 through 9-4). **Bacteria** are microscopic organisms that multiply rapidly. **Protozoa** are tiny one-cell microorganisms. Bacteria and protozoa can live for a long time and continue to multiply in air and water. Many types of bacteria and protozoa exist, but only a few cause diseases. **Viruses** are microorganisms that can live only by feeding on living cells. Most viruses are capable of causing infections.

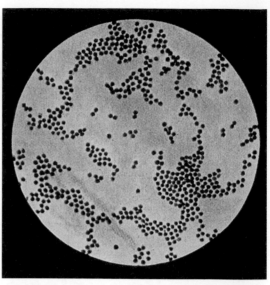

FIGURE 9-2 *Staphylococcus aureus*

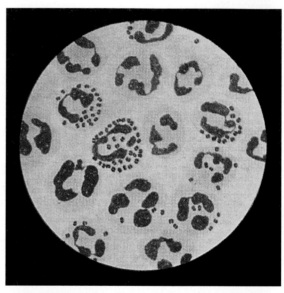

FIGURE 9-3 *Neisseria gonorrheae*

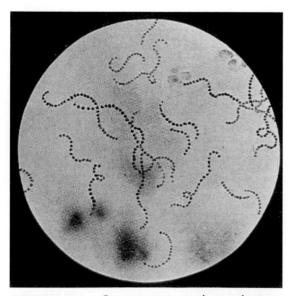

FIGURE 9-1 *Streptococcus hemolyticus*

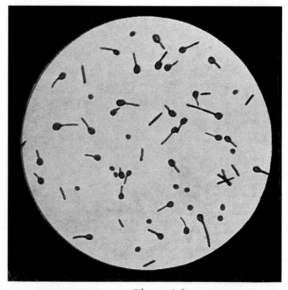

FIGURE 9-4 *Clostridium tetani*

Diseases caused by viruses are flu, colds, acquired immunodeficiency syndrome (AIDS), and hepatitis. **Fungi** include two groups of organisms—yeast and molds—that live normally in the body. Under certain conditions they can cause diseases such as athlete's foot (tinea pedis), ringworm (tinea capitis), thrush, or vaginitis *(Candida albicans)*. Another example of a microorganism that can cause a disease and lives on lice, ticks, fleas, mites, and other insects is called **rickettsiae.** Figure 9-5 lists the ways in which organisms causing various diseases are carried.

Most germs grow and reproduce very rapidly. They spread disease from one part of the body to another. They also may spread disease from one person to another. A home health aide must learn how to keep pathogens from spreading.

Practicing good infection control techniques is the best defense against the spread of germs (Figure 9-6). If there is a possibility of the presence of germs (pathogens) on an article, the article is considered **contaminated.** Articles that are free of all living organisms are **sterile.** The process of sterilization completely destroys microorganisms on objects. **Aseptic techniques** are used to handle sterile articles in the client's home. Many sterile supplies such as gauze dressings, applicators, and instruments come prepackaged in paper for convenience. They must be opened, handled, and used in a special way so that they will not become contaminated. **Disinfection** is the process of destroying disease-producing organisms by using chemicals. For example, if an aide is using a stethoscope that other aides use, the aide must disinfect the earpieces with alcohol before using the stethoscope to prevent transmission of germs from one person to another. A summary of how common infectious diseases are transmitted is given in Figure 9-7.

FIGURE 9-5 Methods by which diseases are carried

Airborne	Animal Carried	Insect Carried
Colds Flu (influenza) Measles Chickenpox Smallpox	Rabies; occurs from bite of infected dog, squirrel, bat Trichinosis; occurs from eating poorly cooked pork of an infected pig Tularemia (rabbit fever); occurs from touching or eating contaminated rabbit	Lyme disease; deer tick Malaria; occurs from bite of Anopheles mosquito Sleeping sickness (narcolepsy); occurs from bite of a tsetse fly Encephalitis; mosquito

Contact	Human Carried	Prenatal
Mononucleosis Venereal diseases (syphilis, gonorrhea, and AIDS) Infectious hepatitis Tuberculosis Conjunctivitis Poliomyelitis	Typhoid fever Mumps Impetigo Whooping cough (pertussis) Diphtheria Poliomyelitis Syphilis and gonorrhea	Syphilis may cause fetal blindness, deafness, malformation, or retardation Rubella (German measles); may lead to fetal blindness, deafness, or malformation

Food Carried	Water Carried	Soil Carried
Dysentery Botulism Worms Salmonella	Typhoid fever Dysentery Poliomyelitis	Tetanus (lockjaw) Dysentery Worms

FIGURE 9-6   Germs can be destroyed or restricted by applying aseptic techniques.

Ways to Kill Germs	Description	Use
Disinfection	The use of chemical products to kill pathogens. Mouthwash, green soap, borax, commercial disinfectants, alcohol, boric acid, chlorine, chlorhexidine. Follow instructions.	Household items Clothes Hands Wounds Thermometers
Sterilization	The application of dry or steam heat under controlled conditions. (Boiled or steamed in pressure cooker or covered pot at 212°—in oven 2–3 hr at 165–170°—aired in sunlight for 6–8 hr)	Baby bottles Dishes and utensils Hypodermic needles Contaminated clothing Bed linens
Incineration	Burning contaminated items such as tissues, etc.	Used tissues Soiled dressings Disposable paper products
Pest control	Use of chemicals and other means to rid area of pests. (Follow instructions carefully to avoid danger of accidental poisoning.)	Rats, mice Flies, roaches Fleas, mosquitos

Ways to Restrict Germs	Description	Use
Waste disposal	Daily removal of nonburnable waste products, double bagging and discarding in covered garbage cans.	Food scraps Tin cans, bottles Contaminated dressings or tissues
Isolation techniques	Keeping client in controlled environment so germs will not spread or new ones enter. Especially important if client has highly contagious disease or is weakened and unable to resist added infections. Using special equipment and supplies such as rubber gloves, apron or coveralls, cap, mask and disposable paper products.	Restrict client's mobility Contaminated dishes Contaminated linen Body discharges Personal and household items
Damp cloth dusting and mopping	Use of wet cloth or sponge to remove germs and dust from surfaces. Prevents raising germs into the air where they can be spread easier.	Furniture surfaces Floors Walls and window sills

Hepatitis B

Infectious **hepatitis B** affects the liver mainly. It is caused by a virus (Figure 9-8), and is transmitted by blood or blood transfusion, by use of contaminated needles or contaminated items, or by sexual contact. The disease comes on suddenly and can be severe and result in a chronic illness. The disease can cause a fever and tiredness, and the client's skin becomes **jaundiced** (yellow). The client may be nauseated and have breathing problems; the liver may become enlarged. A vaccination is available to prevent this disease. Health care workers are at increased risk for contracting hepatitis B, and all home health aides should have

FIGURE 9-7   Common communicable diseases

Disease	How It Enters Body	How It Leaves Body	How It Is Transferred
Hepatitis A	Mouth/intestine	Feces	Direct contact, contaminated water, contaminated food
Hepatitis B	Blood contact, sexual contact	Blood	Blood transfusion, contaminated needles or instrument, sexual contact
Pneumonia	Mouth to lungs	Sputum, nasal discharge	Direct contact, articles used by and around patient, hands
Influenza	Mouth/nose to lungs	As above	As above
Tuberculosis	Mouth/lungs	Sputum	Kissing, coughing, sputum, soiled dressings, hands
Rubella (German measles)	Mouth/nose	Nasal/throat discharges	Airborne, transplacentally
Gonorrhea	Mucous membrane, sexual contact	Body discharges, lesions	Sexual intercourse, birth canal
Syphilis	Sexual contact, blood and tissues through skin breaks	Infected tissues, lesions placenta to fetus	Direct contact, kissing, sexual intercourse
AIDS	Sexual contact, mucous membrane, blood, any discharge containing blood	Placenta to fetus, transfusion, body discharges, blood	Sexual intercourse (anal, oral, and vaginal) needles and syringes, transplacentally

this vaccination. Your employer should provide you with this vaccination at no cost to you. This is important because health care workers never know when they will be exposed to the virus that causes hepatitis B.

Clients with hepatitis B need excellent skin and mouth care. You also will need to supplement their meals with highly nutritious liquid drinks. These clients usually have no appetite and have problems eating.

Tuberculosis

Tuberculosis (TB) is an airborne disease, which means that it is spread by droplets in the air released from deep within the lungs when a TB sufferer coughs. Anyone sharing a poorly ventilated room with an individual with TB can contract the disease. The incidence of TB is on the rise. By 1990, the number of Americans suffering from the disease had increased by 16%. Individuals who live in crowded spaces, have poor nutrition, are substance abusers, are under a high amount of stress, or lack medical care are good candidates for this disease.

When an aide is assigned to care for a client with TB, the aide will need to use standard precautions, especially when handling the client's sputum and nasal secretions. Another important aspect of care is making sure to remind the client to take medication as prescribed. *The medication must be taken on schedule, otherwise the effects of the drugs will be decreased.* TB can be cured if caught in the early stages and if the client takes the medication as ordered usually for 6 months to 1 year. If the client does not take the medication as prescribed, be sure to notify the case manager.

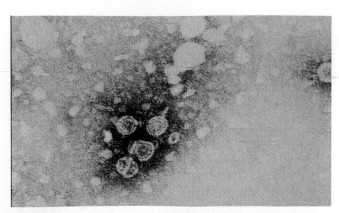

FIGURE 9-8 Electron micrograph of hepatitis B virus

The home health aide also will need to be checked yearly by having a TB skin test or a chest x-ray. The signs and symptoms of TB come on rather slowly. It is common for an individual to have TB for a long time before the signs and symptoms become evident or full blown. The first signs of TB are usually chest pains, tiredness, loss of appetite, and weight loss. Night sweats, shortness of breath, spitting up large amounts of pus-colored sputum develop as the disease progresses. Treatment usually consists of medications and rest.

Common Childhood Diseases

Many children's diseases are communicable and most individuals have experienced them personally. Among these are measles, German measles, mumps, chickenpox, smallpox, and whooping cough. Most children are given immunizations so that they will not get these diseases. See Unit 6, Figure 6-2: Infant and Child Immunization Schedule. Although children may weather these illnesses with few problems, contracting these diseases is more serious for adults. When caring for an ill child use **infection control** precautions to avoid becoming ill yourself.

CONTROLLING THE SPREAD OF ILLNESS

Most everyone practices aseptic techniques for infection control in daily living. Some of the most common practices are:

- Handwashing
- Bathing, brushing teeth
- Changing clothing regularly
- Using fresh towels and washcloths
- Sterilizing baby bottles
- Cleaning bathroom sink, tub, bowl, and floor
- Cleaning kitchen, washing dishes
- Vacuuming and mopping floors
- Laundering clothing and linens

When illness is present, added care must be taken to prevent the spread of germs. An ill person's body is producing pathogens. At the same time, the person is weak and cannot resist other germs. The person's body is so busy fighting one illness that it cannot fight off other germs. The home health aide is responsible for controlling the spread of the client's germs so others in the home will not be harmed. The aide also must help protect the client from the germs carried into the home.

Germs can enter the body in many ways. For example, if the germ that causes a cold enters the respiratory system (the nose, the lungs, etc.) the person would develop a cold because the respiratory system provides just the right climate for the cold germ to grow.

Germs can be spread when others touch contaminated objects or surfaces. Tissues used by the client should be placed in a paper bag at the client's bedside. Dressings or bandages from open cuts or wounds must be double-bagged in plastic and then discarded. Careful cleaning of the client's room is important in stopping indirect spread of germs.

Infectious or contagious diseases are those that spread rapidly and easily from person to person or place to place. Many contagious diseases that once caused many deaths have been largely controlled. Today there are vaccines given to prevent hepatitis, polio, diphtheria, whooping cough, mumps, and measles. Gamma globulin shots may be given to persons exposed to diseases such as hepatitis, measles, and mumps. Although these shots do not always prevent the disease, they cause the client's reaction to be milder.

INFECTION CONTROL MEASURES

A home health aide has a duty to protect clients from unnecessary harm. In addition to keeping the home environment clean and following everyday aseptic practices, the aide also should be in good physical health. An aide who is ill risks carrying germs into the client's environment.

The home health aide's hands are the most common means of carrying infection. To control the spread of germs and to protect the aide and client, the aide's hands must be washed frequently. Just a quick rinse will not do it. The aide should use plenty of warm water and soap, and wash for 15 seconds. If, for any reason, there is no water available, commercially prepared washing pads may be used. To dry the hands, use of disposable paper towels is best. Cloth towels can spread germs when reused. If the hands are dry and chapped, lotion may be used after washing. Hands should be washed:

- On arrival at the client's home
- Before and after each client contact
- Before preparing food
- Before and after each meal
- After blowing the nose or sneezing
- After using the bathroom
- After handling soiled items such as linens, clothing, or garbage
- Before putting on gloves and after using gloves
- After contact with items contaminated with blood, feces, or other body fluids (refer to Procedure 3)

The aide should keep in mind that handwashing is the most important procedure involved in controlling the spread of disease.

CLIENT CARE PROCEDURE

3

Handwashing

PURPOSE

- To prevent the transfer of disease-producing organisms from person to person or place to place

PROCEDURE

1. Collect the items needed for handwashing and bring them to the bathroom or kitchen sink.
   soap
   soap dish
   towel (paper towels preferred)
   washbasin (if needed)
   orange stick (optional)
2. Use a clean paper towel to turn on water and adjust temperature. Wet hands with fingertips pointing down (Figure 9-9).
3. Apply soap—either liquid or bar.
4. With fingertips pointing down, lather well. Rub your hands together in a circular motion to generate friction (Figure 9-10). Wash carefully between your fingers, palms, and back of hands, and rub fingernails against the palm of the other hand to force soap under the nails. Keep washing

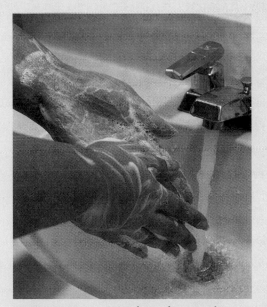

FIGURE 9-9 Wet hands, apply soap, and rub hands to cause lather. Keep hands pointed down so water does not run up arms.

for 15 seconds. Be sure to clean under fingernails (Figure 9-11).

(continues)

CLIENT CARE PROCEDURE **3** ▸ **Handwashing** *(continued)*

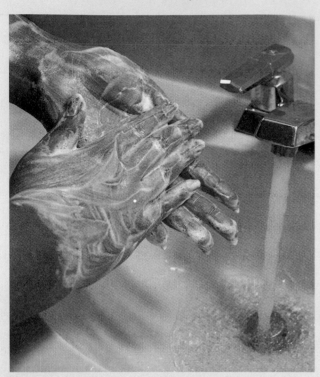

FIGURE 9-10 Use friction between hands to clean well.

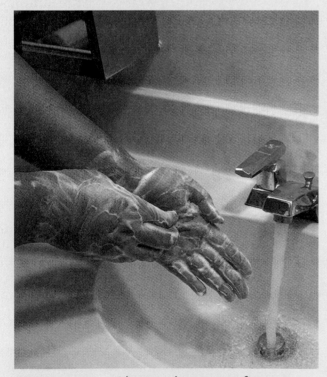

FIGURE 9-11 Always clean your fingernails.

5. With fingertips still pointing down, rinse all the soap off. Be careful not to lean against the side of the sink or touch the inside of the sink because germs are there.

6. With clean paper towel or clean hand towel, dry hands. Use a clean paper towel and turn off faucet (Figure 9-12). Do not turn off faucet with clean hands because the faucet handles are contaminated.

7. Discard the paper towel in the wastebasket. Hand towels can be placed in a laundry hamper.

8. Apply hand lotion if hands are dry or chapped.

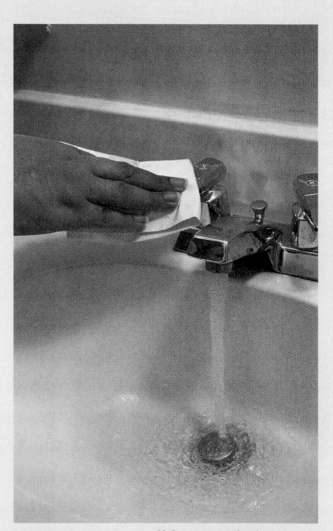

FIGURE 9-12 Turn off faucet with dry paper towel.

Kitchen

In many homes, the kitchen is the center of family life. Most families eat three meals a day and may raid the refrigerator for between-meal snacks. This means that the traffic in and out of the kitchen is heavier than in any other room in the house. The kitchen probably offers the home health aide more challenges than any other room. Keeping the kitchen clean can be a time-consuming job. In some kitchens, the aide will see piles of dirty dishes and garbage. Floors also may be dirty and sticky. Kitchen tasks that are left until the end of the day cause unsanitary and unhealthy conditions. Hours are added to the workload because the dirt has hardened.

Good organization can lighten the workload a great deal. Helpful time-saving tips for keeping a kitchen clean include:

- Wash dirty dishes promptly.
- Let cooked-on dirt soak first to soften it and avoid scrubbing.
- Wipe up spills at once.
- Take garbage out regularly, perhaps once each visit.
- Clean equipment after each use.
- Store supplies properly.

Other infection control tips for the kitchen include:

- Rinse off the tops of cans before opening. After being stored on a grocery shelf or in a pantry the top of the cans may have been contaminated by dirt, insects, or rodents.
- Wash pots, pans, or dishes that have been unused for a long time. They may have been contaminated by roaches, ants, flies, or mice.
- Wash fruits and vegetables before eating or before storing them. If they have been stored, rinse again just before use.
- Cook pork, chicken, and other meats thoroughly. Animal-carried pathogens are killed by proper cooking.
- If sterile water is needed, boil water for 20 minutes. Sterile water that is stored in the refrigerator in a sterile container usually remains sterile for a 36-hour period.

Bathroom and Client's Bedroom

Much of the home health aide's job is to clean the kitchen and prepare meals. However, other important housekeeping duties are to clean the bathrooms and the client's room. The same need for cleanliness applies to these rooms as to the kitchen. Some helpful cleanliness and time-saving tips include:

- Clean bed linens and towels by washing in hot water with a laundry detergent.
- Tissues used by the client should be put in a paper or plastic bag and discarded frequently.
- Clean the bathtub with a disinfecting cleanser after each use.
- Clean the toilet and sink with a disinfectant as needed, at least once a week.
- Change sheets when soiled, or at least once a week.

PREVENTING THE SPREAD OF INFECTION

We cannot tell if people have an infectious disease just from looking at them. Therefore, certain measures must be taken to prevent the spread of infection. These measures are called **standard precautions** and must be used at all times for all patients. Standard precautions are designed to protect the home health aide and the patient. Standard precautions provide guidelines for handwashing, personal protective equipment (PPE) use (gloves, gowns, masks, goggles), patient care equipment, environmental care, linen handling, and safe needle use. See Figure 9-13 for specific guidelines.

TRANSMISSION-BASED PRECAUTIONS

Although the use of special or standard precautions is important to prevent the spread of infection to, or from, a client, keep in mind how odd it must feel to a client to be cared for by a person wearing barriers. Most of us are used to health professionals and paraprofessionals using gloves, gowns, or masks. However, to a person who is feeling isolated or depressed, these protective barriers may increase their feelings of loneliness and sadness. Your tone of voice, what you say, and the gentleness of your touch become even more important.

FIGURE 9-13   Standard precautions guidelines

STANDARD PRECAUTIONS FOR INFECTION CONTROL

Wash Hands (Plain soap)
Wash after touching **blood, body fluids, secretions, excretions,** and **contaminated items.** Wash immediately **after gloves are removed** and **between patient contacts.** Avoid transfer of microorganisms to other patients or environments.

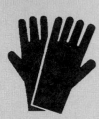

Wear Gloves
Wear when touching **blood, body fluids, secretions, excretions,** and **contaminated items.** Put on **clean** gloves just **before touching mucous membranes** and **nonintact skin.** Change gloves between tasks and procedures on the same patient after contact with material that may contain high concentrations of microorganisms. Remove gloves promptly after use, before touching noncontaminated items and environmental surfaces, and before going to another patient, and wash hands immediately to avoid transfer of microorganisms to other patients or environments.

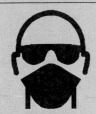

Wear Mask and Eye Protection or Face Shield
Protect mucous membranes of the eyes, nose, and mouth during procedures and patient care activities that are likely to generate **splashes** or **sprays** of **blood, body fluids, secretions,** or **excretions**.

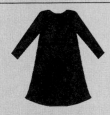

Wear Gown
Protect skin and prevent soiling of clothing during procedures that are likely to generate **splashes** or **sprays** of **blood, body fluids, secretions,** or **excretions**. Remove a soiled gown as promptly as possible and wash hands to avoid transfer of microorganisms to other patients or environments.

Patient Care Equipment
Handle used patient care equipment soiled with **blood, body fluids, secretions** or **excretions** in a manner that prevents skin and mucous membrane exposures, contamination of clothing, and transfer of microorganisms to other patients and environments. Ensure that reusable equipment is not used for the care of another patient until it has been appropriately cleaned and reprocessed and single use items are properly discarded.

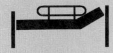

Environmental Control
Follow hospital procedures for routine care, cleaning, and disinfection of environmental surfaces, beds, bedrails, bedside equipment and other frequently touched surfaces.

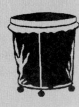

Linens
Handle, transport, and process used linens soiled with **blood, body fluids, secretions,** or **excretions** in a manner that prevents exposures and contamination of clothing, and avoids transfer of microorganisms to other patients and environments.
(continues)

FIGURE 9-13 *(continued)*

STANDARD PRECAUTIONS FOR INFECTION CONTROL

Occupational Health and Bloodborne Pathogens

Prevent injuries when using needles, scalpels, and other sharp instruments or devices; when handling sharp instruments after procedures; when cleaning used instruments; and when disposing of used needles.

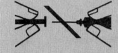

Never recap used needles using both hands or any other technique that involves directing the point of a needle toward any part of the body; rather, use either a one-handed "scoop" technique or a mechanical device designed for holding the needle sheath.

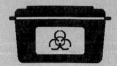

Do not remove used needles from disposable syringes by hand, and do not bend, break, or otherwise manipulate used needles by hand. Place used disposable syringes and needles, scalpel blades, and other sharp items in puncture-resistant sharps containers located as close as practical to the area in which the items were used, and place reusable syringes and needles in a puncture-resistant container for transport to the reprocessing area.

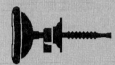

Use **resuscitation devices** as an alternative to mouth-to-mouth resuscitation.

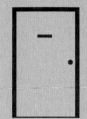

Patient Placement

Use a **private room** for a patient who contaminates the environment or who does not (or cannot be expected to) assist in maintaining appropriate hygiene or environmental control. Consult Infection Control if a private room is not available.

The client with a communicable disease may be placed in **isolation.** This means that the client is kept away from others in the household. Isolation helps prevent family members and the home health aide from getting the client's germs. In such cases home health aides will have to be especially careful in maintaining aseptic conditions. Gloves should be worn for most personal care procedures. Refer to Procedures 4 and 5.

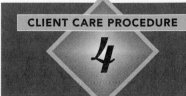

CLIENT CARE PROCEDURE

4

Gloving

PURPOSE

• To prevent the spread of infections

NOTE: Gloves should be worn for most personal care procedures. Always wear gloves when doing procedures in which you have contact with body fluids. Wear gloves when you are giving mouth care, perineal care, handling excretions and body fluids, for example, emptying a bedpan, changing soiled linens, bathing a client with an open skin lesion, and collecting specimens.   *(continues)*

CLIENT CARE PROCEDURE **4** **Gloving** *(continued)*

PROCEDURE

1. Wash your hands.
2. With your dominant hand pull out one glove and slide it onto your other hand.
3. With the gloved hand, pull out another glove and slide your dominant hand into it.
4. Interlace your fingers to make the gloves comfortable and adjust the top of the gloves to stay flat.

Removal of Contaminated Gloves

1. Use your dominant hand to grasp the opposite glove on the palm side, about 1 inch below the wrist (Figure 9-14).
2. Pull the glove down and off so that it is removed inside out and keep hold of that glove with the fingertips of the gloved hand (Figure 9-15).
3. Using your ungloved hand, insert the fingers into the inside of the remaining glove and pull it down and off, inside out, so that the glove you are holding with your fingertips is now inside the glove that you are taking off (Figure 9-16).
4. Drop both soiled gloves together into waste receptacle (which is a double bag) (Figure 9-17).
5. Wash your hands.

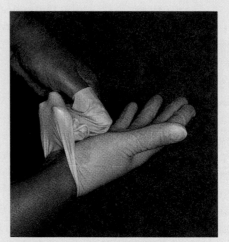

FIGURE 9-16 Use your ungloved hand, insert fingers into inside of remaining glove, turn inside out so glove you are holding is inside glove you're removing.

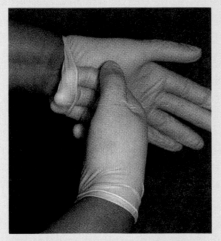

FIGURE 9-14 To remove gloves, grasp glove on the palm side.

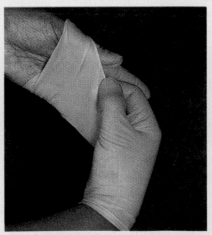

FIGURE 9-15 Pull glove down and off, inside out.

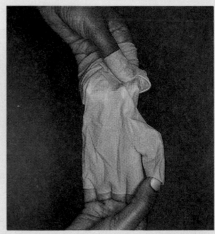

FIGURE 9-17 Drop gloves into proper waste container.

Standard precautions provide guidelines for wearing personal protective equipment such as gowns and masks. Wearing gowns and masks prevents the spread of germs and prevents the contamination of the aide's clothing. Procedure 5 demonstrates the proper method for putting on and removing personal protective equipment.

Isolation is more difficult to arrange in the home than it is in a hospital. Ideally, isolated clients should have a bathroom that only they

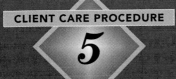

CLIENT CARE PROCEDURE

5

Putting On and Removing Personal Protective Equipment

PURPOSE

- To prevent contaminating the aide's clothing
- To prevent the spread of germs through the respiratory tract

PROCEDURE

1. Assemble personal protective equipment (Figure 9-18).
2. Remove wristwatch and place on clean paper towel.
3. Wash your hands.
4. The first piece of equipment to apply is the mask.
5. Adjust the mask over your nose and mouth. Tie the top strings first and then the bottom strings. Your mask must always be dry, so that droplets are not absorbed into the paper of the mask. If the mask becomes wet, you must replace it.

6. Unfold and open the gown so that you can slide your arms into the sleeves and your hands come right through. Slip the fingers of both hands inside the neckband of the gown and grasp the two strings at the back and tie into a bow, not a knot, so that they can be undone easily after the procedure is completed (Figure 9-19). Reach behind you, overlap

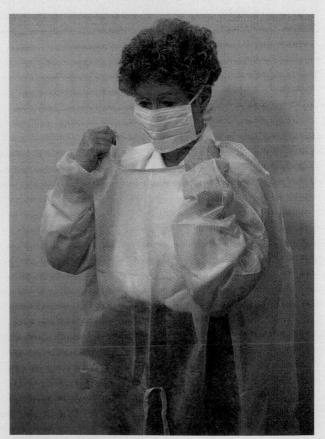

FIGURE 9-19 Putting on gown

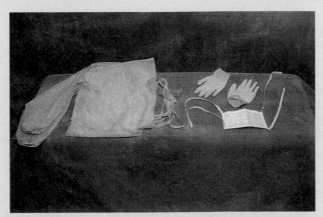

FIGURE 9-18 Protective barriers used in standard precautions: gloves, disposable gown, goggles, and disposable mask

(continues)

CLIENT CARE PROCEDURE ⟨ 5 ⟩ **Putting On and Removing Personal Protective Equipment** *(continued)*

the two edges of the gown so that your uniform is completely covered, and then secure the waist ties (Figures 9-20 and 9-21).

7. **REMEMBER:** Your moisture-resistant gown is only worn once and is then discarded in a container for contaminated linens.

Removing Contaminated Gown and Mask

1. Undo the waist ties of your gown.
2. Remove gloves.
3. Wash hands.
4. Undo your mask, bottom ties first, then top ties. Holding top ties, drop mask in appropriate waste receptacle.

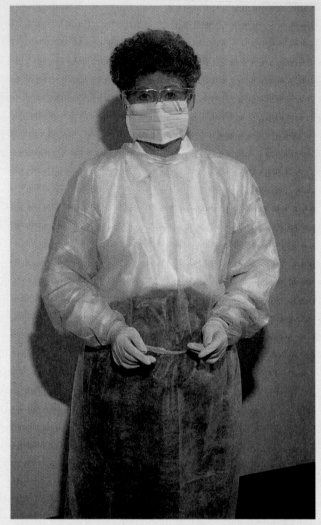

FIGURE 9-21 Properly masked, gloved, and gowned aide

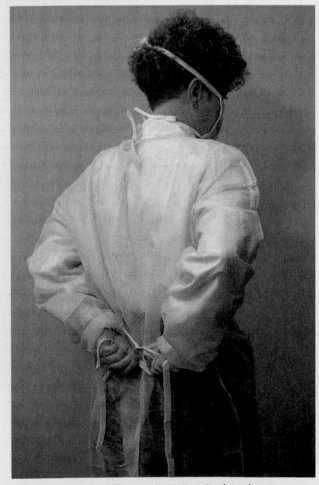

FIGURE 9-20 Tie waist ties in back.

5. Undo neckties and loosen gown at shoulder.
6. Slip finger of right hand inside left cuff without touching outside of gown and pull gown over left hand. With your gown-covered left hand, pull gown down over right hand and then right arm.
7. Fold gown with contaminated side inward and dispose of it into the appropriate receptacle.
8. Wash hands.
9. Remove watch from paper towel and place back on wrist.

may use. However, when this is not possible, the home health aide will have to clean the sink and toilet area each time the client uses it. The aide's hands and the client's hands should be washed often. Handwashing destroys many germs. Disposable dishes, equipment, or tissues should be used whenever possible. The client should use a separate set of dishes and utensils than is used by the family. Combs, brushes, toilet articles, towels, and washcloths used by the client should not be used by others. Keeping these items separate helps prevent indirect spread of infection.

Aides should wear a bib apron or smock over the uniform while in the client's room. Before leaving the room, the cover garment should be placed into a laundry bag or hung inside the door of the client's room. When changing the bed linens, the soiled linens should be held away from the aide's garment. Disposable gloves should be used to pick up soiled linens and place them into a laundry bag. If blood is spilled on the floor, a preparation of 1 part bleach and 10 parts water must be used to clean it up (Figure 9-22). If the spill is on a rug contact a supervisor for cleaning instructions because bleach may remove coloring.

All contaminated materials from the client's room must be discarded by placing them in a double plastic bag and either burned or placed in a covered garbage container. Disposable tissues, dishes, or equipment should be burned if possible. In some cases, linens must be boiled, but most often hot water and soap are adequate. The client's linens and clothing must be washed separately from other family laundry. The client's dishes must be washed separately in hot, soapy

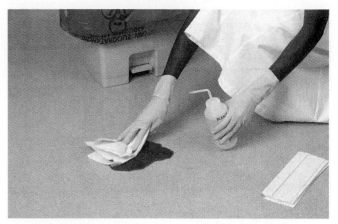

FIGURE 9-22   Solution to clean up blood is 1:10 bleach to water. This solution must be mixed every 24 hours.

water, rinsed, and air-dried. After the isolation period is ended, any items used by the client should be sterilized or disinfected completely. It is important to destroy all germs on the items used before returning to general family use.

Collecting a Specimen From a Client on Transmission-Based Precautions

To collect a specimen from a client on **transmission-based precautions**, it is important to also remember to use standard precautions. Both precautions need to be used because standard precautions alone will not always protect the client and home health aide. For example, if a client is on airborne precautions and you need to collect a urine sample, you must wear gloves (standard precautions) and a mask. Refer to Procedure 6.

CLIENT CARE PROCEDURE

6

Collecting Specimen from Client on Transmission-Based Precautions

PURPOSE

- To obtain and send specimen to laboratory without spreading germs from the client's home

PROCEDURE

1. Assemble equipment:
   clean specimen container, cover, label
   paper towels
   gloves
   plastic transport bag   *(continues)*

CLIENT CARE PROCEDURE **6**
Collecting Specimen from Client on Transmission-Based Precautions *(continued)*

2. Fill in label with client's name, date, time, and type of specimen.
3. Remove cover from the container and place all the equipment on the clean paper towel.
4. Wash your hands and put on gloves.
5. With gloved hands, pick up the specimen and place it in the container so that you do not contaminate any part of the container (Figure 9-23). Replace cover.
6. Remove gloves and wash hands.
7. Using the paper towel, pick up the container without touching it with your bare hands.
8. Place the container in the plastic bag and seal it. Also label the outside of the bag.
9. Send specimen to the laboratory per instruction of your nurse supervisor.

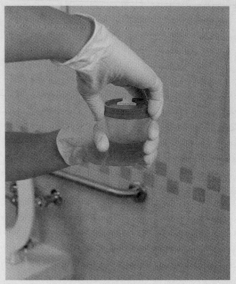

FIGURE 9-23   Collecting a specimen in isolation

REVIEW

1. What is the best defense against germs?

2. Name three infection control procedures commonly practiced in daily living.

3. List the times when the home health aide's hands should be washed.

4. List five ways that diseases can be transferred from one person to another.

5. Name three different types of germs that can cause diseases.

6. Describe three techniques for standard precautions.

7. Give three examples of situations where standard precautions must be followed.

8. A disease-producing microorganism is called:
   a. Contaminated
   b. Contagious
   c. Vector
   d. Pathogen

9. All home health aides should use standard precautions when caring for all clients. The term means:
   a. Wearing gloves when handling body substances
   b. Wiping up blood spills with a solution of bleach and water
   c. Wearing goggles and gloves if required to prevent contact with client's infectious substances
   d. All are correct

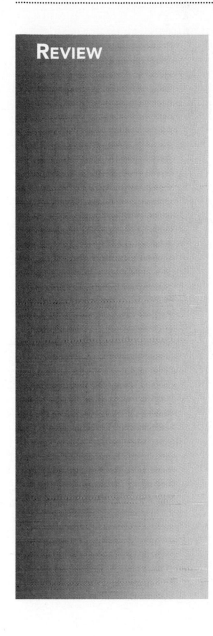

REVIEW

10. An effective method of preventing the spread of infectious diseases in the home is:
    a. Isolating client from family
    b. Soaking clothes in bleach
    c. Handwashing
    d. Hanging clothing of clients outside on clothesline

11. Before using a stethoscope, the aide wipes the earpieces with alcohol—this is an example of
    a. Disinfection
    b. Sterilization
    c. Cross-infection
    d. Contamination

12. Your client, Mrs. Jones is positive for human immunodeficiency virus. After assisting her with a bath, you notice several droplets of blood on the bathroom floor. You make a determination that the blood is a result of Mrs. Jones's menstrual flow. What steps should you take to clean up the blood on the bathroom floor?

13. You have been assigned to a new client, and on your first visit to the home you notice that the kitchen is very dirty. The floors are dirty and sticky, and dishes are piled in the sink. The counters are filled with papers and look like they have not been wiped down in some time. Why is a dirty kitchen a health risk to your client? What steps could you take to organize the workload of keeping the kitchen clean?

14. You are assigned to help your client, who has an open skin lesion, with a bath. Do you need to wear gloves while assisting her with her bath? Under what conditions would you be required to wear gloves when assisting a client? Give specific examples of three procedures where you would be required to wear gloves.

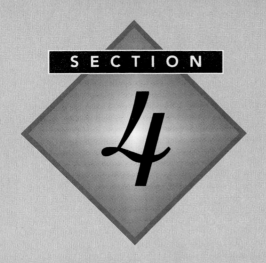
Understanding Health

Units

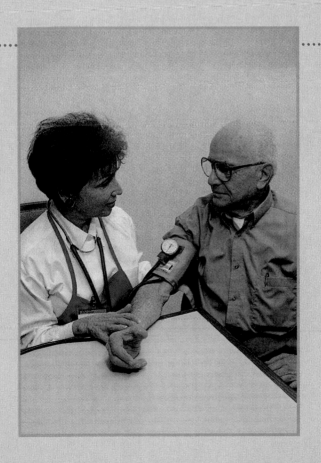

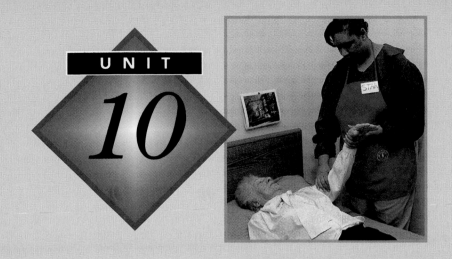

UNIT 10

From Wellness to Illness

activities
acute
apnea
blood pressure
bradycardia
Cheyne-Stokes
chronic
contracture

diastolic
disability
dyspnea
pulse
rales
range of motion exercises
rehabilitation
respiration

sign
sphygmomanometer
symptom
systolic
tachycardia
vital signs

LEARNING OBJECTIVES

After studying this unit, you should be able to:

- Identify the four vital signs and their normal values.
- Name three body sites where temperature is taken.
- Identify four signs that a client may be ill.
- Define disability.
- Define rehabilitation.
- Describe your role in rehabilitation.
- Describe the care given to an unconscious client.
- Demonstrate the following:
  PROCEDURE 7 Taking an Oral Temperature

PROCEDURE 8 Taking a Rectal Temperature

PROCEDURE 9 Taking an Axillary Temperature

PROCEDURE 10 Taking the Radial and Apical Pulse

PROCEDURE 11 Counting Respirations

PROCEDURE 12 Taking Blood Pressure

PROCEDURE 13 Measuring Weight and Height

PROCEDURE 14 Assisting the Client with Self-Administered Medications

(continues)

LEARNING OBJECTIVES

PROCEDURE 15 Performing Passive Range of Motion Exercises

PROCEDURE 16 Assisting the Client to Walk with Crutches, Walker, or Cane

Bodies come in all shapes and sizes. There are records of men who have been as tall as 9 feet and as short as 26½ inches. These statistics are interesting because they show the tremendous contrasts possible within the human body. Just as there are contrasts in size, there are other individual differences. Heredity is the passing of traits from parents to their children. Heredity can determine height, weight, general appearance, skin color, talents and abilities, basic physical wellness, and many other things. All children get half of their heredity from each parent. However, some traits are more dominant than others. This explains why some children are more like one parent than another.

Another factor that helps determine body size, shape, and wellness is environment. Environment is the sum total of the circumstances, conditions, and surroundings affecting the development of an organism. Some environmental factors that may affect growth are nutrition, financial conditions, climate, number of children in the family, and the parents' ages and occupations. The child who is born healthy with good hereditary characteristics is likely to start life as a well person. If the child grows up in a healthy environment where he or she is well fed, clothed, sheltered, respected, and loved, the child will continue to be well physically and mentally. An identical twin with the same heredity would not be as likely to develop into a well person if the twin were raised in an unhealthy environment. Many argue about which is more important, heredity or environment. One side believes that good heredity can overcome poor environment. The other side claims that good environment can rescue a child with poor heredity. It is clear, however, that both contribute to a person's development. Ways to control heredity are limited; however, environment can, to some extent, be controlled. The role of the home health aide is involved in improving environmental conditions for the client.

THE REMARKABLE BODY

Imagine how hard it would be if, each second of the day, you had to consciously perform every body function. Most people take their bodies for granted as long as everything seems to be in good working order. Think of all the activities constantly occurring and all of the things that could go wrong. Maintaining a state of wellness seems miraculous.

The human body is remarkable because it can continue to work when some of its parts break down. Damaged brain cells cannot be "repaired," but there are so many brain cells that new ones can be trained to take over. Many body structures are in "pairs." A body has two arms, two legs, two kidneys, two eyes. In the well body all of the parts work together.

What happens when one of a pair becomes diseased? In the case of kidneys, one can be removed surgically and the other will take over the work. The person with only one kidney must be more careful with diet and generally take more health precautions than the average person, yet a person can return to a state of wellness with even one kidney. The human body and mind are able to adapt. The home health aide's efforts are important in helping a client adapt physically, mentally, and emotionally. Human beings have often been compared to machines. When functioning perfectly, the body operates as smoothly as a well-oiled machine. The human body, however, is much more efficient than any machine. Unlike a machine, the human body often can repair itself, for example, new skin can grow over a wound. When the body functions at its peak efficiency with all of its parts working like a finely tuned engine, it is in a state of wellness.

The body is a complex organism. It is made up of millions of cells, which are the smallest structural units of the body. Many cells make up a tissue and tissues make up organs (Figure 10-1).

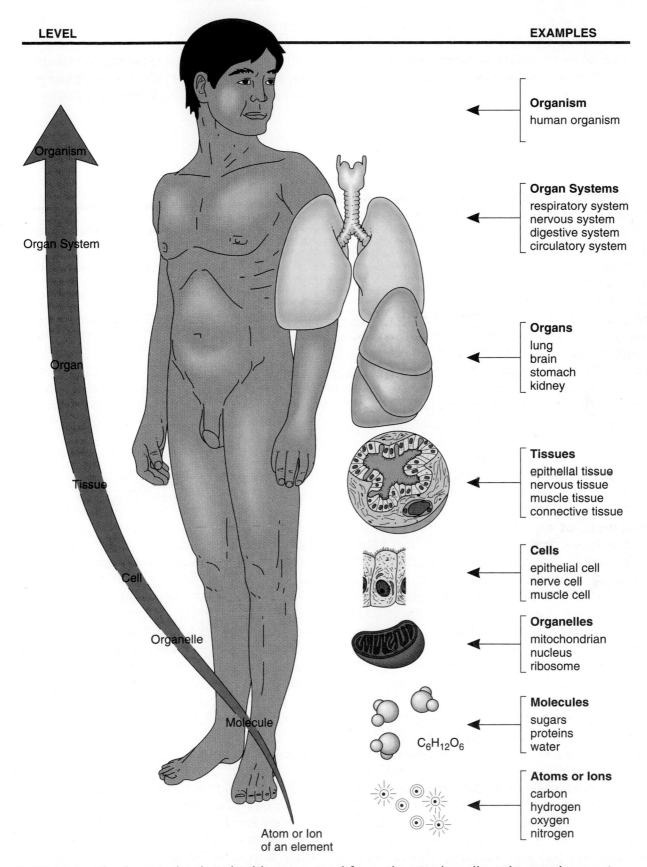

LEVEL

Organism

Organ System

Organ

Tissue

Cell

Organelle

Molecule

Atom or Ion
of an element

EXAMPLES

Organism
human organism

Organ Systems
respiratory system
nervous system
digestive system
circulatory system

Organs
lung
brain
stomach
kidney

Tissues
epithellal tissue
nervous tissue
muscle tissue
connective tissue

Cells
epithelial cell
nerve cell
muscle cell

Organelles
mitochondrian
nucleus
ribosome

Molecules
sugars
proteins
water

$C_6H_{12}O_6$

Atoms or Ions
carbon
hydrogen
oxygen
nitrogen

FIGURE 10-1   The human body is highly organized from the single cell to the total organism.

Organs act together in making the total body function. All of these separate units interact within the body in systems. There are nine body systems, each one performing a necessary function in the body (Figure 10-2).

INTERNAL HEALTH

Wellness is the normal state of the human body. Illness occurs when the body machinery is not working properly. This may be caused by exter-

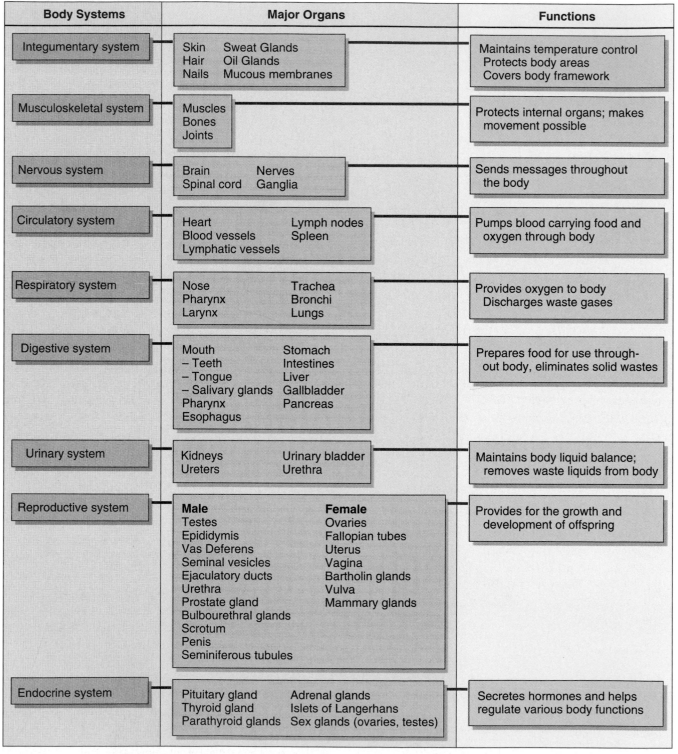

Body Systems	Major Organs	Functions
Integumentary system	Skin Sweat Glands Hair Oil Glands Nails Mucous membranes	Maintains temperature control Protects body areas Covers body framework
Musculoskeletal system	Muscles Bones Joints	Protects internal organs; makes movement possible
Nervous system	Brain Nerves Spinal cord Ganglia	Sends messages throughout the body
Circulatory system	Heart Lymph nodes Blood vessels Spleen Lymphatic vessels	Pumps blood carrying food and oxygen through body
Respiratory system	Nose Trachea Pharynx Bronchi Larynx Lungs	Provides oxygen to body Discharges waste gases
Digestive system	Mouth Stomach – Teeth Intestines – Tongue Liver – Salivary glands Gallbladder Pharynx Pancreas Esophagus	Prepares food for use throughout body, eliminates solid wastes
Urinary system	Kidneys Urinary bladder Ureters Urethra	Maintains body liquid balance; removes waste liquids from body
Reproductive system	**Male** **Female** Testes Ovaries Epididymis Fallopian tubes Vas Deferens Uterus Seminal vesicles Vagina Ejaculatory ducts Bartholin glands Urethra Vulva Prostate gland Mammary glands Bulbourethral glands Scrotum Penis Seminiferous tubules	Provides for the growth and development of offspring
Endocrine system	Pituitary gland Adrenal glands Thyroid gland Islets of Langerhans Parathyroid glands Sex glands (ovaries, testes)	Secretes hormones and helps regulate various body functions

FIGURE 10-2 The body systems and their major organs and functions

nal factors or it may result from an internal disorder (abnormality). Internal problems occur when some part of the body is not working correctly. Accidents and environmental hazards are examples of external causes of illness.

Some external environmental factors that may affect people's health are air and water. Particles or organisms present in the air and water can enter the body and cause illness. People who have asthma and lung disorders have great difficulty breathing when the air quality is poor. Coal miners may breathe in coal dust, which harms the lungs. These particles can seriously damage the respiratory system. Viruses are external organisms carried through the air in water droplets. When they enter the nose or mouth they can cause infectious diseases. Flu, the common cold, and measles are examples of virus infections.

Illnesses may be either acute or chronic. An **acute** illness is one that begins suddenly, usually is severe, and is usually followed by complete recovery. A **chronic** illness is one that continues to affect a person for a long period of time and from which recovery is incomplete or full recovery is unlikely.

Illness, an accidental injury, a birth defect, or the normal sensory losses of aging may be the cause of a disability. A disability may involve impaired mental or emotional functioning or involve an impaired body function, such as eyesight or ambulation (walking). The Americans with Disabilities Act (a national law protecting the rights of people with disabilities) defines a person with a **disability** as someone who:

- Has a physical or mental impairment that substantially limits one or more major life activities
- Has a record of such an impairment
- Is regarded as having such an impairment

Because the home health aide will be caring for clients who are ill or disabled or who are recovering from an illness, it is important for the aide to understand the basic principles and terms related to disorders and diseases and to their treatment.

Internal Disorders

Internal disorders may happen at any age. However, they are more likely to occur as the body grows older and becomes more prone to breaking down. Usually young people recover more quickly from accidents and diseases because their body tissues and cells repair and grow at a faster rate. It takes longer for recovery in older persons because the growth rate of new cells is slower. The circulatory system often becomes less efficient as people age. Heart disease, stroke, diabetes, and hypertension are major physical disorders of the aged.

Emotional Disorders

An internal disorder that can happen at any age is an emotional breakdown. Some mental disorders are so severe that the client must be hospitalized. Many times, a person who normally functions well suffers an emotional breakdown when external stress becomes too great. Depression is a normal response to illness. Illness, pain, and physical trauma put stress on the body and the person's emotions. On the other hand, physical care such as proper nutrition, exercise, companionship, and relief from pain can do much toward lifting depression and relieving mental stress. The aide must recognize that mentally ill clients, young or old, need just as much care and consideration as the ones with heart conditions or other physical disorders.

Emotional and physical health depend on one another. Emotional illness may sometimes cause a physical illness. For example, a client who believes that there is poison in the food will refuse to eat. This can lead to severe malnutrition. Physical illness can bring on emotional problems, too. Some clients seem more able to cope with illness than others. A person who is ill or suffering from a disability caused by an accident, illness, or aging has to cope with an increase in physical and emotional pain as well as many losses. The individual who is ill experiences a decrease in physical and emotional energy, an increase in physical discomfort, and perhaps chronic pain. Medications may cause drowsiness or confusion. The ability to make decisions for oneself may be impaired. A person who is disabled or ill may experience many changes and losses that have to do with their jobs and other important roles they have with their family and in their community. Sometimes, adjusting to these changes and losses can be difficult.

Family members who have counted on the individual to perform certain tasks at home, or play a certain role in their lives will have a hard time adjusting to the new needs of the person who is ill or injured. A daughter who is used to looking toward her father as a pillar of strength now has to be the strong one. A son who depends on his mother to nurture and take care of him may need to learn how to take care of her. This shift in roles can bring out the best in people as they experience a new ability of their own, but the stress can bring out anger, fear, and tension, too. A home health aide must be able to recognize and deal with the emotional and psychological effects of an illness on both the client and the client's family. See Unit 11 for a detailed discussion on mental health.

OBSERVING SIGNS AND SYMPTOMS

In later chapters, individual medical conditions are discussed. For each condition, the home health aide will be told the signs and symptoms that may arise during the illness. The aide must be able to recognize, record, and report significant signs and symptoms. A **sign** is a change that can be observed or measured. Signs of emotional stress might include wringing of the hands and unusual or sudden changes in behavior. Signs of a physical change include changes in the client's appearance. For example, the client may become flushed, turn pale, break into a heavy sweat, or turn blue (cyanotic). With experience, the home health aide learns which signs should be reported to the supervisor. Irregular eating patterns, swelling of lower limbs (edema), and a deep yellow complexion (jaundice) are also physical signs that may be observed. **CAUTION:** Medical signs that should be reported at once are bleeding, vomiting, unusual coldness, flushing and heavy perspiration, loss of consciousness, or severe shortness of breath.

A home health aide also should be alert to the client's symptoms. **Symptoms** are changes that cannot be observed but are experienced by the client. Examples of symptoms are pain and discomfort. A pain can be described as dull or sharp. It may be localized (in one area) or generalized (all over). The aide should have the client describe how the pain feels so that the pain can be reported accurately to the supervisor. As a home health aide becomes more familiar with a client, the aide can better observe signs of stress and recognize symptoms. After the aide has seen the normal reactions of the client, deviations (change), which could be serious, can be recognized.

VITAL SIGNS

Vital signs are signs obtained by use of an instrument; they indicate the status of a person's life functions. They include temperature, pulse, respiratory rate, and blood pressure. Vital signs must be measured accurately and regularly. Changes outside the normal range must be reported to the supervisor. The home health aide will be given exact instructions as to when to take these measurements for each assigned client.

Temperature

The difference between the heat produced and the heat lost is the body temperature. Temperature is measured with a thermometer. An oral thermometer is used to take oral and axillary temperatures. When the temperature must be taken in the rectum, a rectal thermometer with a rounded end is used. Today the glass thermometer is often replaced with a digital thermometer. Figure 10-3 shows the normal body temperatures taken by various methods. Refer to Procedures 7, 8, and 9 for the proper ways to take temperatures. Each home health aide must be able to take and record a temperature accurately.

FIGURE 10-3 Temperature variations in the same person			
	Oral	**Axillary**	**Rectal**
Average Temperature	98.6°F	97.6°F	99.6°F
Range	97.6–99.6°F (36.5–37.5°C)	96.6–98.6°F (36–37°C)	98.6–100.6°F (37–38.1°C)

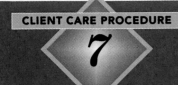

Taking an Oral Temperature

PURPOSE

- To measure the client's body temperature in the most appropriate way
- To routinely check the temperature to note any significant change

NOTE: Using an oral thermometer is the most convenient way to obtain a person's temperature. However, it is not the most accurate method. If the client has taken a cold or hot drink within 15 to 20 minutes, the temperature of the mouth changes. In addition to accuracy, the aide must consider safety because it is possible that the thermometer might break in the client's mouth. [CAUTION: The oral thermometer can be used only when the client is able to hold it in the mouth properly. If for any reason the client cannot keep the thermometer in the mouth, call the supervisor for instructions.] In some of these cases, a rectal temperature may need to be taken with a rectal thermometer.

PROCEDURE

1. Ask the client not to drink any liquids or to smoke 15 minutes before the temperature is taken. Otherwise an inaccurate reading could result.
2. Gather the equipment needed:
   disposable gloves
   oral thermometer (Figures 10-4A and B)
   tissues
   pad and pencil
   watch with second hand
   alcohol
3. Wash your hands thoroughly and put on gloves.
4. Ask the client to find a comfortable position, either in a chair or in a bed.
5. Hold thermometer by stem end and read mercury column. It should register 96°F or lower (35.5°C). If it does not, shake down the thermometer with a snap of the wrist (Figure 10-5). Shake the thermometer down until it reads 94°F (34.4°C).

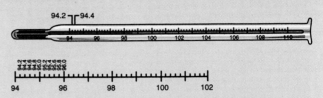

FIGURE 10-4A Glass thermometer for oral use

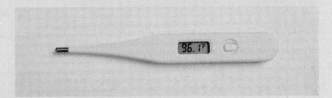

FIGURE 10-4B Inexpensive digital thermometer may be used instead of a glass thermometer.

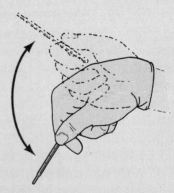

FIGURE 10-5 Shake mercury down in column by holding thermometer by the stem and snapping the wrist. Check the reading. Repeat until the reading is below 96° Fahrenheit.

6. Insert bulb end of thermometer under client's tongue (Figure 10-6). Slant it toward the side of the mouth. Ask the client to close the mouth and keep the thermometer under the tongue.
7. Be sure the client holds the thermometer under the tongue for a minimum of 3 minutes and then remove the thermometer.

(continues)

CLIENT CARE PROCEDURE **7 Taking an Oral Temperature** *(continued)*

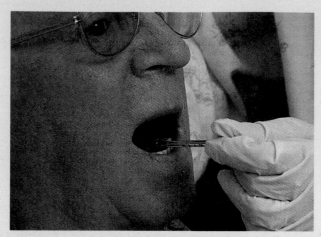

FIGURE 10-6 The bulb end of the thermometer is inserted under the tongue, left 3 minutes, then removed.

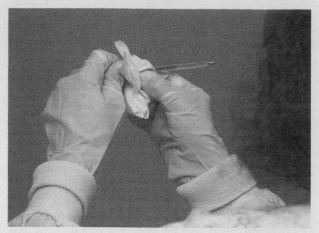

FIGURE 10-7 Wipe thermometer after removing it from client's mouth.

8. Gently wipe the thermometer with a tissue from the stem to the bulb end (Figure 10-7). Discard the contaminated tissue. If using a thermometer cover, discard it.

9. Hold the thermometer at eye level (Figure 10-8) and record the measurement. Normal oral temperature is 98.6°F (37°C). Mark down the time the reading was made and the temperature reading. Report any temperature that reads above 101°F (38°C).

10. Clean the thermometer by washing it with a small amount of mild soap and cold water. Rinse all soap from the thermometer. A tissue wet with alcohol also may be used to clean the thermometer. Wipe from stem end to the front, bulb end (clean to dirty).

11. The client may have an electronic thermometer. These thermometers emit a beeping sound when the temperature has been obtained, and give a digital readout (see Figure 10-4B).

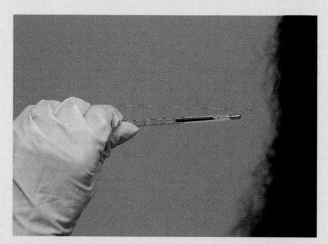

FIGURE 10-8 Hold the thermometer at eye level. Locate the column of mercury and read closest line.

12. Return thermometer to the proper storage place.

13. Remove gloves and wash your hands after the procedure.

Pulse and Respiratory Rates

Two other vital signs that a home health aide is required to take and record are the pulse and respiratory rates. These two readings are usually taken one after the other. After taking the pulse, the client's arm is held in the same position and the respirations are counted. It is better if the client does not realize that respirations are being counted. The results are more accurate if the client thinks that only the pulse rate is being checked.

CLIENT CARE PROCEDURE

8

Taking a Rectal Temperature

PURPOSE

- To obtain the most accurate measure of the client's temperature
- To obtain the temperature of a person who cannot hold an oral thermometer in the mouth
- To routinely check the temperature to note any significant change

NOTE: A rectal temperature is sometimes taken instead of an oral temperature. At times this is done because the rectal temperature is more accurate. If a person breathes through the mouth or uses oxygen, an oral temperature would not give an accurate reading. Drinking fluids or smoking before a reading also alters it. In these situations clients must have rectal temperatures taken. A rectal temperature is necessary for those who cannot hold a thermometer in the mouth—infants, small children, and adults who are seriously ill, mentally confused, unconscious, or those who cannot hold a thermometer properly. In addition, rectal temperatures are taken for any person with a history of convulsions. Do not take a rectal temperature if the client has hemorrhoids or surgery in the rectal area.

The rectal thermometer is shaped differently from the oral thermometer. The bulb end of the rectal thermometer is thicker and more rounded. This shape adds to the safety and comfort of the client. The normal rectal temperature (99.6°F) is 1° higher than the normal oral temperature (98.6°F).

PROCEDURE

1. Gather the equipment needed:
   disposable gloves
   rectal thermometer
   lubricant
   tissues
   pad and pencil
   watch with second hand
   alcohol

2. Wash your hands thoroughly and apply gloves.
3. Tell the client that you plan to take a rectal temperature. Provide for privacy. Do not expose the client unnecessarily.
4. Shake down the thermometer to 96°F (35.5°C).
5. Position client on left side, Sims' position. Cover the client with a sheet or blanket and remove the client's clothing from the rectal area of the body.
6. Lubricate the bulb tip of the thermometer with water-soluble jelly on a tissue. This makes insertion easier and more comfortable for the client.
7. Fold back the sheet or blanket to expose the client's buttocks. Raise top buttock with your hand and, with the other hand, gently insert bulb end of thermometer into the client's rectum about 1 to 1½ inches (Figure 10-9).
8. Redrape the client and hold the thermometer in place for 3 to 5 minutes. **CAUTION:** Do not let go of the rectal thermometer.

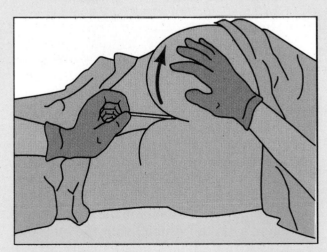

FIGURE 10-9 The rectal thermometer is lubricated and then inserted 1½ inches into the rectum.

(continues)

CLIENT CARE PROCEDURE **8** **Taking a Rectal Temperature** (continued)

9. Remove the thermometer; wipe it from stem to bulb end (clean to dirty) with a tissue wet with alcohol.
10. Discard contaminated tissue.
11. Read the thermometer and record the temperature. Record the time, and place the letter *R* (rectal) beside the temperature reading.

12. Return the client to a comfortable position.
13. Clean the thermometer using soap and cold water or alcohol. Rinse it thoroughly. Store properly.
14. Remove gloves and wash your hands thoroughly after the procedure.

CLIENT CARE PROCEDURE

9

Taking an Axillary Temperature

PURPOSE

* To obtain the client's temperature reading when a rectal or oral reading is not possible

NOTE: The axillary temperature is not the most accurate method of taking a temperature. However, it may be ordered by the nurse supervisor when an oral reading is not possible. Taking an axillary temperature is more convenient than taking a rectal temperature and is less embarrassing for the client. An axillary temperature is usually 0.5° to 1.0°F (0.28° to 0.56°C) lower than an oral temperature.

PROCEDURE

1. Wash your hands before beginning the procedure.
2. Rinse the thermometer in cold water and wipe it dry with a tissue to clean it.
3. Shake down the thermometer so the mercury is below 96°F (35.6°C).
4. Provide privacy. Remove clothing from shoulder and arm. Dry the client's armpit with a tissue.
5. Place the thermometer in the center of the client's axilla (armpit) with the bulb end toward the client's head (Figure 10-10). This position rests the bulb end against the blood vessel and a more accurate reading can be obtained.
6. Position the client's arm closer to the body and place the client's forearm over

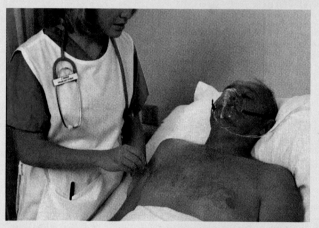
FIGURE 10-10 To take an axillary temperature, place glass thermometer in center of the client's axilla.

the client's chest. This position enables the arm to hold the thermometer in place.
7. Leave the thermometer in place for 10 minutes.
8. Remove the thermometer and wipe it clean of any perspiration.
9. Read the temperature indicated on the thermometer. (A normal axillary temperature is 97.6°F.)
10. Record the temperature. An axillary temperature is recorded with an *Ax* (axillary) beside the number, e.g., 97.6°F Ax.
11. Shake down the thermometer, clean it, and return it to its proper place.
12. Wash your hands following the procedure.

Pulse. The **pulse** is the force of the blood pushing against the artery walls. Movement of the blood through the arteries is initiated by the heart's contraction. Thus, the pulse rate should be the same as the heart rate. The pulse may be felt at any of the sites shown in Figure 10-11. The most common site for checking the pulse is the radial artery, which can be felt inside the wrist on the thumb side (Figure 10-12). Procedure 10 demonstrates how to take a radial and apical pulse.

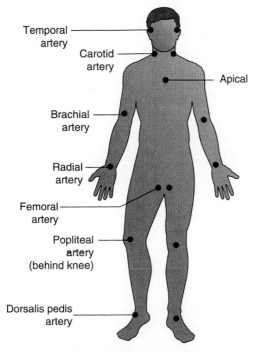

FIGURE 10-11 The pulse may be taken at any of the places shown.

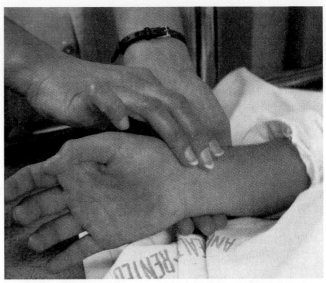

FIGURE 10-12 Position for taking client's pulse

Respiration. **Respiration** is the sum total of processes that exchange oxygen and carbon dioxide in the body. However, respiration is most commonly known as breathing. The act of inhaling and exhaling once is counted as one respiration. Difficult or labored breathing is called **dyspnea.** Sometimes respirations stop for a few moments. This absence of breathing is called **apnea.** The bubbling sound may be heard when fluid or mucus gets caught in the air passages. This condition is called **rales,** and can often be heard in clients with pneumonia or emphysema. The normal rate of respirations for adults is 16 to 20 per minute. In adults, respiration rates of 25 or more are called accelerated.

CLIENT CARE PROCEDURE

10

Taking the Radial and Apical Pulse

PURPOSE

- To measure, record, and observe the character and rate of the client's pulse
- To report changes to the supervisor, nurse, or doctor

NOTE: A pulse is taken to determine its regularity, strength, and rate. Regularity is de-scribed as either regular or irregular. An irregular pulse may indicate skipped heartbeats or changing rhythm patterns. An irregular pulse should always be reported.

Strength is described as bounding, strong, weak, or thready. If the strength has changed, the aide should call the supervisor.

(continues)

CLIENT CARE PROCEDURE **10** **Taking the Radial and Apical Pulse** *(continued)*

Pulse rate is described as the number of beats per minute. The age, size, and sex of the client may influence the rate. Normal ranges in pulse rates are:

60–100 adults
70–110 children over 6 years of age
80–120 children under 6 years of age
100–140 infants

PROCEDURE FOR DETERMINING PULSE RATE

1. Gather the equipment needed:
   wristwatch with a second hand
   notepad and pen or pencil
2. Wash your hands before beginning the procedure.
3. Tell the client that you are going to check the pulse rate. Ask the client to help by remaining quiet and still while you are counting.
4. Have the client sit in a comfortable chair or lie in bed with arms resting gently on the chest.
5. Place the tips of your first two fingers on the pulse site. The radial pulse on the inner wrist is most often used (Figure 10-13). **CAUTION:** Do not use your thumb to feel the client's artery. Using the thumb can result in an inaccurate reading.
6. Count the pulse beats for 1 full minute.
7. Record the pulse rate, regularity, and strength. Also record the time the pulse was taken. If irregular, take apical pulse for 1 minute and record apical pulse.

PROCEDURE FOR TAKING APICAL PULSE

1. Assemble equipment:
   stethoscope
   watch with second hand
2. Tell client what you plan to do.
3. Clean stethoscope earpieces and bell with disinfectant (Figure 10-14).
4. Place stethoscope earpieces in your ears.
5. Place the stethoscope diaphragm or bell over the apex of the client's heart, 2 to 3 inches to the left of the breastbone, below the left nipple.

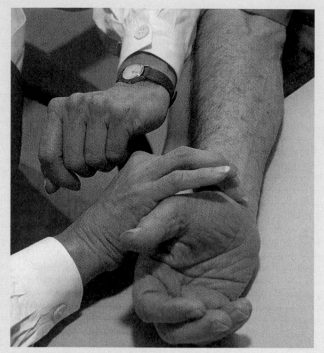

FIGURE 10-13 Locate the pulse on the thumb side of the wrist with the tips of your fingers.

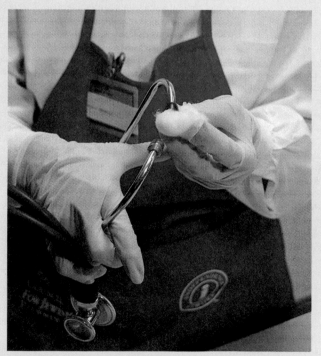

FIGURE 10-14 Carefully clean earpieces of the stethoscope before use.

(continues)

CLIENT CARE PROCEDURE **10** **Taking the Radial and Apical Pulse** *(continued)*

6. Listen carefully for the heartbeat. It will sound like "lub-dub."

7. Count the louder sound for 1 complete minute.

8. Check radial pulse for 1 minute. The best way to obtain these numbers is to have an aide count the apical pulse. Another aide may take the radial pulse at the same time the apical pulse is being counted (Figure 10-15).

9. Compare the results and note the numbers on a pad.

10. Clean earpieces and bell or diaphragm of stethoscope with alcohol wipe.

11. Document both pulse rates, i.e.:

　　Apical pulse = A 100 @ 10:00 AM
　　Radial pulse = R 92
　　Pulse deficit: 8 (100 – 92 = 8)

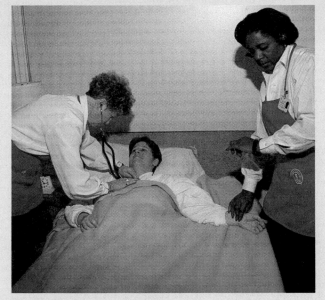

FIGURE 10-15 If another aide is present, it is better to take the apical and radial pulses at the same time.

FIGURE 10-16 Average pulse rates		
Adults	60–100	beats per minute
Children over 6	70–110	beats per minute
Children under 6	80–120	beats per minute
Infants	100–140	beats per minute

Pulse rates differ depending on age, sex, size and physical condition of the client (Figure 10-16). An extremely slow heartbeat is called **bradycardia.** An extremely rapid heartbeat is called **tachycardia.** A sudden change to either condition must be reported immediately to the supervisor. Pulse readings show the rate, rhythm, and volume of blood pulsing through the artery. Rate is the times per minute. Rhythm is the evenness or regularity of the beat. Volume is the fullness of the beat. An example of how a normal pulse would be recorded is 70 (rate), regular (rhythm), and full (volume). An abnormal pulse for an adult might be over 100 (rate), irregular (rhythm), and weak or thready (volume).

Weak respirations, which are characterized by only slight chest movements, are described as being shallow. Breathing characterized by many large breaths is described as being deep. **Cheyne-Stokes** is a term used to describe respirations that are very rapid and then stop and then start again. This type of breathing pattern occurs prior to the client's death. Procedure 11 demonstrates how to count respirations.

Blood Pressure. **Blood pressure** is measured in two parts—systolic and diastolic—by using an instrument called a **sphygmomanometer** (Figures 10-17A and B). Blood pressure is the amount of force the blood exerts against the walls of the arteries as it flows through them. It is expressed in numbers, with the higher number (**systolic**) representing the pressure while the heart is beating, and the lower number (**diastolic**) representing the pressure when the heart is resting between beats. The systolic number is always stated first and the diastolic second; for example: 134/72 (134 over 72); systolic = 134, diastolic = 72. Although this procedure requires concentration and demands accuracy, the home health aide should become familiar with the technique. Refer to Procedure 12.

Counting Respirations

PURPOSE

• To count the rate and observe the character of respirations

NOTE: Character of respirations is described as regular or irregular; labored, difficult, shallow, or deep; and noisy or quiet.

A normal respiratory rate for adults is 16 to 20 breaths per minute.

PROCEDURE

1. Gather equipment needed.
   wristwatch with a second hand
   notepad and pen or pencil
2. After client's pulse has been taken, leave the fingers in position on the wrist. By doing this, the client is not aware that you are counting respirations.
3. One rise and fall of the chest counts as one respiration. Count the number of respirations during a full 1-minute period.
4. Note how deeply the client breathes. Also check the regularity of the rhythm pattern. Note the sound of the breathing.
5. Record the number of respirations occurring in 1 minute. Record the character of the client's breathing.
6. Report changes from the client's usual way of breathing. Report any difficulty in breathing to the supervisor at once.
7. Wash your hands following the procedure.

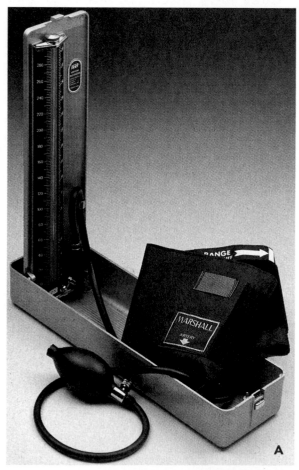

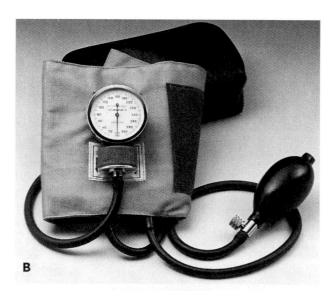

FIGURE 10-17 A. Aneroid sphygmomanometer   B. Mercury sphygmomanometer

12   Taking Blood Pressure

PURPOSE

- To take blood pressure correctly
- To accurately report blood pressure readings to the case manager, nurse, or doctor

NOTE: Blood pressure is taken by the use of a sphygmomanometer (an instrument with a cuff, rubber bulb, and dial gauge for recording pressure) and a stethoscope (a listening device that magnifies sound).

Two readings are recorded. The systolic pressure is recorded first. This is the pressure that is felt in the artery when the heart contracts. The diastolic pressure is recorded second. This is the pressure that is felt in the artery when the heart is in the relaxation stage. The systolic rate is always higher than the diastolic rate. Normal blood pressure for an adult is about 120/80, although it may vary depending on age, sex, emotional state, fitness, and weight.

The cuff should be the right size for the client's arm; otherwise an incorrect reading may be obtained. Cuffs come in various sizes: child, normal adult, and extra large. It is important to read the mercury at eye level; therefore, it is best to take the readings while you are sitting down, next to the client.

PROCEDURE

1. Gather equipment needed:
   sphygmomanometer
   stethoscope
   alcohol sponges or cotton balls
2. Wash your hands before beginning the procedure.
3. Explain to the client what you plan to do. Have the client sit or lie in a comfortable position with one arm extended at the same level as the heart. The palm should be upward. The arm should be in resting position. The arm should not be dangling by the hip because you may get an inaccurate reading. Locate brachial pulse.

4. Pick up the stethoscope. Wipe the earpieces. Place the stethoscope around your neck.
5. Pick up the cuff and wrap it securely around the client's arm, 1 inch above the elbow (Figure 10-18). The cuff must be placed at the level of the client's heart. Fasten. (Some cuffs have a Velcro fastener; others have hooks at the end of the cuff.) The center of the rubber bladder should be directly over the brachial artery. If the cuff is marked with an arrow, place cuff so that the arrow points over the brachial artery.
6. Attach the manometer (the dial gauge) to the top of the cuff so you can read it (Figure 10-19).
7. Tighten the small round valve that is located along the side of the rubber bulb. (This valve controls the pumping you will do later.)
8. With the tips of your fingers, locate the artery on the inside of the client's elbow

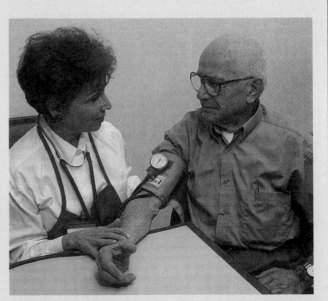

FIGURE 10-18   Apply cuff snugly to arm at least 1 inch above the elbow.

(continues)

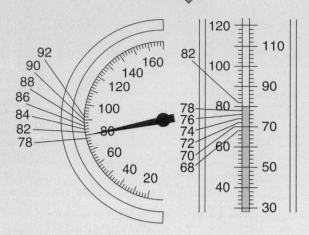

FIGURE 10-19 The aneroid gauge (left) and the mercury gravity gauge (right). Take a reading at the closest line.

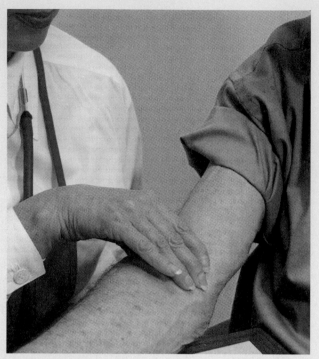

FIGURE 10-20 Locate and feel the brachial pulse.

(Figure 10-20). When you feel a throbbing beat, you have located the artery. Keep your fingers on the spot. Never use your thumb because it, too, has a pulse beat.

9. Place the round disk of the stethoscope over the artery you located on the client (using your fingers to hold it in place) (Figure 10-21). With your other hand, insert the earpieces in your ear.

10. Take the rubber bulb in your hand. Look at the dial gauge while you pump air into the cuff by squeezing the bulb. Pump until the reading on the dial gauge is about 180 to 200.

11. Listen with the stethoscope placed in your ears and the disk over the artery. You should not hear any sound.

12. While listening, slowly release the air by opening the valve located beside the bulb, using the thumb and forefinger, deflating the cuff at the rate of 2 to 3 mm Hg per second. (This will cause air to escape from the cuff and the reading on the manometer will drop.) You may have to tighten the bulb valve if the air escapes too fast.

13. Listen carefully. When the first sharp thump is heard, remember the number seen on the dial gauge. This is the systolic pressure.

14. Watch the dial continue to fall as the air escapes. When the last loud beat be-

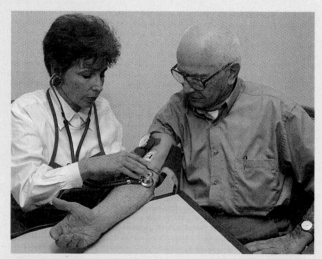

FIGURE 10-21 Place stethoscope diaphragm or bell right over the brachial artery.

comes a muffled sound, remember the number. This is the diastolic pressure.

15. Release the remainder of the air from the cuff and remove it, leaving the valve open.

16. Record the two readings (Figure 10-22). Blood pressure reading is written as a

(continues)

CLIENT CARE PROCEDURE **Taking Blood Pressure** *(continued)*

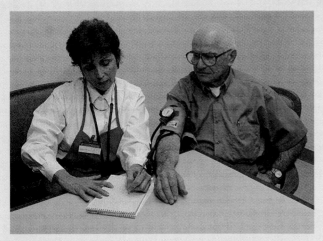

FIGURE 10-22   Record your reading right away. If repeat procedure is necessary, wait at least 1 minute.

fraction with the systolic (top) listed first and the diastolic (bottom) written under the line; for example,

$$\text{BP} \frac{120}{80} \quad \begin{array}{l}\text{(systolic pressure)}\\ \text{(diastolic pressure)}\end{array}$$

17. **CAUTION:** Be careful not to pump the pressure too high. Remember that the pressure of the cuff can cause the client discomfort, so it is important to release the air and work quickly when taking the blood pressure. If it is necessary to repeat the procedure, wait 1 or 2 minutes before inflating the cuff; this allows the circulation to return to normal.

18. If you are unsuccessful in obtaining a blood pressure reading after the first attempt, move to the client's other arm and try again, repeating the same procedure. (A second reading taken immediately, in the same arm, would probably be inaccurate and the client would become uncomfortable.) Never guess. If a blood pressure is hard to take or you are not sure, tell the nurse. Record reading.

19. Wash your hands following the procedure.

PRECAUTIONS

- If you are taking the blood pressure of a stroke client or a client who has had a mastectomy, use the unaffected arm only.
- If your client is having home dialysis (as part of a kidney treatment), or is receiving intravenous (IV) fluids, take the blood pressure on the unaffected arm.
- Do not inflate cuff unnecessarily high.

Unusually high blood pressure readings can be extremely dangerous and are often life threatening. Studies to date link obesity with hypertension (high blood pressure) as common physiologic problems. Careful attention must be given to this growing health condition. High blood pressure can lead to serious medical problems. Blood pressure varies with age, sex, race, altitude, muscular development, and the state of mind or tiredness. It is usually lower among women than men. It is also generally low in childhood, becoming higher with advancing age. African Americans and Native Americans have a greater incidence of high blood pressure than Caucasians. Refer to Figure 10-23 for blood pressure guidelines.

In some areas of the country, taking and recording blood pressure is considered to be too technical for the home health aide to perform. Other areas expect home health aides to be able to take and record blood pressure accurately. Home health aides should check with their particular agencies to determine if they are permitted or expected to obtain blood pressure readings.

Height and Weight.   Occasionally it is necessary to obtain a client's height. You will need a tape measure to do this. You have the client stand to do it. Be sure the client is standing as straight as possible and that the client is not wearing shoes. Another task that may need to be done monthly, weekly, or daily is weighing a client. Refer to Procedure 13.

FIGURE 10-23 Blood pressure guidelines

Category	Systolic (mm Hg)	Diastolic (mm Hg)
Normal	<130	<85
High normal	130–139	85–89
Hypertension		
STAGE 1 (Mild)	140–159	90–99
STAGE 2 (Moderate)	160–179	100–109
STAGE 3 (Severe)	180–209	110–119
STAGE 4 (Very Severe)	≥210	≥120

(Courtesy of National Heart, Lung, and Blood Institute, NIH Publication No. 93-1088, January 1993.)

CLIENT CARE PROCEDURE

13

Measuring Weight and Height

PURPOSE

- To determine if unusual weight gain or loss has occurred
- To routinely check height

NOTE: Weight changes can make a difference in medical prescriptions and should be reported to the case manager. For instance, some medication amounts are determined by the weight of a client and a sudden or gross weight loss would require a lesser dosage.

PROCEDURE FOR WEIGHT

If the client is bedbound and cannot stand to be weighed, the case manager can bring a chair scale into the house. If the client is mobile, weight can be checked daily or weekly on a bathroom scale (Figure 10-24). Guidelines to follow:

1. Client should be weighed at the same time of day.
2. Client should be wearing the same amount of clothing each time.
3. Scale should be checked to see if it is balanced correctly.
4. Record and document weight.

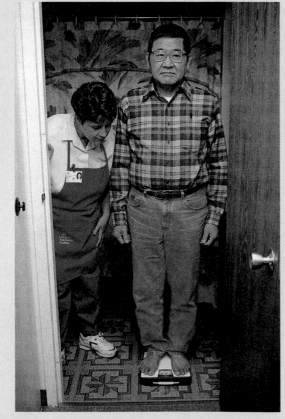

FIGURE 10-24 Weighing client using a portable bathroom scale

(continues)

CLIENT CARE PROCEDURE **Measuring Weight and Height** *(continued)*

NOTE: Height is not a common measurement for the elderly. As individuals age, there is some "settling" and a loss of height of perhaps an inch or two. If you need to take the height of an immobile client, you need a tape measure and a pad and pencil.

PROCEDURE FOR HEIGHT

1. Have client positioned in bed flat on his back with arms and legs straight.
2. Make a small pencil mark at the top of the client's head on the sheet.
3. Make a second pencil mark even with the bottom of the heels.
4. Using the tape measure, measure the distance between the two marks.
5. Record the height on the paper and record in client's record.
6. If client can stand, have the client stand with his back to the wall. Mark the wall with a small pencil mark on top of client's head. Client should not wear shoes.
7. Measure from floor to small pencil mark with tape measure.
8. Record on paper and then on client's chart.

ASSISTING WITH MEDICATIONS ··········

Some clients will need medications prescribed by doctors to relieve pain and other symptoms, to help the body fight infections, and to treat diseases. Although home health aides do not give medications, they can remind clients when to take the prescribed medication and assist clients in checking to see if the dosage and amount of medicine are correct. In some instances clients may also take over-the-counter medications. It is a good idea to report to your nurse supervisor what over-the-counter medications your client is taking. Procedure 14 describes how to assist the client with self-administered medications.

CLIENT CARE PROCEDURE
14
Assisting the Client with Self-Administered Medications

PURPOSE

- To relieve pain and other symptoms, to help the body fight infections, and to treat diseases
- To encourage the client to take the prescribed medication at the right time, in the right dose, in the right amount, and in the right manner
- The following information should be made available to you by your nurse supervisor and clearly written down:
  —Name of each medicine
  —What each medication is for
  —Description of medicine—color, form
  —What time(s) of day or night when each medicine is to be taken
  —How long the medicine should be taken
  —Whether the medicine should be taken with food or other liquid
  —Possible side effects
- The home health aide should be aware of common reactions to medications so the nurse supervisor can be called if symptoms appear.

NOTE: The aide must take special care in assisting blind clients with their medications. Be sure that medications are coded so that the

(continues)

CLIENT CARE PROCEDURE **Assisting the Client with Self-Administered Medications** (*continued*)

client can find the correct bottles when they are needed. Medications for the blind client must be kept in exactly the same spot so that an error will not be made. Special arrangements should be made by the pharmacist or nurse supervisor in setting up the coding.

PROCEDURE

1. Have the nurse supervisor or pharmacist prepare a list of medications prescribed and the time they are to be given. Some medications are given 3 times a day (tid), usually before (ac) or after (pc) each meal. Others may be ordered 4 times a day (qid) or every 6 hours (q6h). A medication taken every 6 hours could be given at 6 AM, noon, 6 PM, and midnight. The pharmacist usually informs the client at which times the medications should be taken.

2. The nurse supervisor will set a schedule to be followed daily. After each medication has been taken, check it off. This informs both the aide and the client that the medicine has been taken. Refer to the schedule and remind the client when medicine is due. Your nurse supervisor may prepare your client's medication in special containers that have all the medication needed for a specific time (Figure 10-25).

3. Check with the client each time to make sure the medicine is the correct one listed on the schedule.

4. Make sure the correct method of taking the medication is followed. For example, some medicines are taken with juice or milk instead of water. Others are taken on an empty stomach, still others with food.

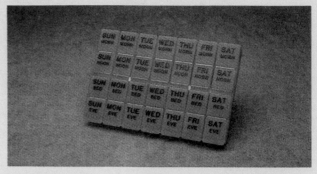

FIGURE 10-25 Special medication container

5. Certain medications such as nitroglycerin tablets must be within the client's reach at all times. When the client has chest pain, the client needs to place these tablets under the tongue immediately.

6. Be sure sleeping and pain medication bottles are kept in a safe place after each use. They should only be taken as often as the doctor has ordered.

7. Review the times with the client when the prescribed medicines are to be taken. Leave the medication within easy reach of the client. Remind the client to take the nighttime dose in a well-lit room.

8. If the client has questions about the medications, encourage the client to ask the pharmacist, nurse supervisor, or doctor. The client should be knowledgeable about medications that he or she is taking.

9. As a home health aide, you are not allowed to pour the client's medication from the bottle; the client needs to do this himself/herself.

CONSCIOUS AND UNCONSCIOUS CLIENTS

In most cases, a home health aide will be assigned to care for clients who are conscious. Consciousness is the normal state of awareness. Conscious people are responsive and know who and where they are. Normal consciousness varies in intensity throughout the day.

Have you had the experience of going to look for an item only to forget what it was when you got into the room? Have you ever been talking to someone and at some point lost the purpose of the conversation? These examples show that different levels of consciousness exist. While doing routine work, thoughts may wander and daydreaming may occur. At other times, a person may be extremely aware and sensitive of surroundings and events.

Just as there are varying levels of awareness or consciousness, there are different levels of unconsciousness (Figure 10-26). Sleep is a temporary state of unconsciousness. Other types of unconsciousness are due to a body malfunction or an injury. Fainting is an example of a temporary loss of consciousness. The blood supply to the brain is decreased; the person feels dizzy and may black out. When the head is lowered, the blood rushes back to the brain and the faintness disappears.

The deeply unconscious client is totally helpless and the home health aide must follow a supervisor's instructions carefully. The client's bed should be comfortable and kept clean and dry. The client should also be given frequent mouth care. Two of the greatest potential problems for an unconscious client are pressure sores and contractures. **Contracture** is the abnormal shortening of muscle tissue. When contractures occur, the muscles become inelastic and fixed. The hands may curl into tight fists and become locked into that position. The arms and legs also become stiff. In some cases, the entire body curls into the fetal position. Exercising the client's limbs can help prevent contractures. Exercises done to prevent contractures and the loss of motion in the joints are called **range of motion exercises.** Refer to Procedure 15.

An unconscious client must have special care. Figure 10-33 indicates the special needs of the unconscious client and how to meet those needs.

FIGURE 10-26 Levels of unconsciousness

Level	Physical Signs and Client Reactions
Somnolence	Client can answer questions but is confused and fades in and out of sleep.
Stupor	Client is restless and can only be aroused by continuous stimulation. Must be protected from falling out of bed. Responds to bright lights, loud sounds, and can locate painful site.
Semicoma	Client can only be aroused with difficulty. May groan or mutter, reacts to painful stimuli (when pinched or stuck with needle). Usually loses control of bowel and bladder (is incontinent).
Coma	Responds only to painful stimuli, if at all. In a deep coma, all responses are lost. Must be turned and repositioned or will remain in one position. Client is incontinent.

CLIENT CARE PROCEDURE

15 Performing Passive Range of Motion Exercises

PURPOSE

- To increase muscle tone and strength in the client's body
- To restore function to injured parts of body
- To prevent joint stiffness and contractures

NOTE: Do not perform the exercises until you have received instructions specific for your client's joints. When possible, support the extremity above and below the joints being exercised. If the client shows pain or discomfort, stop the exercise and document it. The head can be exercised if specifically ordered by the physical therapist. Exercises can be done in

(continues)

CLIENT CARE PROCEDURE ⟨15⟩ **Performing Passive Range of Motion Exercises** *(continued)*

bed or in the chair. It is important to keep the client covered or clothed to prevent unnecessary exposure during the procedure.

PROCEDURE

1. Wash your hands.
2. Read any special instructions for these exercises for your client.
3. Tell client what you plan to do. Ask client to assist as much as possible.
4. Exercise the shoulder.
   Supporting the upper and lower arms, exercise the shoulder joint. Abduct (away from the body) the entire arm out at right angles to the body (Figure 10-27A) and then adduct (bring back to the midline of the body) the arm back to the center of the client's body (Figure 10-27B).
5. Exercise the elbow.
   Bend elbow, keeping the arm close to the body. Bring the fingers to touch the

shoulder. Lower the fingers to touch the bed (Figures 10-28A and B).
6. Exercise the forearm.
   Bring the arm out to the side. Rest it on the bed. Take the client's hand and rotate the arm, palm up and palm down (Figures 10-29A and B).
7. Exercise the wrist and fingers.
   Take the client's hand and move the hand forward and back (Figures 10-30A and B). Move the hand side to side. Curl the client's fingers and straighten them (Figures 10-30C and D). Spread the fingers apart and rotate the thumb. Touch all fingers to thumb (Figure 10-30E).
8. Exercise the knee and hip while the client is lying on the back.
   Bend the knee and raise it to the chest (Figure 10-31). Bring the leg out to the side and back. Cross one leg over the other leg. Allow the leg to rest on the bed with the

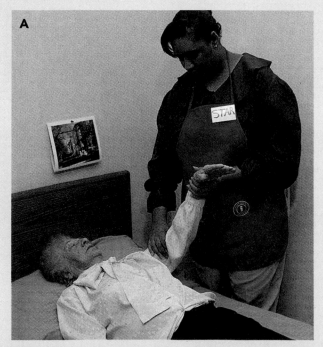

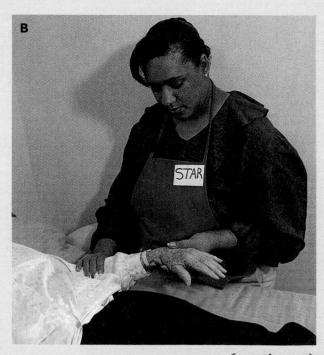

FIGURE 10-27 Exercising the shoulder joint

(continues)

15 Performing Passive Range of Motion Exercises *(continued)*

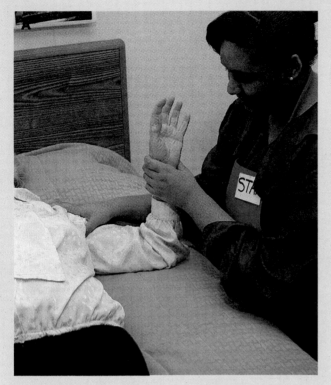
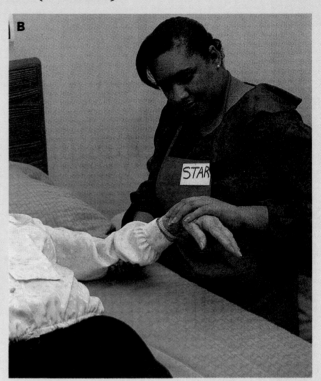

FIGURE 10-28   Exercising the elbow

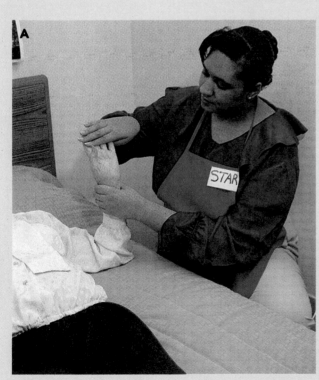
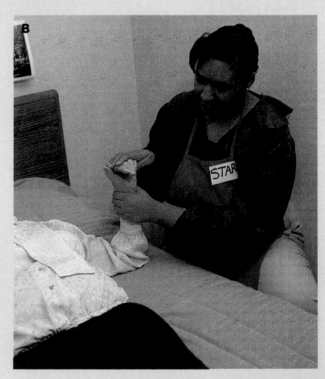

FIGURE 10-29   Exercising the forearm   *(continues)*

CLIENT CARE PROCEDURE **15** **Performing Passive Range of Motion Exercises** *(continued)*

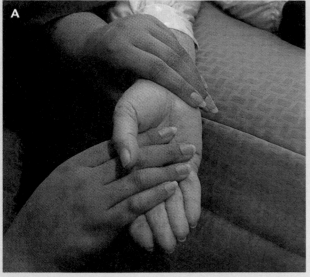

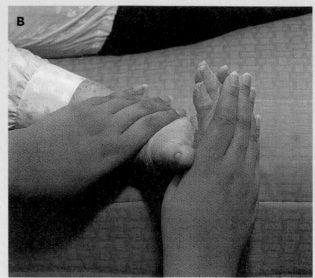

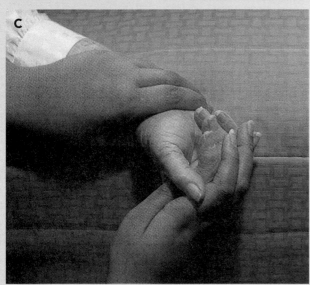

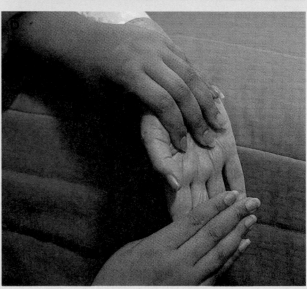

FIGURE 10-30 Exercising the wrist and fingers

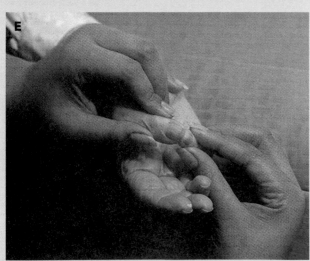

(continues)

CLIENT CARE PROCEDURE **Performing Passive Range of Motion Exercises** *(continued)*

knee straight and the heel resting on the bed. Rotate the leg inward and outward.

9. Exercise the ankle.
   Bend client's knee slightly and support lower leg with one hand. With other hand, bend client's foot downward (plantar flexion) and then bend client's foot toward client's body (dorsiflexion) (Figures 10-32A and B). With client's legs extended on bed, place both hands on client's foot and move foot inward and then outward.

10. Exercise the toes.
    Bend (flexion) and straighten (extension) each toe. Do abduction and adduction with each toe as you did with the fingers.

11. Go to other side and repeat movements for each joint.

12. Wash hands.

13. Document the completion of the exercises and client's reactions.

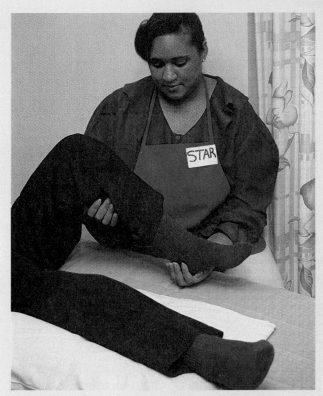

FIGURE 10-31 Exercising the knee and hip

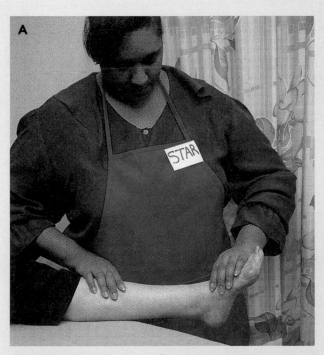

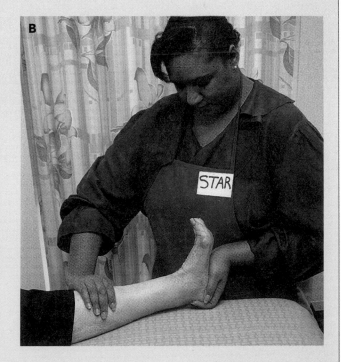

FIGURE 10-32 Exercising the ankle and foot

FIGURE 10-33 Meeting the special needs of the unconscious client

Care Required	Frequency	What to Do
Mouth care	Every 2 hours	Wipe tongue, lips, gums, and teeth with gauze pad or cotton swab moistened with water or mouthwash. Lubricate and moisten mouth tissues with glycerin or vegetable oil. Wipe away saliva as it dribbles from the mouth.
	When client vomits	Turn client to side at first sign of vomiting. Catch vomitus in a bowl or basin held to the side of the mouth. Wipe mouth with gauze pads or clean damp cloth.
Eye care	Wipe clean in AM and PM	Cover eyelids with soft cloth moistened in water. (Prevents eye cavity from becoming dry because eyes may not close or blink.)
Repositioning	At least every 2 hours	Turn from back to side, and side to front, etc. (This prevents pressure sores from forming.)
Range of motion (ROM) exercises	As ordered by doctor	Exercise all client's body parts if permitted. (Keeps blood circulating, prevents contractures, and prevents loss of motion in joints.)
Body massage with lotion	At least daily	Rub skin firmly but gently. Rub in a circular motion around bony prominences.
Care of bowel and bladder drainage	At least every hour	Check perineal area and bed linens to see if they are clean and dry. If client has not voided for 8 hours, report it to the supervisor. If client has not had bowel movement for 2 days, report it to the supervisor.
Accident prevention	At all times	Put up guardrails or place chairs beside bed to prevent falls. Observe for signs of vomiting and keep saliva wiped away; client may choke or inhale fluids into the lungs. Keep blankets and pillows away from the client's nose and mouth to avoid smothering.
Easy access to client	At all times	Safety and ease of working with client. Place the bed away from the wall so both sides of the bed are accessible.
Room ventilation	Open windows or vent daily	Keep temperature between 66–70°, keep drafts from client. Open windows or vents to circulate air.
Tender loving care (TLC)	At all times	Talk to the client as if the client were conscious. Client may be able to hear and understand. (Communication gives client link with reality.) Use gentle touch often; if time allows, hold the client's hands and run fingers across forehead.

NEED FOR REHABILITATION ....

Part of the care plan for a client may include **rehabilitation,** which is the restoring of physical abilities to the highest level possible. Most rehabilitation is planned and carried out by a specialist such as the physical or occupational therapist. When physical ability or skill has been lost, the client must relearn it or adjust to coping without it. A blind client must be taught self-feeding and learn how to become more independent. A stroke victim must learn again to use parts of the body that may be paralyzed. Range of motion exercises, speech therapy, and other kinds of rehabilitation may be needed. In some cases the home health aide will be able to assist in the rehabilitation program.

The home health aide may be expected to assist a client with walking. A physical therapist will determine when the client is ready to begin walking again and what types of assistive devices may be necessary to maintain the client's safety. Procedure 16 demonstrates how to assist the client to walk with crutches, a walker, or a cane.

CLIENT CARE PROCEDURE

16

Assisting the Client to Walk with Crutches, Walker, or Cane

PURPOSE

- To provide support and maintain balance as client walks

NOTE: There are three basic walking patterns: nonweight-bearing, partial weight-bearing, and weight-bearing. With a nonweight-bearing pattern, all the weight is placed on the arms and uninvolved leg. A partial weight-bearing pattern means that minimal weight is placed on the toes. However, most weight is still on the arms and the uninvolved leg.

To walk in a nonweight-bearing pattern the client uses crutches (Figure 10-34). The physical therapist measures the client to select the correct length of crutches. The therapist also teaches the client how to walk with the crutches.

To walk in a partial weight-bearing pattern, the client can use crutches but often uses a walker. The walker is a curved metal frame with four legs. It is a walking aid that gives maximum stability as the client moves. The client steps forward while holding onto the walker with both hands. Some walkers have wheels so that the client does not have to lift up the walker between steps (Figure 10-35).

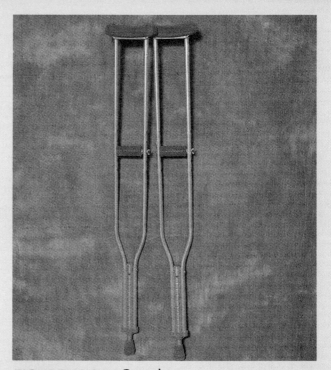

FIGURE 10-34 Crutches

A cane is used when the client is strong enough to bear full weight on both legs. A standard cane should not be used as a weight-bearing aid. A special cane with four ***(continues)***

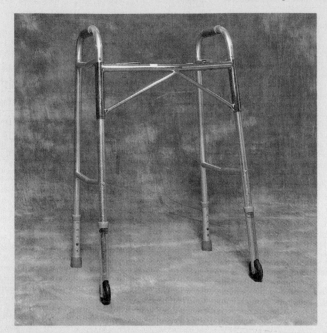

FIGURE 10-35 Walker with small wheels

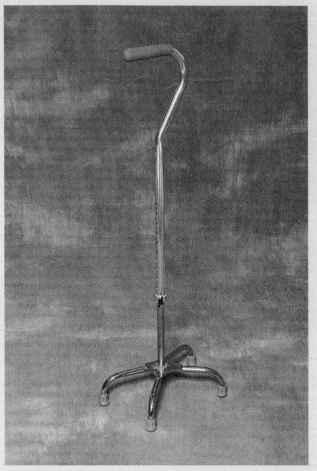

FIGURE 10-36 Four-point (quad) cane

short legs, called a quad cane, is designed to bear a small amount of weight only (Figure 10-36). A cane is primarily used for balance. Check rubber tips on the canes, walkers, and crutches because they wear out quickly if used on sidewalks.

Always have client wear good supportive shoes with nonskid soles. Instruct clients to pick up their feet and not to look at their feet, but to look straight ahead.

PROCEDURE

1. Wash your hands. Apply transfer belt unless instructed not to.
2. Always walk on the client's weak side.
3. Walk slightly behind the client holding onto the transfer belt from behind.
4. For the client using crutches, hold onto the transfer belt if the client feels uncomfortable using the crutches (Figures 10-37A and B).
5. For the client using a walker, instruct the client to place the walker firmly before walking. If the client is strong enough, the walker and the weaker leg can be moved forward at the same time.
6. For the client using a cane (Figures 10-38A and B), instruct the client to hold the cane in the hand opposite the weaker leg. If the right ankle has been injured, the client should hold the cane in the left hand.
7. Balance is a judgmental situation. If the client has poor balance, the aide should support the weak side. If the client has good balance and can walk without assistive devices, the aide should use a transfer belt for safety reasons.
8. Wash your hands at completion of the procedure.
9. Document how far the client walked and client's reaction.

(continues)

CLIENT CARE PROCEDURE **Assisting the Client to Walk with Crutches, Walker, or Cane** (continued)

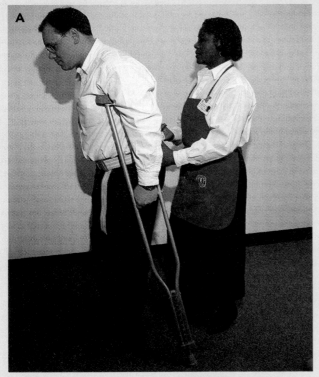
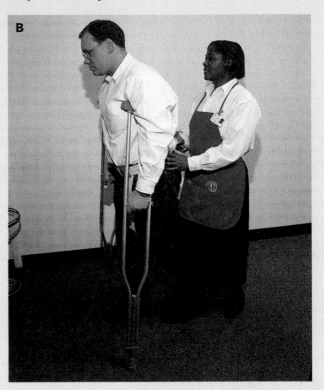

FIGURE 10-37   Crutch walking

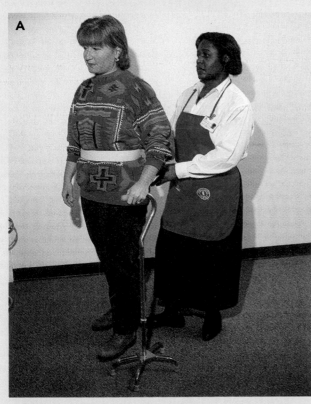
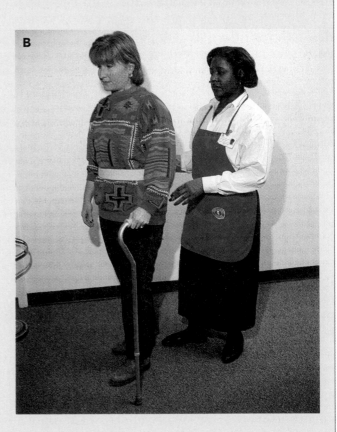

FIGURE 10-38   Using various types of canes

While recovering from an illness, clients sometimes become discouraged and depressed and fear they will never feel better. A home health aide must encourage the client, but not raise the client's expectations beyond a reasonable level. It is better to emphasize the client's "abilities" rather than "disabilities." It is important to set realistic daily goals while at the same time working toward a long-term level of physical rehabilitation that can be reasonably expected. If, for instance, a client is relearning to walk after an accident or stroke, the client should be praised and consistently given positive feedback for being able to take one more step than the client took the day before. The aide and client could set a goal of walking from the chair to the door by the end of the week, for example. If that goal is reached, the client will be very happy. If, on the other hand, the goal is not quite reached, the aide can point out how much closer the client is than the client had been the week before. This is an example of positive reinforcement.

If an aide were working with a young person recovering from a fractured leg and the client claimed the exercises planned by the physical therapist were too painful and refused to do them, what would the aide do? A home health aide's job is to encourage the client and explain that although there is pain, it is best to follow a daily plan. Let the client know that he or she is responsible for his or her own recovery. Suggest that a little pain now is better than permanent stiffness, which can lead to permanent disability. Severe pain should be reported to the case manager.

EMOTIONAL ASPECTS OF REHABILITATION

A person with a disability may have lost an ability many of us take for granted. However, he or she can be quite capable in other areas. The loss of sight, which makes assistance with bill paying necessary, for example, does not mean that a person cannot make correct decisions about her money. A person unable to walk is still quite capable of making choices or to direct his or her own care. The home health aide should treat every client, no matter his or her ability, with dignity and respect, enabling the client's right to make decisions, to maximize and support the physical, cognitive, and emotional abilities that do exist.

The aide should report to the case manager, supervisor, or physical therapist the client's lack of motivation or interest. This may be a sign of depression that can be treated by the appropriate therapist. The case manager may have some tips on ways to motivate this individual or may want to involve family members in supporting and motivating the client.

The important fact to know about rehabilitation is that the client's condition will determine the extent of rehabilitation possible. A blind person will probably never be able to see again. A client with crippling arthritis will probably never have the full use of the hands or feet. The aide's job is to assist clients to regain as much use of their body as is possible under a given set of circumstances. The aide should remember to give honest praise when a client is making progress and encourage a client who is reluctant to even try to help himself or herself.

REHABILITATION AND ACTIVITIES

The care plan is developed to make the client comfortable and to work toward recovery or to regain as much ability as possible. Several factors influence the care that is planned. The case manager and the home health aide must consider the person's age, condition, abilities, areas where assistance is needed, and personal interests before the accident or illness occurred. The personal habits and the client's personality also enter into the total care plan.

The value of activity must not be overlooked. **Activities** are useful in helping a person relearn skills that may have been lost because of the illness or accident. They also provide meaningful activity to a person who may be depressed due to the illness. An appropriate activity reminds a person of what he or she is still able to do. Activities are not just structured arts and crafts, or music, but are also sorting socks, washing dishes, planning a meal, dictating a letter, reading a newspaper together, or sorting photos for a photo album. An activity can be used to stimulate reminiscence, to aid in regaining verbal skills after a stroke, or to enhance a relationship.

The possibilities for activities are unlimited. A recreational or activity therapist can recommend activities geared to the abilities and interests of the client (Figure 10-39).

FIGURE 10-39. 101 ways to use capabilities

Lower Level

1. Read a story
2. Start cards
3. Review family photographs
4. Read poetry
5. Hold hands and share a special moment
6. Read a newspaper aloud
7. Exercise
8. Take a walk
9. Arrange a drawer
10. Clean a closet
11. Let client or patient help sort and fold clean socks
12. Put on makeup and give a manicure
13. Make an indoor garden
14. Take a car ride
15. Listen to some favorite records
16. Share a family recorded message
17. Make a scrapbook
18. Share a sack lunch or box dinner from home
19. Play horseshoes—inside or out
20. Make another person smile
21. Join an activity program together
22. Bible study
23. Clip coupons
24. Paint a picture
25. Catalog shop
26. Reminisce
27. Have a spell down
28. Bring something from home to share
29. Sort buttons
30. Watch a balloon sail away
31. Take family pictures
32. Read your horoscopes
33. Repot a plant
34. Make a grocery list—discuss prices—now and then
35. Make a Christmas list
36. Decorate a small tree
37. Give a back rub
38. Set hair or let client or patient set yours
39. Make a no-bake recipe
40. Taste something new on the market, i.e., soda, candy
41. Play trivia
42. Practice buttoning a shirt, tying a shoe
43. Roll up skeins of yarn for future project
44. Color a picture
45. Look through a magazine
46. Start a collection to work on together
47. Have a party
48. Make a birdhouse or small project to paint
49. Review the date, time, place
50. Make a mobile for client or patient's room
51. Bird or animal watch
52. Tear newspaper for garden mulch
53. Make a collage
54. Make ice cream
55. Pray together
56. Polish nails
57. Work on service project
58. Make some homemade lemonade
59. Pass out hugs
60. Have a tea party
61. Press flowers
62. Make holiday decorations
63. Have a picnic with all the trimmings
64. Dictate a letter
65. Finger paint

Higher Level

66. Play cards
67. Work a jigsaw puzzle
68. Work on a family tree
69. Play checkers
70. Write poetry
71. Plan the holiday meal
72. Do crossword puzzles
73. Talk about television show you have in common
74. Go for a walk
75. Make craft project
76. Make family recipe book
77. Make phone call to someone you haven't spoken with in a while
78. Polish shoes
79. Wrap a gift
80. Crochet together
81. Make party favors
82. Ask for some good old-fashioned advice
83. Sing
84. Watch and play television game show
85. What about those (name your favorite sports team)?
86. Play cribbage or poker
87. Play lotto
88. Go over activity calendar, help make selections for the week
89. Make list of things you like to do
90. Write letter or card
91. Play tic-tac-toe
92. Quilt a lap blanket
93. Play bingo
94. Write an article for a newsletter
95. Travel, learn about a country through a book
96. Stencil some stationery
97. Give a book report
98. Share talent with group
99. Write your autobiography
100. Think of 101 more things to do
101. Set a date—make plans for an outing

(From Glantz, Coralie, H., OTR/L, FAOTA and Richman, Nancy, OTR/L, FAOTA, Glantz Richman Rehabilitation Associates, Ltd. Reprinted with permission.)

REVIEW

1. List the vital signs.

2. Indicate the normal values of each vital sign.

3. What is the difference between a sign and a symptom?

4. Describe the care given to an unconscious client.

5. Explain rehabilitation.

6. List three sites where a person's temperature can be taken.

7. List four signs that a client may be ill.

8. Explain the role of a home health aide in restoring skills lost by disease or accidents.

9. When counting a client's pulse rate:
   a. Place your thumb over the client's artery.
   b. With your fingers, use light pressure on the wrist on the thumb side.
   c. Count the beats over any vein.
   d. Check the artery on the right side of the wrist.

10. You have just recorded a blood pressure as 130/72. The bottom number stands for the:
    a. Systolic pressure
    b. Diastolic pressure
    c. Mercury pressure
    d. Pulse deficit

11. The top number of a recorded blood pressure stands for the:
    a. Systolic pressure
    b. Diastolic pressure
    c. Mercury pressure
    d. Pulse deficit

12. Blood pressure above normal is called:
    a. Hypotension
    b. Rales
    c. Dyspnea
    d. Hypertension

13. T F There are three basic walking patterns: nonweight-bearing, partial weight-bearing, and weight-bearing.

14. T F With a nonweight-bearing person, all of the weight is placed on their arms and the uninvolved leg.

15. T F Partial weight-bearing means that all of the person's weight should be placed on their toes, rather than on the foot.

16. A person who is weight bearing:
    a. Has enough strength to bear full weight on both legs
    b. Should not use a standard cane as a weight-bearing aid
    c. May use a quad cane for balance purposes only
    d. All of the above

17. Your client, Miss F, is a 23-year-old woman who has been injured in a motorcycle accident, resulting in paralysis from the waist down. Miss F has been reluctant to do her physical ther-

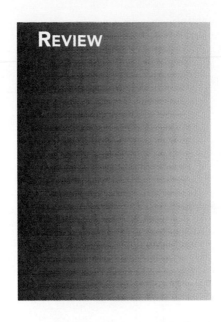

REVIEW

apy exercises. She will cooperate with the therapist, but not with you when you attempt to assist her on the days the therapist does not come.

What are some possible reasons why Miss F would not want to do her physical therapy exercises? Why is it important for you to reposition her legs and feet? What should you be watching for?

18. Your client, Mr. R, a 68-year-old man, has had a stroke resulting in weakness on his left side. Since your last visit he has lost weight. You notice that his face is flushed, and his breathing appears labored. You check his pulse and temperature, finding both elevated. When you ask Mr. R how he feels, he replies that he is chilled, has lost his appetite again, and is having chest pain. Which of the facts above are signs of illness? Which are symptoms? What could be happening with this client? What should you do?

11

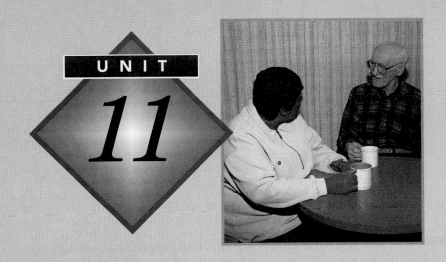

Mental Health

KEY TERMS

adjustment
delirium
dementia
depression
emotions

empathy
external stimulus
internal stimulus
mental disorder
optimist

pessimist
psychology
psychosis
stress

LEARNING OBJECTIVES

After studying this unit, you should be able to:

- Identify several common emotions.
- Identify how a physical response can result from an emotional reaction.
- Define mental illness.
- Define psychology, mental health, and adjustments.

- Differentiate between external and internal stimuli.
- Identify the major symptoms of depression.

Psychology is the science of human behavior. It is the study of the way the mind works and how emotions and feelings affect human behavior. Just as no two bodies are exactly alike, no two minds react in the same way. **Adjustment** is the change a person makes in behavior to deal with a situation. A person is mentally healthy if he or she can see reality as it is, respond to its challenges, and develop a reasonable strategy for living. A mentally healthy person has compassion or feelings for other people. A mentally healthy person can accept limitations and possibilities of reality. When chronic illness occurs, a well-adjusted person may feel stressed, even overwhelmed at times. A well-adjusted person is able to handle the daily problems of living, taking bad times in stride and coping with crises. The well-adjusted person has a good self-image and can be flexible when meeting new or difficult obstacles. It takes less time for a well-adjusted person to recover from a difficult situation. People can adjust easily to some situations and not to others. A person does not have to be strong all the time. The mentally healthy person is able to make life work in a way that is both personally and socially acceptable.

To understand basic psychology it is necessary to review the nervous system. The brain acts as the body's communication center. All messages (called stimuli) from the five senses are carried to the brain, where they are received and acted on. There are both internal and external stimuli. For example: The stomach is empty, so the nerve endings in the stomach send a message to the brain. The brain translates the impulses, and the individual thinks, "I'm hungry," and looks for food. This is an **internal stimulus.** On the other hand, on entering a room where food is being cooked, a person might smell a pleasant aroma or see an attractive piece of fruit. The sight and smell of the food can stimulate the nerve endings and the person might think, "I'm hungry," and eat the food even though it was not mealtime. This is an **external stimulus.**

Internal stimuli cause automatic or unconscious reactions within the body. External stimuli come from outside the body and bring about a conscious reaction. Psychology relates to both internal and external stimuli. In some conditions, chemical imbalances within the body or brain and nerve cell damage can cause changes in behavior. In other cases, environmental conditions may have a direct effect on emotional health.

UNDERSTANDING EMOTIONS

Emotions are common to all people and are neither good nor bad. An **emotion** is a strong, generalized feeling. The way a person shows emotion may be healthy or unhealthy. There is a wide range of acceptable levels of emotional behavior. Well-adjusted people most often use emotions in a healthy way to serve their purposes; they can control emotions so as not to harm themselves or others. There are a wide range of emotions that are regarded as normal, including fear, anger, grief, and others. Whether emotional behavior is healthy depends on whether a person can express these emotions in a manner that is socially acceptable.

Emotions may cause physical reactions. Anger and fear sometimes cause the heart to beat faster, respirations to increase, and chemical changes to occur within the body. The mouth may become dry; the person may become pale and may start to shake. Such physical changes are common and usually of short duration. Emotions can trigger the release of hormones and produce unusual results. For example, it is not unusual for those experiencing a shocking or traumatic event to find that they are physically capable of functioning at unusually high levels of strength and energy.

Individuals develop a pattern of emotional response. This may be a hereditary characteristic although environment also can influence mental health. Some babies, for instance, seem calmer and happier than others. The social environment of a family can influence whether a baby's early experiences are pleasant or unpleasant. As years pass, the child's successes and failures in daily life influence the child's emotional patterns. The child who is healthy and who is given tender, loving attention from birth has a good chance of growing up to be well adjusted. The stages of personality development are listed in Figure 11-1.

The type of emotion (pleasant or unpleasant) that a person feels most of the time is referred to as his or her disposition. A disposition is the usual mood of an individual. An **optimist**

FIGURE 11-1   Tasks of personality development according to the stages defined by Erikson

Physical Stage	Year of Occurrence	Tasks to Be Mastered
Oral-sensory	Birth–1 yr (Infant)	To learn to trust (Trust)
Muscular-anal	1–3 yr (Toddler)	To recognize self as an independent being from mother (Autonomy)
Locomotor	3–5 yr (Preschool years)	To recognize self as a family member (Initiative)
Latency	6–11 yr (School-age years)	To demonstrate physical and mental skills abilities (Industry)
Adolescence	12–18 yr	To develop a sense of individuality as a sexual human being (Identity)
Young Adulthood	19–35 yr	To establish intimate personal relationships with a mate (Intimacy)
Adulthood	35–50 yr	To live a satisfying and productive life (Generativity)
Maturity	50+ yr	To review life's events and examine how they have influenced the development of a unique individual (Ego integrity)

probably feels more pleasant emotions and, therefore, has a brighter outlook than a pessimist. The aide who has a cheerful outlook may transfer this pleasant mood to the client. Words, tone of voice, actions, and facial expression show how a person looks at life. This often exposes the person's inner feelings. **Pessimists** may be just as well adjusted as optimists but their viewpoints differ. Pessimists tend to take a negative view of situations. A classic example showing the difference between an optimist and a pessimist is to consider a glass filled half-way with water. An optimist would be more likely to regard the glass as half full, whereas the pessimist may regard the glass as half empty.

People have mood changes or emotional cycles. It is normal to feel high or low from time to time. In some people, this mood swing is more noticeable than in others. Emotional cycles can be affected by the time of day, season of the year, or the weather. An emotionally healthy person can function in both high and low emotional cycles. For example, some people are happiest and function best early in the day. Others, who are sometimes called "night people,"

are more alert in the evening hours. Some people find that the season affects their feelings. Some dislike the winter and feel down, others dislike the summer months.

Mentally healthy people learn to make their emotions work for them. One can deal with negative emotions in a positive way. When a home health aide feels angry with a client, the aide cannot have a tantrum. Strong outbursts of emotion are not acceptable while on duty. Sometimes anger must be expressed, but it should be done in a way that is constructive. A home health aide must not only deal with her own emotional needs, but must also be aware of the emotional needs and reactions of the client. This requires a great deal of self-control and self-discipline. The home health aide must be sensitive to the emotions of the client. Clients are often frightened and worried about their health. The home health aide must be kind and understanding and think of the client's needs first. Illness can cause temporary changes in the client's personality. This often requires the client to make many adjustments. It takes time to accept the physical changes caused by a disease. The home health aide must be willing to allow clients to express their emotions. The well-adjusted aide will be able to endure the client's strong emotional feelings without becoming a part of them.

STRESS

Stress is a mentally or emotionally disruptive or upsetting condition that occurs in response to adverse external stimuli.

Handling stress effectively is an important component of mental health and is essential for avoiding both physical and mental illness. Stress can make the body more vulnerable to physical illnesses such as colds, ulcers, headaches, and high blood pressure. In severe and prolonged cases, stress can lead to emotional illness.

Although no one can avoid stress all the time, steps should be taken to either eliminate the stressor or to diminish its negative effects. Regular exercise and adequate sleep will help to strengthen the body's resistance to stress. Relaxation is another useful technique to diminish stress and may include participation in hobbies, quiet meditation, or some other activity that an individual enjoys. It is often helpful to talk about stressful situations with a trusted friend (Figure 11-2). If these measures are not enough, it may be necessary to consult with a professional.

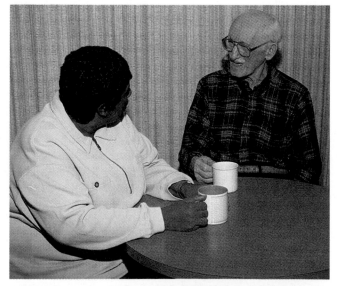

FIGURE 11-2 Often it is helpful to talk about stressful situations with a trusted friend.

MENTAL DISORDERS

Emotions play an important role throughout our lifetime. Although there is a broad range of feelings that are considered normal reactions to everyday life, other feelings or behaviors may signal a problem that requires medical attention. A person is said to have a **mental disorder** if he or she is having difficulty functioning satisfactorily in society as a result of changes in thoughts, behavior, personality, or emotion. A mental disorder can be temporary or permanent and can affect people of all backgrounds and economic levels. Mental disorders can be caused by physical or chemical changes in the brain, genetics, and social and psychological factors. Mental illness is never caused by a character weakness. Most people with mental illness require special treatment from a mental health professional. The most common treatments used today are drug therapy, talk therapy (or "counseling"), or a combination of both. There are different kinds of mental disorders. These are dementia, delirium, mood disorders, commonly known as depression, and psychotic disorders.

Dementia

Dementia is a loss of intellectual functions, such as thinking, remembering, and reasoning. It can become so severe that it interferes with a person's daily life. Dementia is either reversible or irreversible. Some examples of reversible dementia would be those caused by medications, some infections, and poor nutrition. An irreversible cause of dementia is Alzheimer's disease. Alzheimer's disease is the most common and serious form of dementia, causing memory loss, disorientation, personality changes, impaired judgment, and the loss of language and planning skills. Refer to Unit 22 for more information on Alzheimer's disease.

Delirium

Delirium is a disturbance of consciousness, making it difficult for a person to focus or shift his or her attention. A person who is delirious often looks confused or intoxicated. Delirium is a disorder of brain functioning often seen in patients with multiple diseases and is regarded as the final stage of a severe disease process.

Mood Disorders

Mood disorders are the most common mental disorders for people of all ages. Mood disorders include depression, and its opposite, mania (extreme happiness and hyperactivity). **Depression** is a term that is used to describe a range of emotions from blue feelings to a severe clinical condition.

Depression. People who are depressed show signs of feeling extremely sad, worthless, or hopeless. They may become forgetful or seem unfocused. They can become angry easily or are constantly irritable. Anxiety is another sign of depression. Also, depressed people often express feelings of guilt. Figure 11-3 gives a comprehensive list of symptoms caused by depression.

People suffering from clinical depression are unable to enjoy any aspect of their lives and have great difficulty focusing or paying attention. Although a person may not complain about feeling depressed, he or she does frequently complain about things that can add up to depression. For example, many older people have physical problems, but people who are preoccupied with their physical illnesses may be depressed. They may say things like "I don't know what's the matter with me. I just don't feel right." These complaints may be covering up their depression.

Depression can also affect the way a person thinks. Depressed people can have false beliefs about themselves. They often believe they are worthless and that nothing they do is right. Depressed people can be irritable, disagreeable, and at odds with everything.

People with depression think nothing will ever get better, and they are overwhelmed by guilt. They put themselves down and cannot see

FIGURE 11-3   Signs of depression checklist

Signs of Depression	
FEELINGS CAUSED BY DEPRESSION	
• Extreme sadness • Hopelessness	• Worthlessness • Inability to enjoy life
NEGATIVE THOUGHTS CAUSED BY DEPRESSION	
• Fear nothing will ever get better • Overwhelming guilt • Low self-esteem	• Difficulty in paying attention • Forgetfulness
BEHAVIORAL CHANGES CAUSED BY DEPRESSION	
• Excessive crying • Slowness in walking, talking, and moving • Low energy • Poor personal appearance	• Jittery, unsettled manner • Anxiety • Excessive anger • Sleep disorders
PHYSICAL CHANGES CAUSED BY DEPRESSION	
• Too much or too little appetite • Weight loss	• Headaches, shortness of breath, stomachaches
SUICIDAL TENDENCIES CAUSED BY DEPRESSION	
• Thoughts about wanting to kill oneself	• Suicide • Suicide attempts

(From *The Paraprofessional in Home Health and Long-Term Care*, Health Professions Press, 1995. Reprinted with permission.)

anything good about themselves. A depressed person may have difficulty paying attention and also may be forgetful. Encourage the client to seek help for his or her depression. Many home health agencies can provide mental health services by a licensed professional, so be sure to alert your supervisor if you believe that your client is depressed.

Depression as a Cause of Difficult Behavior. It can be hard for an aide to decide whether a client is just being difficult or is suffering from depression. These three questions may help identify the problem:

1. Has the person changed dramatically?
2. Has the change been constant for 2 weeks or longer?
3. Is the change interfering with the person's day-to-day functioning?

If the answer to all three questions is "yes," then the person may be depressed.

If depression is suspected, the aide should tell a supervisor. Friends and family members of the client should be asked if they have noticed changes in the client's mood. The three questions listed above are useful in this context also.

When working with the client, do not tell the client to "shape up" or to "snap out of it," or ask "What's wrong with you?" Do not be critical of the client's new behavior, difficult as it may be to deal with. It is important for the home health aide to avoid blaming the client. Recognize that depressed people are often unable to control the way they feel or behave.

The aide should listen with empathy to a depressed client. Depressed people need someone to talk to who will listen and understand. **Empathy** involves being able to look at the world through the other person's eyes. Home health aides need to communicate in a way that shows they understand how the depressed person feels and the experiences behind these feelings.

Getting the person to talk and listening carefully to what the person says can offer the client hope. Although depressed clients will say that they do not believe things will get better, they still need to hear that there is hope. Unit 3 discusses communication strategies in greater detail.

A home health aide's job is to help clients do things that they may no longer be able to do for themselves. However, this increased dependency may be a factor behind the depression. A worker should encourage clients to use their remaining capabilities. Clients can be involved in tasks if activities are structured in small, simple steps so that they do not feel overwhelmed. Emphasize doing things *with* clients rather than doing things *for* them. Doing everything for those who are depressed can increase their feelings of helplessness and inadequacy.

A client who feels out of control can be rigid and uncooperative. There are often ways to regain control. The home health aide can allow the client to make some decisions about what to eat, when to bathe, and what activities to do. However, avoid giving depressed people too many choices. They may feel overwhelmed and unable to choose. A choice between two simple items is best. Instead of "What would you like for lunch?" ask "Would you like tomato soup or a tuna sandwich for lunch?" When looking in the closet, ask "Would you like to wear the blue dress or the red one?"

The client has the right to privacy and independence, including the right to make a bad decision. A worker may have a hard time watching a client do something that seems clearly incorrect. However, the best way to intervene is to share one's observations and concerns. The decision rests with the client.

The home health aide must have keen observation and listening skills. Most importantly, a worker must be watchful for signs of suicide. Home health aides are in a unique position—they can be the eyes and ears of the family and the employer. It is imperative that aides be able to recognize changes in the depressed client and know when to report them.

There are usually warning signs if a depressed person is considering suicide. Some people will talk about their plan, others will behave in certain ways. The home health aide will want to watch for the following warning signs of suicide:

- Client expresses feelings of depression and hopelessness.
- Client makes statements expressing the desire to end his or her life (i.e., "I can't go on anymore," or "I just want to relieve the pain" etc.).
- Client has thought of a method of suicide—the more specific the plan, the higher the risk of suicide.
- Client has the ability to carry out the plan and has a method available (i.e., guns, pills, car).

- Client has sudden or dramatic changes in behavior (may begin giving things away or clear up personal affairs).
- Client becomes isolated.

If a home health aide recognizes any of the above signs or symptoms in a client, he or she should contact the supervisor immediately.

Psychotic Disorders

Psychosis is a serious condition in which the thinking process is distorted by hallucinations, delusions, or both. The most common form of psychotic disorder is schizophrenia. Generally, people with severe psychotic episodes will be treated in a hospital to ensure their safety. In less severe cases, antipsychotic medications are prescribed to decrease excitement and agitation and to improve the thought processes. Supportive psychotherapy may also be helpful for those with psychotic disorders to improve functioning in everyday life.

EFFECTS OF EMOTIONS ON HEALTH

Sometimes a physical illness can aggravate a mental illness; but a person's emotional health may also affect his physical health. Wellness means different things to different people; people feel better on some days than on others. Temporary discomforts are not necessarily a health hazard or danger. After a very hard day at work, an argument with a close friend, or the death of a loved one, people may feel unwell. A tension headache caused by an emotional crisis can make a person feel ill for a short time. When the upset is resolved, the person forgets the pain and feels well again. Persons who are acutely or chronically ill also have good and bad days. To a great extent these changes are related to their emotional outlooks. When routines have gone smoothly or when a special friend has called or visited, a person may feel very well despite physical problems. On a day when the home health aide comes late and is in a bad mood, the client may complain of feeling much worse than the physical condition warrants.

No two people react the same to external stimuli. The stress situation causing one person to feel unwell may have no effect on another person. People react to personal crises in their own ways. It has been proven that an emotionally depressed person is more likely to catch a cold or develop a physical disorder. Wellness may be described as freedom from discomfort—both physical and mental. Emotional health may strongly influence a person's state of wellness.

The home health aide can help the client by being aware of the client's mental health status and responding to the client in a supportive and nonjudgmental way. The aide should be aware of the signs of depression, and report any changes to a supervisor. *An aide must take all suicidal threats expressed by the client seriously and report these immediately to a supervisor.* In addition, the home health aide must pay close attention to his or her own stress level and find constructive ways to cope with stressful situations on the job.

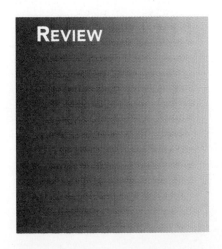

REVIEW

1. List four common emotional reactions.
2. What is the difference between an internal stimulus and an external stimulus?
3. Explain how a physical response can result from an emotional reaction.
4. Define mental health and adjustment.
5. Characteristics of a mentally healthy person are:
   a. Sees reality as it is
   b. Responds to change
   c. Sets reasonable strategies for living
   d. All are correct

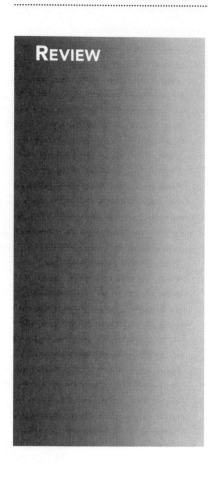

REVIEW

6. List four behavioral changes caused by depression.

7. List two physical changes caused by depression.

8. Fill in the blank: In severe and prolonged cases, _____ can lead to emotional illness.

9. List three constructive ways to manage stress.

10. Fill in the blank: A person is said to have a _____ _____ if he or she is having difficulty functioning in society as a result of changes in thoughts, behavior, personality or emotions.

11. You arrive at Mrs. Smith's home in the middle of the afternoon. She is still wearing her pajamas. She tells you she hasn't eaten much the last several days; she appears lethargic and uncommunicative. What steps could you take to determine if she is depressed? What should you do to help Mrs. Smith?

12. One of your clients, an elderly man with multiple health problems, also has a history of depression. During one of your visits he seems particularly depressed and irritated about his chronic health problems, which cause him a great deal of pain and restrict his independence. He tells you "I've had it!" and "Sometimes I think it just would be easier if I weren't around anymore." What steps should you take to help your client? Should you call your supervisor?

SECTION 5

Body Systems and Common Disorders

Units

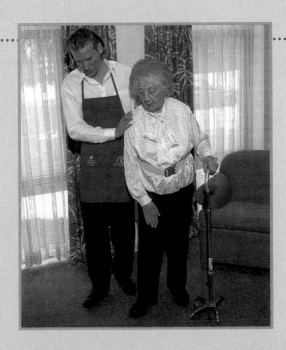

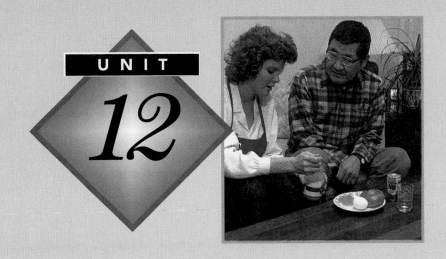

Digestion and Nutrition *Exme*

KEY TERMS

bland diet	feces	malnutrition
calorie-controlled diet	fiber	Meals on Wheels
clear liquid diet	food allergy	metabolism
degenerative diseases	food guide pyramid	nutrition
diabetic diet	full-liquid diet	peristalsis
diuretic	high-fiber diet	pureed diet
emesis	impacted	soft diet
empty calorie	low-residue diet	stool
enzymes	low-sodium diet	vegetarians

LEARNING OBJECTIVES

After studying this unit, you should be able to:

- List the six food groups on the food guide pyramid.
- Identify the special diets used for at least five medical conditions.
- Name six things to keep in mind when planning and preparing meals.
- Name eight special diets that may be prescribed for your client, and describe the types of foods that are usually permitted for each.
- Identify the special diet a client with acquired immunodeficiency syndrome (AIDS) would require.
- Demonstrate the following:
  PROCEDURE 17 Feeding the Client

Nutrition is the sum of a combination of processes by which the body receives and uses food and nutrients. The body needs food for energy, cell growth, and comfort and satiety. The single most important use of food is to provide proper nutrition to the body. The digestive system changes food into a form that can be used by all the cells of the body. Those parts of food that cannot be used by the body are expelled as waste products, called **feces** or **stool.**

DIGESTIVE SYSTEM

Food is the fuel burned by the digestive system to provide energy for the entire body. This use of food can be compared to gasoline in a car that burns to give power to the car or oil in a furnace that produces heat. In the body, the fuel is food; the process of burning this fuel is called **metabolism.**

Metabolism depends on the proper functioning of each organ of digestion (Figure 12-1). The digestive process begins the moment food is taken into the mouth. The teeth and tongue tear the food into small pieces and mix it with saliva so that it can be swallowed easily. In the saliva, chemical substances called **enzymes** start to break down the starchy foods into products that can be used by the rest of the body. From the mouth the partially processed food is swallowed, moving into the esophagus. An involuntary wavelike muscle action called **peristalsis** moves food through the esophagus and then into the stomach. Sometimes the body rejects or refuses food during the digestive process. When this occurs, the voluntary and involuntary muscles work together to force the food backward. This is called vomiting or **emesis.**

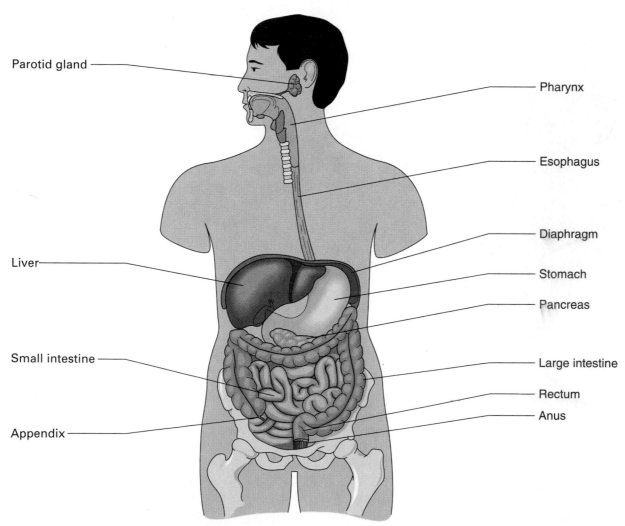

FIGURE 12-1 The digestive system

The stomach is an elastic, muscular organ that holds the food and secretes and mixes in gastric juices. The stomach passes the food into the small intestine. Enzymes in the intestinal juice are especially important in the digestive process. The liver produces bile, which is necessary to absorb fat. Bile is produced in the liver but is stored in the gallbladder. Bile enters the small intestine and breaks up fats in the duodenum so they can be digested and absorbed. The duodenum is the first 10 inches of the 19- to 20-foot small intestine. The jejunum is the second portion of the small intestine. It is about 9 feet long. The ileum is the third portion and is about 9 feet. The pancreas also releases digestive enzymes into the duodenum. Insulin, which controls sugar metabolism, is also released into the bloodstream from a specific area within the pancreas.

The digestive juices work together to break down food into a simpler form. The usable products of this breakdown are called nutrients. The nutrients are absorbed through the walls of the small intestine. The nutrients are then carried by the bloodstream to all parts of the body. Some portion of food remains in the small intestine because it cannot be broken down or absorbed. This remaining material moves into the large intestine in a semiliquid state. The large intestine, also called the colon, is about 5 feet long. In this area, much of the liquid from the food is absorbed into the body. This helps maintain the balance of fluids in the body. Peristalsis moves the remaining solid material into the lower part of the colon. When enough waste has collected, the voluntary muscles expel it through the anus. This is a normal bowel movement.

COMMON DISORDERS OF THE DIGESTIVE SYSTEM

Constipation, diarrhea, and heartburn are common disorders of the digestive system. Constipation and diarrhea are affected by diet and exercise. Heartburn is caused by the backflow of digestive juices into the esophagus.

Constipation

A common problem with the bowels is constipation. This is a condition in which bowel movements are hard and difficult to pass. Prevention might include exercise, increased fluid consumption, and eating more foods enriched with **fiber,** such as whole grain cereals, raw fruits, and vegetables. Prolonged or long-lasting constipation can cause feces (the technical name for the waste material of the body) to become lodged in the rectum (**impacted**). It may then be necessary for the person to receive an enema or a laxative, or have disimpaction done by the nurse.

Stools may have blood on the outside surface, which may be the result of bleeding hemorrhoids or rectal cancer. If the stool looks dark, black, or tarry, the cause may be medications or internal bleeding in the gastrointestinal system. Brighter colored blood in the stool may result from bleeding in the lower part of the intestinal tract.

Diarrhea

Diarrhea is a condition in which feces are watery and frequent. Constipation and diarrhea may result from a number of causes. Proper diet, fluid consumption, adequate exercise, and regular elimination of wastes help prevent both constipation and diarrhea.

Heartburn

So-called heartburn results from a backflow of the digestive juices into the lower portion of the esophagus. These juices, because of their high acid content, cause irritation of the lining of the esophagus. Those affected experience a burning sensation. It is unrelated to heart disease.

NUTRITION

Because the field of nutrition is complex, home health aides should take in-service courses to learn more about this vital health area. One of the most rapidly growing fields in health care is nutrition. Hospitals have nutritionists on staff as do other health care facilities such as nursing homes. It is becoming a common practice for hospitals and nursing homes to provide a nutritionally sound plan to patients as part of their discharge instructions. The nutritionist considers the age, weight, sex, and medical condition of the patient when setting up a food plan. It is the responsibility of the home health aide to follow this plan.

Some dietitians recommend that the average diet consist of the following:

- 20% fat
- 15% protein
- 10% simple sugars (such as fruits)
- 45% complex carbohydrates

They further suggest that the amount of fiber, found in whole grains, leafy vegetables, fruits, beans, and peas, be increased in the daily diet. Fiber flushes out food wastes and may help to prevent constipation and cancer of the colon.

In addition, nutritionists believe that the average individual should have a regular exercise program. A half-hour walk three times a week would be beneficial to keep the body trim. Nutritional therapists know that individual diets must consider a person's ethnic background and food likes and dislikes. Also to be considered is any physical condition that prevents a client from eating certain foods and requires certain foods as part of the care plan.

FOOD GUIDE PYRAMID

The foods recommended in the food pyramid are the fruit group; vegetable group; milk, yogurt, and cheese group; bread, cereal, and rice group; meat, poultry, and fish group; and the fats, oils, and sweets group. Each individual needs the nutrients that can only come from a proper balance of the **food guide pyramid** (Figure 12-2).

Dietary Guidelines for Americans

- Eat a variety of foods.
- Maintain a healthy weight.
- Choose a diet low in fat, saturated fat, and cholesterol.
- Choose a diet with plenty of vegetables, fruits, and grain products.
- Use sugars only in moderation.
- Use salt and sodium only in moderation.
- If you drink alcoholic beverages, do so in moderation.

These guidelines call for moderation in balance and variety, avoiding extremes in diet. Both eating too much and eating too little can

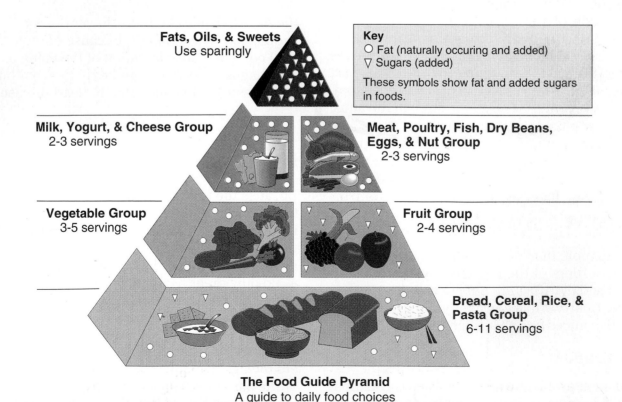

The Food Guide Pyramid
A guide to daily food choices

FIGURE 12-2 Food pyramid—a guide to daily food choices. (Courtesy U.S. Department of Agriculture)

be harmful. Also, be cautious of diets based on the belief that a food or supplement alone can cure or prevent disease.

The foods Americans have to choose from are varied, plentiful, and safe to eat. These guidelines can help you choose a diet that is both healthful and enjoyable.

Eat a Variety of Foods

You need more than 40 different nutrients for good health. Essential nutrients include vitamins, minerals, amino acids from protein, certain fatty acids from fat, and sources of calories (protein, carbohydrates, and fat).

These nutrients should come from a variety of foods, not from a few highly fortified foods or supplements. Any food that supplies calories and nutrients can be part of a nutritious diet. The content of the total diet over a day or more is what counts.

Many foods are good sources of several nutrients. For example, vegetables and fruits are important for vitamins A and C, folic acid, minerals, and fiber. Breads and cereals supply B vitamins, iron, and protein; whole-grain types are also food sources of fiber. Milk provides protein, B vitamins, vitamins A and D, calcium, and phosphorus. Meat, poultry, and fish provide protein, B vitamins, iron, and zinc.

No single food can supply all nutrients in the amounts needed. For example, milk supplies calcium but little iron; meat supplies iron but little calcium. To have a nutritious diet, people must eat a variety of foods.

One way to ensure variety—and with it, an enjoyable and nutritious diet—is to choose foods each day from the six food groups described in the food guide pyramid (see Figure 12-2). Individuals who do not eat foods from one or more of the food groups may want to contact a dietitian for help in planning how to meet nutritional needs.

A Daily Food Guide

Eat a variety of foods daily, choosing different foods from each group. Most people should have at least the lower number of servings suggested from each food group. Some people may need more because of their body size and activity level. Young children should have a variety of foods but may need small servings.

Food Group	Suggested Servings per Day
Vegetables	3–5 servings
Fruits	2–4 servings
Breads, cereals, rice, and pasta	6–11 servings
Milk, yogurt, and cheese	2–3 servings
Meats, poultry, fish, dry beans and peas, eggs	2–3 servings
Fats and sweets	Use sparingly

People who are inactive or are trying to lose weight may use the lower number of suggested servings. They need to choose nutrient-rich foods lower in calories illustrated in the food pyramid. They also need to eat less of foods high in calories and low in essential nutrients, such as fats and oils, sugars, and alcoholic beverages.

Diets of some groups of people are notably low in some nutrients. Many women and adolescent girls need to eat more calcium-rich foods, such as milk and milk products, to get the calcium they need for healthy bones throughout life. Young children, teenage girls, and women of childbearing age must take care to eat enough iron-rich foods, such as lean meats, dry beans, and whole-grain and iron-enriched breads, cereals, and other grain products.

Vitamins and minerals taken regularly in large amounts can be harmful. If you use the food pyramid as a guide and eat a variety of food that is well balanced and taken in moderation, vitamins, minerals, and supplements are not necessary. Exceptions in which your doctor may recommend a supplement are:

- Pregnant women often need an iron supplement. Some other women in their childbearing years may also need an iron supplement to help replace iron lost in menstrual bleeding.
- Certain women who are pregnant or breast-feeding may need a supplement to meet their increased requirements for some nutrients.
- People who are unable to be active and do not eat properly may need supplements of special formulas that may be enriched with vitamins and minerals.
- People, especially the elderly, who take medicines that interact with nutrients may need supplements.

Choose a Diet Low in Fat, Saturated Fat, and Cholesterol

Most health authorities recommend an American diet with less fat, saturated fat, and cholesterol. The American diet, which is high in fat and cholesterol, leads to a higher prevalence of heart disease in this country.

A diet low in fat makes it easier for you to include the variety of foods you need for nutrients without exceeding your calorie needs, because fat contains more than twice the calories of an equal amount of carbohydrates or protein.

A diet low in saturated fat and cholesterol can help maintain a desirable level of blood cholesterol. For adults this level is below 200 mg/dL. As blood cholesterol increases above this level, greater risk for heart disease occurs. Risk can also be increased by high blood pressure, cigarette smoking, diabetes, a family history of premature heart disease, obesity, and being a male.

The way diet affects blood cholesterol varies among individuals. Excessive weight leads to higher cholesterol levels in the bloodstream. The blood cholesterol level increases with a diet high in saturated fat and cholesterol and excessive in calories. Of these, dietary saturated fat has the greatest effect; dietary cholesterol has less.

Suggested goals to reduce fats in American diets are as follows:

Total Fat. Intake should be 30% or less of total calories consumed. Thus, the upper limit on the grams of fat in your diet depends on the calories you need. For example, at 2000 calories per day, your suggested upper limit is 600 calories from fat (2000 × .30). This is equal to 67 grams of fat (600 ÷ 9, the number of calories each gram of fat provides). The grams of fat in some foods are shown in Table 12-1.

TABLE 12-1   Plan for a Diet Low in Fat, Saturated Fat, and Cholesterol

Fats and Oils

- Use fats and oils sparingly in cooking.
- Use small amounts of salad dressings and spreads, such as butter, margarine, and mayonnaise. One tablespoon of most of these spreads provides 10 to 11 grams of fat.
- Choose liquid vegetable oils most often because they are lower in saturated fat.
- Check labels on foods to see how much fat and saturated fat are in a serving.

Meat, Poultry, Fish, Dry Beans, and Eggs

- Limit your portion of meat, poultry, and seafood to 6 ounces, 2–3 servings per day. A 3-oz portion is a piece of meat, the size of a deck of cards, or ¾ cup of flaked fish.
- Trim fat from meat; take skin off poultry.
- Eat cooked dry beans and peas instead of meat occasionally.
- Reduce the use of egg yolks, 3–4 per week.
- Select luncheon meats with fewer than 3 grams of fat per ounce, such as lean roast beef, turkey breast, lean ham, or turkey pastrami.

Milk and Milk Products

- Consume at least 2 or 3 servings daily. (Count as a serving: 1 cup of milk or yogurt or about 1½ oz of cheese.)
- Select skim or low-fat dairy products, nonfat or low-fat yogurt, and nonfat or low-fat cheese most of the time. One cup of skim milk has only a trace of fat, 1 cup of 2% milk has 5 grams of fat, and 1 cup of whole milk has 8 grams of fat. Cheese or any other dairy product with 5 grams of fat or fewer per ounce can be considered a good choice.

Saturated Fat.   Saturated fatty acids should be less than 10% of calories consumed (less than 22 grams at 2000 calories per day). All fats contain both saturated and unsaturated fat (fatty acids). The fats in animal products are the main sources of saturated fat in most diets, as are tropical oils (coconut, palm kernel, and palm oils) and hydrogenated fats such as margarine.

Cholesterol.   Animal products are the source of all dietary cholesterol. Eating less fat from animal sources will help lower cholesterol as well as total fat and saturated fat in your diet.

These goals for fats are not for children under 2 years, who have special dietary needs. As children begin to eat with the family, usually at about 2 years of age or older, they should be encouraged to choose diets that are lower in fat and saturated fat and that provide the calories and nutrients they need for normal growth. Older children and adults with established food habits may need to change their diets gradually toward the goals.

These goals for fats apply to the diet over several days, not to a single meal or food. Some foods that contain fat, saturated fat, and cholesterol, such as meats, milk, cheese, and eggs, also contain high-quality protein and are the best sources of certain vitamins and minerals. Low-fat choices of these foods are lean meat and low-fat milk and cheeses.

DEVELOPING GOOD EATING HABITS

Is it possible to look at a person and tell whether that person's body is well nourished? A well-nourished person usually has shiny hair, clear skin, good posture, and firm flesh. The person also appears alert and energetic. To be well nourished, people must select the correct foods. Lower forms of animals seem to have a natural body wisdom. They eat only those foods that are good for them and they do not overeat. People, however, have so many foods to choose from that they often make mistakes and overconsume.

Often people living alone do not get the proper nourishment. They may not have the desire to eat, or they may not have the knowledge or energy to purchase and prepare nutritious meals.

Empty-Calorie Foods

Favorite foods are often oversalted, oversweetened, or high in fat content. Examples of such favorite foods are potato chips, candy, soda, and french fries. Teenagers especially have a tendency to eat these foods. In everyday language, these foods are called junk foods, but the proper descriptive name for them is **empty calorie.** Empty-calorie foods are high in sugars and fats; they are very low in proteins, minerals, and vitamins. Overindulgence in these empty-calorie foods leads to poor nutrition and overweight.

Refer to Figures 12-3 and 12-4. Figure 12-3 provides definitions of important nutritional terms. Knowing these terms will help you understand the value of meal planning for a balanced diet. Figure 12-4 lists vitamins, their important food sources, and their functions.

Overeating

Another dietary problem is overeating. Normally, the body can only burn or use a certain number of calories every day. Calories not used are turned into fat tissue. In the United States, it has been estimated that 60% of the population is 10 pounds or more overweight. Excess weight forces the heart to work harder and is a major cause of heart disease.

Degenerative Diseases

Many degenerative diseases can be traced directly to the kinds and amounts of food eaten. **Degenerative diseases** cause tissues or organs to weaken and become diseased. Included in this category are diabetes and arteriosclerosis. The most common of all degenerative diseases is tooth decay. Strong, healthy teeth are important for the proper digestion of food. Eating too much sugar is a main cause of tooth decay.

FIGURE 12-3 Knowing terms used in nutrition helps us to understand how the body uses food.

Word	Definition	Examples
Carbohydrates	Sugars or starches that are made up of carbon, hydrogen, and oxygen and deliver quick energy to the body	Found in grains, potatoes, corn, fruits, and sweets
Proteins	Compounds composed of amino acids needed for growth and tissue repair	Found in meats, fish, milk, eggs, nuts, dried beans
Fats	Oily substances made up of glycerin and fatty acids, which provide stored energy to the body, and protect vital organs	Present in meats, butter, milk, peanuts
Minerals	Inorganic elements essential in tissue building and in regulation of body fluids	Iron, calcium, sodium, and zinc
Vitamins	Organic substances vital to certain metabolic functions and needed to prevent deficiency disease. Vitamins are needed only in small amounts but must be obtained from food sources since they are not produced in the body.	Vitamins A, C, B$_{12}$
Water	A tasteless, odorless liquid compound of hydrogen and oxygen necessary in the digestive process and to regulate body processes	
Calorie	A measure of heat produced by the body when using a specific portion of food	
Metabolism	Sum total of processes needed for the breakdown of food and absorption of nutrients	

FIGURE 12-4 Many foods contain more than one vitamin.

Vitamins	Best Sources	Functions
Fat-Soluble Vitamins		
Vitamin A	Vegetables (dark green and deep yellow) Fish liver oils Liver Egg yolk Fruits (yellow) Milk	Essential for: Growth Health of eyes Structure and functioning of the cells of the skin and mucous membranes
Vitamin D	Sunshine Fish liver oil Milk (irradiated) Egg yolk Liver	Essential for: Growth Regulating calcium and phosphorus metabolism Building and maintaining normal bones and teeth *(continues)*

FIGURE 12-4   *(continued)*

Vitamins	Best Sources	Functions

Vitamin E	Wheat germ and wheat germ oils
	Vegetable oils
	Margarine
	Legumes
	Nuts
	Dark green, leafy vegetables
		Not conclusively defined in humans;
		  may affect the red blood cells
		Recommended for middle-aged
		  women as it helps in the metabo-
		  lism of calcium

Vitamin K	Spinach Kale Cabbage Cauliflower Pork liver	Essential for: Normal clotting of blood

Water-Soluble Vitamins

Vitamins	Best Sources	Functions

Vitamin C
(Ascorbic acid)
	Citrus fruits, pineapple
	Melons and berries
	Tomatoes
	Broccoli
	Green peppers
		Essential for:
		  Maintaining strength of blood
		  vessels
		Health of the teeth and gums
		Aids in wound healing

Thiamine (B_1)	Wheat germ
	Lean pork
	Yeast
	Legumes
	Whole grain and enriched cereal
	  products
	Liver, other organ meats
		Essential for:
		  Carbohydrate metabolism
		  Healthy appetite
		  Functioning of nerves

Riboflavin (B_2)	Milk, cheese
	Enriched bread and cereals
	Yeast
	Green, leafy vegetables
	Eggs
	Liver, kidney, heart
		Essential for:
		  Health of skin, eyes, and mouth
		  Carbohydrate, fat, and protein
		  metabolism

Niacin
(Nicotinic acid)
	Meats (especially organ meats)
	Poultry and fish
	Yeast
	Enriched breads and cereals
	Peanuts
		Essential for:
		  Prevention of pellagra
		  Carbohydrate, fat, and protein
		  metabolism

Vitamin B_6 (Pyridoxine)	Wheat germ Liver and kidney Meats Whole grain cereals Soybeans and peanuts	Essential for: Metabolism of proteins
Pantothenic Acid	Heart, liver, kidney Eggs Peanuts Whole grain cereals	Aids various steps in metabolism

(continues)

FIGURE 12-4 *(continued)*

Vitamins	Best Sources	Functions
Biotin	Organ meats Yeast Mushrooms Peanuts	Aids various steps in metabolism
Vitamin B$_{12}$ (Cobalamin)	Liver, kidney Muscle meats Milk, cheese Eggs	Essential for: Metabolism Healthy red blood cells Treatment of pernicious anemia
Folacin (Folic acid)	Dark green, leafy vegetables Liver, kidney Yeast	Essential for: The blood-forming system Metabolism

Malnutrition

Malnutrition is poor nourishment, which most often occurs when the body does not get a full, balanced diet. Early signs of malnutrition include muscle weakness and a constant feeling of tiredness or fatigue. Later symptoms include a distended or swollen abdomen, a dull film over the eyes, hair that is dry and brittle, and bones that become deformed. A state of malnutrition may occur after a person has gone on a severe weight-reducing diet. This condition is most often found among teenage girls who diet. After a time the lack of nutrients causes serious body fluid imbalances. It can reach a point where the dieter is unable to eat at all, and the body rejects all foods. It may be necessary to hospitalize the person and provide liquid nourishment through intravenous feedings. A long time may be needed before the body systems are again in balance.

The Importance of Water

One item that many people overlook in their daily diet is water. It is generally recommended that each individual drink 6 to 10 glasses of water daily. This is necessary for proper digestion; it also helps to maintain proper elimination. Wastes are eliminated from the body by the kidneys. This flushing process is helped by the amount of water taken into the body. Water keeps feces from becoming hardened and decreases chances of constipation. Water also prevents dehydration.

GENERAL GUIDELINES FOR MEAL PLANNING

There are some general rules to follow when planning nutritious meals for clients. In addition to the general rules listed, the aide should see that an emergency food supply is on hand. The home health aide should consider the ethnic and regional preferences of the client when planning a menu.

Eating Patterns

Generally, people expect to have three meals a day—breakfast, lunch (dinner), dinner (supper) (Figure 12-5). The midday and evening meals are a cultural choice. For example, farmers who work hard during planting and harvesting often expect and need a hot, full meal at noon. They expend so much effort in the morning that they need to replace energy at noon so they can go back to work. Office workers usually do not need nor want more than a light lunch. They usually prefer to have their main meal in the evening in the comfort of their homes. This gives them a chance to be with their families as they all enjoy a hot meal.

Some older people find that eating the main meal in the evening makes them uncomfortable. They find that they feel better having their main meal at midday and then eating a light meal in the evening. This relieves the feeling of heaviness and discomfort when they go to bed.

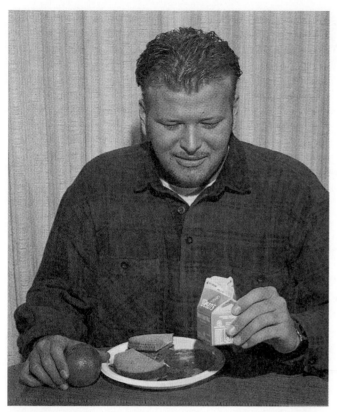

FIGURE 12-5 A man eating a balanced meal in a restaurant

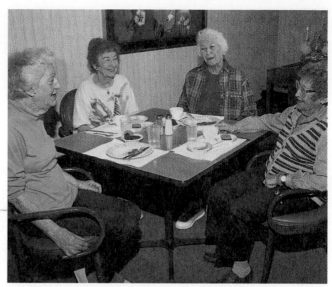

FIGURE 12-6 Many older adults enjoy a daily meal at their local senior citizens center.

Meals on Wheels (a service that brings hot meals to shut-ins and the elderly) usually provides the food at midday for this reason.

Some elderly who can ambulate prefer the companionship of a meal shared with friends at a local senior citizen center (Figure 12-6).

Some people prefer to have five or six smaller meals that can be divided into a light breakfast, an early light lunch, a midafternoon snack, a small dinner, and a late-night snack. Cancer patients are often encouraged to follow this practice. The aide should also remember that persons who are ill may lose their appetites as a result of their condition. Six small meals may be more comfortable for someone with this condition.

Food Allergies

The incidence of food allergies varies widely, from as little as 0.2% of the population to up to 50%. Food reactions are most common in infancy, diminishing in childhood and adulthood.

Food allergies can produce a range of symptoms including skin rashes, digestive tract problems, and respiratory disorders. Limited evidence suggests that food allergies can also affect a person's mood. However, most of the reactions people may experience from food are not allergies at all, but rather an intolerance to a particular food. A true **food allergy** is any negative reaction to a food, or a food component, that involves the immune system. The reaction can be immediate (within minutes to hours of eating the food), or delayed (symptoms do not appear for 6 to 24 hours after eating the food). Symptoms from a food allergy can be mild to life-threatening, depending on a person's tolerance and the amount of the food or food component ingested. Symptoms may include hives, rashes, breathing difficulties, sores in the mouth, bloating, and diarrhea.

Any food item can cause an allergic reaction; however, some of the food categories associated with an allergic response include chocolate, cow's milk, corn, eggs, fish, nuts, strawberries, tomatoes, and wheat. A person who cannot tolerate wheat must avoid all commercial products that contain wheat, including cakes, cookies, noodles and rice, breads, cereals, crackers, and canned soups. Dealing with allergies to basic foods such as milk, corn, or wheat requires the help of a dietitian to make sure that the diet remains nutritionally balanced.

Sometimes a person is allergic to a raw food, but has no difficulties with the same food if it is cooked. Those with a food allergy may also have an allergic reaction to foods in the same food family (Figure 12-7).

FIGURE 12-7   If you are intolerant or allergic to a food, you also may react to other foods in the same food family.

Food Families and Allergies
Plant Families
Apple: apple, crab apple, loquat, pear, quince *Citrus:* quince, grapefruit, lemon, orange, tangerine *Cola nut:* coffee, chocolate, cola drinks, tea *Goose foot:* beet, spinach, Swiss chard *Gourd:* cantaloupe, cucumber, melon, pumpkin, winter squash *Grass:* barley, corn, oats, rice, rye, wheat *Heath:* blueberry, cranberry, huckleberry, loganberry *Laurel:* avocado, bay leaf, cinnamon *Lily:* asparagus, garlic, leek, onion, sarsaparilla *Mint:* basil, bergamot, marjoram, peppermint, oregano, sage, savory, thyme *Cruciferous:* broccoli, cabbage, cauliflower, mustard, Brussels sprouts, turnip *Pea:* bean, soybean, lentil, pea, peanut, alfalfa, tamarind *Plum:* almond, apricot, blackberry, cherry, peach, plum *Rose:* blackberry, raspberry, strawberry *Sunflower:* artichoke, chamomile, chicory, endive, lettuce, sunflower *Walnut:* walnut, hickory nut, pecan
Animal Families
Birds: chicken, egg, duck, goose, pheasant, turkey *Crustaceans:* crab, crayfish, lobster, prawn, shrimp *Fish:* catfish, cod, flounder, halibut, mackerel, salmon, sardine, snapper, sole, trout, tuna *Mammals:* cow (milk), goat, lamb, pork, rabbit, sheep *Mollusks:* abalone, clam, cockle, oyster, scallop, mussel

(From *Food & Mood: The Complete Guide to Eating Well and Feeling Your Best* by Elizabeth Somer. Copyright © 1995 by Elizabeth Somer. Reprinted by permission of Henry Holt and Co.)

Some people, although not allergic to food per se, are allergic to the molds that grow on some foods. Mold allergies produce milder symptoms, such as headaches, fatigue, or nasal congestion. Beer, wine, canned tomato products, cheese, dried fruits, and certain types of breads are potential mold accumulators.

Food Preparation and Appeal

Foods may be prepared in a number of ways. They may be eaten raw. Some can be broiled, baked, fried, boiled, or steamed. Overcooking causes the loss of minerals, vitamins, and other nutrients. Some meats, particularly pork, ground beef and chicken, must be thoroughly cooked to kill any bacteria that may be present in the meat.

When planning and preparing food the home health aide must always remember that a menu should provide proper nutrition. This is the most important rule. Foods selected must fall within the limits of those foods allowed by the client's medical condition.

When planning and preparing meals, a home health aide should keep the following in mind:

- Variety
- Appearance
- Flavor and aroma
- Satiety (hunger satisfaction)
- Individual preferences (Figure 12-8)
- Food costs
- Balance

FIGURE 12-8 Traditional ethnic, regional, and racial food patterns

Ethnic Group	Bread and Cereal	Eggs, Meat, Fish, Poultry	Dairy Products	Fruits and Vegetables	Seasonings, Etc.
Chinese	Rice, wheat, millet, corn, noodles	Little meat and no beef, fish, including raw fish, eggs of hen, duck, pigeon	Water buffalo milk occasionally, soybean milk, cheese	Soybeans, soybean sprouts, bamboo sprouts, soy curd cooked in lime water, radish leaves, legumes, vegetables, fruits	Sesame seeds, ginger, almonds, soy sauce, sesame, soybean and peanut oils
African American	Hot breads, cookies, pastries, cakes, cereals, white rice, corn breads	Chicken, salt pork, ham, bacon, sausage, salted salmon, salt herring, fish	Milk and milk products, little cheese	Kale, mustard, turnip greens, cabbage, hominy grits, dandelion greens	Molasses, Deep frying
Jewish	Noodles, crusty white seeded rolls, rye bread, pumpernickel bread, challah, bagels	Koshered meat (from forequarters and organs from beef, lamb, veal), milk not eaten at same meal (not a rule for all Jewish people), fish, chicken	Milk and milk products, cheese	Vegetables (sometimes cooked with meat), fruits, cooked fruits (compote)	Salt, garlic, dill, parsley
Italian	Crusty white bread, cornmeal and rice (northern Italy), pasta (southern Italy)	Beef, veal, chicken, eggs, fish	Milk in coffee, cheese (many different kinds)	Broccoli, zucchini, other squash, eggplant, artichokes, string beans, tomatoes, peppers, asparagus, fresh fruit	Olive oil, vinegar, salt, pepper, garlic, basil, wine
Puerto Rican	Rice, beans, noodles, spaghetti, oatmeal, cornmeal	Dry salted codfish, meat, salt pork, sausage, chicken, beef	Coffee with hot milk	Starchy root vegetables, green bananas, plantain, legumes, tomatoes, green peppers, onions, pineapples, papayas, citrus fruits, corn	Lard, herbs, oil, vinegar, hot peppers

(continues)

	FIGURE 12-8 *(continued)*				
Ethnic Group	**Bread and Cereal**	**Eggs, Meat, Fish, Poultry**	**Dairy Products**	**Fruits and Vegetables**	**Seasonings, Etc.**
Near Eastern	Bulgur (wheat)	Lamb, mutton, chicken, fish, eggs	Fermented milk, sour cream, yogurt, cheese	Nuts, grape leaves	Sheep's butter, olive oil
Greek	Plain wheat bread	Lamb, pork, poultry, eggs, organ meats	Yogurt, cheeses, butter	Onions, tomatoes, legumes, fresh fruit	Olive oil, parsley, lemon, vinegar, olives
Mexican	Lime-treated corn, rice	Little meat (ground beef or pork), poultry, fish	Cheese, evaporated milk as beverage for infants	Pinto beans, tomatoes, potatoes, onions, lettuce	Chili pepper, salt, garlic, herbs

Variety. Variety is necessary to avoid dulling the appetite. People become bored with the same menu day after day. This can cause a loss of interest in food. It is important for sick people to receive appealing meals. The same nutrients can usually be obtained from a variety of foods. Variety in the menu helps improve the client's interest in eating.

Appearance. Appearance is the way food looks when it is served. Nicely arranged food adds to the pleasure and enjoyment of eating. When foods are overcooked they become mushy and unappetizing. At the same time, overcooking destroys many of the nutrients. Overcooked meats become tough and lose flavor. Foods that appeal to the eye perk up the appetite. Properly cooked vegetables, for example, retain their natural color. The color enhances the appearance of the vegetables on the plate. The attractiveness of the meal can be illustrated by two examples. Imagine a plate of food consisting of a chicken breast, mashed potatoes, white bread, and cauliflower. This meal would be nutritious but it would look dull and colorless. If the potatoes or cauliflower were replaced by a garden salad and string beans, the meal would look much brighter and more appealing.

Flavor and Aroma. Flavor and aroma set the digestive juices into action. Seasonings most of-

ten used are salt, pepper, and garlic. However, many herbs, such as thyme, rosemary, parsley, sage, and basil, can be added to bring out the aroma and sharpen the flavor. Often these herbs and spices can be used when a client is on a salt-free diet. Fresh lemon juice can be squeezed over meat and vegetables also. Because both sight and smell affect the appetite, proper use of seasonings can be of value in planning a menu.

Satiety. Satisfying the pangs of hunger is another reason people eat. Some foods make the stomach feel full but not uncomfortable. This feeling is called satiety. If daily menus are well planned, the satiety value will be provided. Bulk foods such as bread, macaroni, beans, and spaghetti are good fillers.

Individual Preferences. An important factor in meal planning is providing foods the client likes to eat. There is no logic to explain why some people like certain foods and dislike others. Some individuals want steak served rare; others will only eat it well done. Some people dislike spinach, cabbage, beets, or mushrooms. The home health aide must try to prepare foods the client likes, cooked as the client likes them.

Food Costs. In most homes, it is necessary to work within a budget. Therefore, it is important to check newspaper ads for daily specials, coupons, and seasonal bargains. Fresh fruits and vegetables are lower in price during the summer and fall. At other times it is more economical to purchase frozen, canned, or dried items. If money is a consideration, then planning and purchasing must balance. All six food groups that appear in the food pyramid should be included daily, although oils, fats, and sweets should be used sparingly. Careful planning makes it possible to meet nutritional needs while keeping costs at a minimum.

DIET THERAPY

Certain medical conditions require special diets. The home health aide must carefully follow directions in preparing special diets. The aide should try to vary the menus and make the food look attractive. Flavor and aroma of the food should be maintained. Meals should satisfy hunger while considering the client's food preferences. However, it may not always be possible to meet all of these conditions. Occasionally the client may beg the home health aide for "just a little taste" of a forbidden food. At such times, the aide should gently and kindly refuse the client's request. An answer to such a plea might be, "I know you would rather have something else, but it would not be wise to go off your special diet. See if the dietitian will add new foods." An attractively arranged tray may stimulate the appetite of a client whose diet is limited.

Special Diets

Special diets may be ordered by the doctor to meet a client's specific health needs. A description of some special diets follows. Figure 12-9 lists recommended foods and foods to avoid for these special diets.

Low-Fat (Low-Cholesterol) Diet. A low-fat diet is required for those with heart disease and gallbladder conditions.

FIGURE 12-9	Special diets		
Diet	**General Use**	**Foods Allowed**	**Foods to Limit/or Avoid**
Low-calorie	Overweight	Skim milk, fresh fruits, lean meat or fish, vegetables, 1–2 servings of cereal per day	Fried foods, rich gravies and sauces, jams, jellies, rich desserts
High-calorie	Underweight	Peanut butter, eggnog, jellies, ice cream, desserts, frequent snacks, milk shakes	None
Bland	Stomach or intestinal precaution; ulcers	Eat three well-balanced meals.	Highly seasoned, fried foods, raw vegetables and fruit, whole grains and cereals, spices such as chili peppers or powder, black pepper, red pepper, caffeinated and alcoholic beverages. Decaffeinated coffee or tea will be served according to individual tolerance.

(continues)

FIGURE 12-9 *(continued)*

Diet	General Use	Foods Allowed	Foods to Limit/or Avoid
Diabetic	Diabetes	Canned fruits in natural juices, fresh fruits, regular meat, vegetables, bread, sugarless gelatin, custards	Foods containing sugar, alcoholic beverages, gravy, sauces, chocolate; sweetened carbonated beverages
Low-sodium	Fluid retention; heart problems; high blood pressure	Foods cooked without salt, regular meat, vegetables, fruits, salt substitute (are not recommended in renal conditions)	Smoked, cured, canned fish and meats, cold cuts, cheese, potato chips, pretzels, pickles, bouillon, prepared mustard, catsup, commercial salad dressings, soy sauce
Low-fat, low cholesterol	Heart disease; liver disease; gallbladder	Veal, poultry, fish, skim milk, buttermilk, yogurt, low-fat cottage cheese, fat-free soup broth, fresh fruits and vegetables, cereals, gelatin, angel cake, ices, carbonated beverages, coffee, tea, jams, jellies	Fatty meats, bacon, butter, whole milk, cheese, kidney, liver, heart, fried foods, rich desserts, sauces
Clear-liquid	Preoperative or postoperative	Tea or black coffee with sugar, apple juice, plain gelatin (no fruit), clear broth or bouillon	Solid foods
Full-liquid	Gastrointestinal problems; chewing problems	All foods in clear-liquid diet, strained juices, milk, cream, buttermilk, eggnog, strained cream soups, strained cereal, cocoa, carbonated beverages, ices, ice cream, gelatin, custard puddings, sherbets, milk shakes, bouillon, yogurt	Solid foods
Soft, mild	Gastrointestinal conditions; chewing problems	Milk, cream, butter, mild cheeses (cottage, cream cheeses), eggs (not fried), soup, broth, strained cream soups, tender cooked vegetables, fruit juices, cooked fruits, bananas, grapefruit and oranges peeled with all section skins removed, white bread, cereals, cooked cereals, spaghetti, noodles, macaroni, pasta, tea, coffee, carbonated beverages, sherbets, ices, sponge cake, tender chicken, fish, ground beef or lamb, only small amounts of salt and spices	Fibrous meat, coarse cereals, fried foods, raw fruits and vegetables, rich pastries

(continues)

FIGURE 12-9 *(continued)*			
Diet	General Use	Foods Allowed	Foods to Limit/or Avoid
Pureed	Difficulty or discomfort in swallowing	All semisolid foods, foods put through a blender, and liquids of a viscous nature such as nectars	Sticky foods such as peanut butter or melted cheese, thin liquids such as water
Low-residue	Postoperative; colitis; diverticulitis	Milk, buttermilk, butter, mild cheeses, tender chicken, fish, ground beef, ground lamb, soup broths, fruit juices, breads and cereals, macaroni, noodles, custards, sherbet, vanilla ice cream, sponge cake, plain cookies, strained and cooked vegetables	Fried foods, fresh fruits and vegetables, fibrous meats, nuts, seeds
High-fiber	Constipation	Whole grain breads and cereals, raw and cooked vegetables, fruit juices, dried beans, bran or bran flakes, nuts, seeds, and dried fruits	
High-potassium	Potassium loss due to medication	Fresh fruits and vegetables, especially bananas and raisins	Canned tomato juice, raw clams, sardines, frozen lima beans, frozen peas, canned spinach, canned carrots

NOTE: This chart is a general guide to special diets. Always follow the dietitian's prescribed diet plan.

Diabetic Diet. A **diabetic diet** calls for using measured amounts of the foods allowed on the food pyramid. All foods must be carefully measured. Sugar or foods high in sugar such as sugar-cured ham and many sweetened, dry cereals must be limited or avoided. A special diet list is supplied by the dietitian. Refer to Unit 20 for a detailed discussion of diabetes.

Calorie-Controlled Diet. A **calorie-controlled diet** may be ordered for an obese person or a malnourished person. The calorie count is very low for the obese person and high for the person who is underweight. The individual client's needs and characteristics (age, sex, height, type of work done, and weight) determine the size of the portion served and the total intake of calories. For example, very active children burn more calories per day than an aging person who is confined to bed. Whatever the size of the servings or the prescribed caloric

intake, proper selections must be made from the food pyramid.

Bland Diet. A person with a peptic ulcer is kept on a **bland diet.** The foods allowed are served without strong spices; caffeinated and alcoholic beverages should be limited or avoided.

Low-Residue Diet. A **low-residue diet** is one in which tough fiber foods are kept at a minimum. It is low in vitamins and is used only as long as needed to clear up a condition in the intestinal tract. Clients with colitis or diverticulitis may be on low-residue diets. There is very little waste product in this diet. Examples of food allowed in the low-residue diet are strained and cooked vegetables, custards, mild cheeses, and tender meats.

High-Potassium Diet. Persons with high blood pressure are treated with a drug called a **diuretic.** A diuretic helps to lower blood pressure by washing salt from the body. However, it may cause potassium to be flushed from the body. The loss of potassium may cause muscle cramps and muscular weakness. Some older persons taking diuretics or persons taking the drug digitalis may also need added potassium in their diets. Very often this can be provided by eating foods high in potassium. Most fruits are high in potassium; bananas, oranges, and raisins are especially high in potassium. Fresh vegetables, raw or cooked, are also good sources of natural potassium and are included in a high-potassium diet.

Liquid Diet. A person recovering from an illness, injury, or a surgical operation may require a light, easily digested diet. Especially after surgery, the body needs to be treated very carefully. Postsurgical patients are usually put on a **clear liquid diet.** Liquids that one can see through and are easy to digest such as broth, tea, and apple juice are given. As the client becomes better, a **full-liquid diet** is prescribed. Milk, pudding, and strained cream soups are added to the clear liquid diet.

Soft Diet. After the client is able to tolerate a full liquid diet, the **soft diet** is prescribed. Soft-boiled eggs, toast, and other easily digested foods are added. As the body heals, the client can gradually return to eating a regular diet. Clients with chewing problems or gastrointestinal conditions may also be on a soft diet.

Pureed Diet. A diet for an individual with difficulty or discomfort in swallowing. A **pureed diet** consisting of thickened liquids is designed to facilitate the ease of swallowing and reduce the risk of aspiration.

High-Fiber Diet. Another special diet is the **high-fiber diet.** Elderly clients or clients on bed rest are often prescribed high-fiber diets. Fiber is helpful for providing good bowel elimination.

Vegetarian Diet. **Vegetarians** (people who eat only vegetables, fruit, grains, eggs, dairy products, and nuts) are increasing in number in the United States, especially among the young adults. (Some vegetarians omit dairy products, others omit just red meats.) People become vegetarians for many different reasons including religious, ethical, cultural, and financial considerations. If you have a client who requires this type of diet, more time will be required for meal planning and preparation than for a regular diet.

AIDS Diet. Clients with AIDS generally need a nutrient-dense diet high in protein and calories. An extra liquid nutritional supplement (special concentrated drink that contains all the essential nutrients) is often included. Using liquid nutritional products to supplement regular food intake can offset the client's decreased intake of calories (Figure 12-10). The AIDS client will need more frequent meals and regular snacks. As a home health aide, you will need to be aware of the client's likes and dislikes. In general, highly seasoned and spicy foods and very hot or very cold foods should be avoided. In some cases, bland or dry food may be more readily tolerated. A few AIDS clients may request low-fat foods rather than foods high in fat content. Fad diets should be discouraged. The goal is to provide a balanced, nutrient-packed diet that allows for individual food preferences with an adequate intake of protein and calories for the body needs.

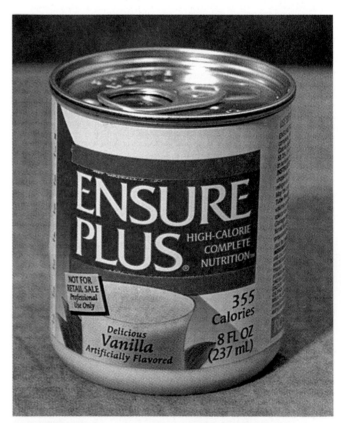

FIGURE 12-10 Extra nourishment can be obtained by the use of special nutrient drinks.

Low-Sodium (Sodium-Restricted) Diet. Low-sodium diets are prepared without salt. They may be prescribed when the client has a heart condition, kidney disease, or hypertension. Some clients on a low-sodium diet are able to use salt substitutes with the doctor's permission.

Experts recommend that the daily intake of sodium (salt) be limited to 2400 to 5000 mg. This amount includes sodium that is added to processed foods or that occurs naturally in foods.

Salt Use. Table salt contains sodium and chloride—both are essential in the diet. However, most Americans eat more salt and sodium than they need. Food and beverages containing salt provide most of the sodium in our diets, much of it added during processing and manufacturing.

In populations with diets low in salt, high blood pressure is less common than in populations with diets high in salt. Other factors that affect blood pressure are heredity, obesity, and excessive drinking of alcoholic beverages.

In the United States, about one in three adults has high blood pressure. If these people restrict their salt, sodium, and chloride, usually their blood pressure will fall.

Some people who do not have high blood pressure may reduce their risk of getting it by eating a diet with less salt and other sources of sodium. At present there is no way to predict who might develop high blood pressure and who will benefit from reducing dietary salt and sodium. However, it is wise for most people to eat less salt and sodium because they need much less than they eat and reduction will benefit those people whose blood pressure rises with salt intake.

To Moderate Use of Salt and Sodium.
- Use salt sparingly, if at all, in cooking and at the table.
- When planning meals, consider that
  —Fresh and plain frozen vegetables prepared without salt are lower in sodium than canned ones.
  —Cereals, pasta, and rice cooked without salt are lower in sodium than ready-to-eat cereals.
  —Milk and yogurt are lower in sodium than most cheeses.
  —Fresh meat, poultry, and fish are lower in sodium than most canned and processed ones.
  —Most frozen dinners and combination dishes, packaged mixes, canned soups, and salad dressings contain a considerable amount of sodium. Condiments such as soy and other sauces, pickles, olives, catsup, and mustard are also high in sodium.
- Use salted snacks, such as chips, crackers, pretzels, and nuts, sparingly.
- Check labels for the amount of sodium in foods. Choose those lower in sodium most of the time.

FEEDING THE CLIENT

On occasion, it may be necessary for the aide to assist with feeding the client to provide the proper nutrition for the client who is unable to feed him or herself, or who needs assistance with feeding. Eating should be a pleasant and enjoyable experience for a client. The foods should be served with "hot foods hot, and cold foods cold." Food should be served attractively. If possible, have the client eat in a pleasant environment (Figure 12-11) and preferably not in the bedroom. Procedure 17 demonstrates the proper way to feed the client.

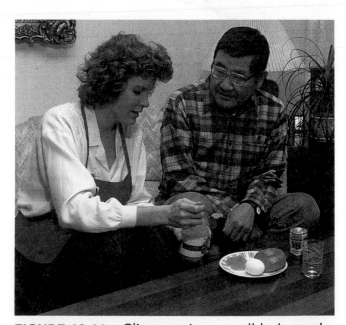

FIGURE 12-11 Client eating a well-balanced meal prepared by the home health aide. The environment is made as pleasant as possible to promote enjoyment of the meal.

CLIENT CARE PROCEDURE

17

Feeding the Client

PURPOSE

- To provide proper nutrition for clients who are unable to feed themselves or who need assistance in feeding
- To provide suitable food, based on client's condition, meeting standards of the food guide pyramid
- To provide a pleasurable experience for the client
- To encourage client to use adaptive devices for feeding

If the client needs to be fed, it is desirable that the client be sitting up in a chair (Figure 12-12). If this is not feasible, you can position the client up in bed with the use of a few pillows. The food will be digested better if the client is in a sitting position. It is recommended that the aide sit while feeding and be at the eye level of the client.

Most clients will prefer to feed themselves if possible. Many different feeding devices available today make this possible (Figure 12-13).

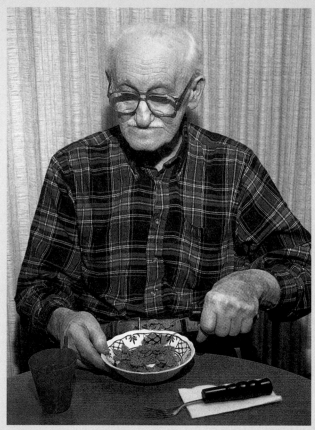

FIGURE 12-13 Client feeds himself using special feeding devices.

The feeding device will need to be chosen according to the client's disability.

If your client chokes easily, it may be recommended to mix a thickener in the liquid foods (see Pureed Diet, Figure 12-9). Clients do choke more readily on thinner liquids than thick liquids. If the client has a poor appetite and is becoming malnourished, it is advisable to offer high-calorie and high-protein drinks often throughout the day.

Some clients are fed through a feeding tube inserted through an opening in the abdominal wall (Figure 12-14A). A special control apparatus monitors the rate at which fluid nourishment is supplied to the client (Figure 12-14B). It is the nurse's responsibil-

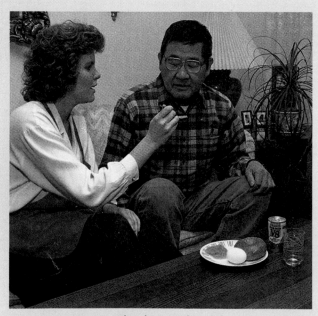

FIGURE 12-12 The home health aide should feed the client slowly, one food at a time.

(continues)

CLIENT CARE PROCEDURE **Feeding the Client** *(continued)*

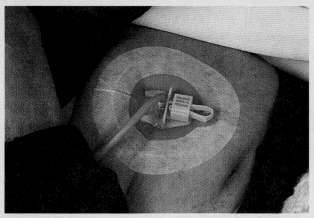

FIGURE 12-14A If the client is unable to eat, a feeding tube may be inserted into a client's stomach to maintain proper nutrition. The nurse inserts the feeding tube into the client's stomach.

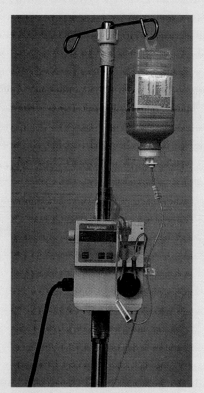

FIGURE 12-14B The feeding tube is regulated with a special monitor placed on a pole. It is the nurse's responsibility to teach the family how to administer and monitor a tube feeding.

ity to teach the family how to administer and monitor a tube feeding.

PROCEDURE

1. Wash your hands.
2. Prepare the client to eat. Wash the client's face and hands. Position client in sitting position in bed or sitting up in a chair. Make environment as pleasant as possible. If necessary, do mouth care before to increase the client's desire to eat. Place large napkin over client's chest.
3. Bring food to client. Tell client what foods you have prepared.
4. How you feed or assist your client depends on the handicap or physical problem the client has. If the client is blind, you need to tell the client where each food is on the plate in relation to a clock. If the client has use of only one hand, a suction plate or plate guard may be used. If the client cannot chew food, the food will need to be soft in consistency.
   CAUTION: The client should never be given cause to be embarrassed because of any physical disability.
5. Ask the client which food is desired first. (Getting the client's cooperation and participation is important.)
6. If the client must be fed by the aide, remember:
   - Check to see if dentures are in place.
   - Feed slowly; let the client set the pace. Thermal bowls and cups will assist in keeping foods at proper temperature.
   - Feed small amounts of food at a time.
   - Make sure the consistency of the food is appropriate.
   - Do not use a syringe to feed the client. A child's feeder cup or plastic glass works well in this situation.
   - If possible, have client hold finger foods or bread.

REVIEW

1. List the six groups of food on the food guide pyramid.

2. Name four considerations for making the client's meals appealing.

3. Name six special diets that may be ordered to meet a client's specific health need.

4. A client with a gallbladder problem may be placed on what type of special diet? *Lot Fat – Low Chol*

5. Foods cooked without salt are to be included in what type of special diet? *Blood pressure*

6. What type of foods should be omitted in a diet for a client with hypertension?

7. A client's appetite may be increased when (s)he is:
   a. Served food (s)he likes
   b. Eating alone
   c. Smelling bad odors
   d. Inactive
   e. Experiencing pain

8. One guide for adequate nutrition is the food pyramid plan. The type of foods included in the six groups are:
   a. Milk, meat, vegetables-fruit, and bread-cereals
   b. Bread-cereal, fruit, vegetables, milk-cheese, meat-poultry, oils-sweets
   c. Bread-cereal, milk, protein, vegetables, and fruits
   d. Milk, bread, cereal, meat, and vegetables

9. Identify, by circling, the two items on each tray that should *not* be on the listed special diet:

   Low Cholesterol
   batter-fried fish fillets
   baked potatoes with sour cream
   steamed green beans
   angel food cake with
      fresh raspberries

   Clear Liquid
   apricot nectar
   beef broth
   cherry gelatin cubes
   apple juice
   coffee with cream and sugar

10. Clients with heart problems are usually placed on:
    a. Low-sugar diet
    b. Low-salt diet
    c. Low-protein diet
    d. None of the above

11. Clients with AIDS need to be on a diet that is _____ and _____ .

12. Place a letter, which best represents the nutrient function in Column II, with the appropriate nutrient name in Column I.

Column I	Column II
___ 1. vitamin B_{12}	a. essential for normal blood clotting
___ 2. vitamin K	b. regulates calcium and phosphorus metabolism
___ 3. vitamin C	c. use in treatment of pernicious anemia

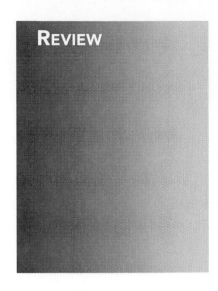

REVIEW

___ 4. vitamin D

___ 5. vitamin B$_1$

d. essential to maintain strength of blood vessels

e. essential for carbohydrate metabolism

13. A client with severe hypertension asks you to prepare soup and a salami sandwich for lunch. Is this a good idea? What steps could you take to encourage your client to make healthy food choices?

14. You are making a visit to a new client who appears to be quite thin. You notice that there is not much food in her cupboard or in the refrigerator. In her freezer are several packages of frozen dinners. Is this client at risk for malnutrition? What steps could you take to ensure that your client receives adequate nutrition?

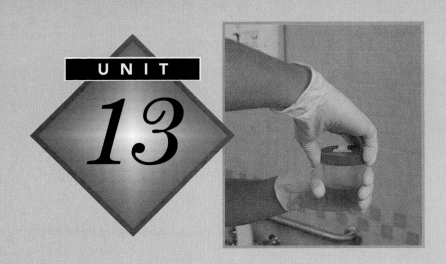

UNIT 13

Elimination

KEY TERMS

bladder
clean-catch specimen
constipation
cystitis
detrusor instability
enema

impaction
incontinent
kidney
kidney stones
ostomy bag
perineum

stoma
suppository
urinary catheter
ureters
urethra

LEARNING OBJECTIVES

After studying this unit, you should be able to:

- Identify the structures of male and female urinary tracts.
- Describe three types of urinary incontinence.
- Demonstrate the following:

URINARY SYSTEM

The urinary system consists of the kidneys, ureters, bladder, and urethra (Figure 13-1). The **kidneys** are the primary organs of this system. Their function is to filter waste material from the bloodstream. As the blood passes through the kidneys, it undergoes a purifying and recycling process; waste material and excess water are filtered from it. As the blood continues through the kidneys, much of the filtered water and some minerals are reabsorbed into the bloodstream. This reabsorption is necessary to maintain the body's liquid balance. The waste material and excess water (now called urine) pass from the kidneys into the bladder through tubes called **ureters.** The **bladder** is a muscular organ for storing urine. When the bladder has accumulated about a pint of urine, nerves sense discomfort. Involuntary muscle contractions of the bladder then empty the urine into the **urethra**, a tube that empties urine from the bladder. These muscular contractions can be controlled and do become voluntary to a large extent. The normal daily output of urine is 1500 to 2000 mL (1½ to 2 quarts).

COMMON DISORDERS OF THE URINARY SYSTEM

Incontinence, cystitis, and kidney stones are three common disorders of the urinary system.

Incontinence

Some individuals have no voluntary control of their bladder muscles. This causes them to be **incontinent,** or to expel urine unexpectedly. Incontinence occurs in babies before toilet training because they have not yet developed control over the muscles in the urethra.

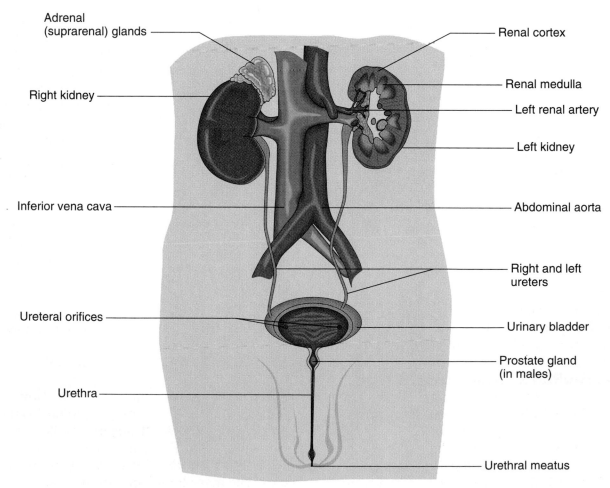

Adrenal (suprarenal) glands
Renal cortex
Right kidney
Renal medulla
Left renal artery
Left kidney
Inferior vena cava
Abdominal aorta
Right and left ureters
Ureteral orifices
Urinary bladder
Prostate gland (in males)
Urethra
Urethral meatus

FIGURE 13-1 The urinary system

According to Newman and Jakovac-Smith:

Stress incontinence refers to the involuntary loss of small amounts of urine during activities that increase intra-abdominal pressure, such as coughing, running, laughing, or lifting heavy objects. Typically caused by weakened pelvic floor muscles or a weakened or damaged urethral sphincter, stress incontinence is most common in women but may affect men following prostate surgery.

Urge incontinence refers to the involuntary loss of urine because of the inability to reach the bathroom in time. Most common in older adults, this type of incontinence usually is caused by weakened pelvic floor muscles, tumor, kidney or bladder stones, or diverticula. **Detrusor instability** (unstable bladder) is associated with disorders of the lower urinary tract or neurologic system, including multiple sclerosis and diabetes.

Overflow incontinence refers to the continuous or periodic dribbling of urine because of an atonic bladder [bladder that has lost tone], or an anatomic obstruction, such as an enlarged prostate or a urethral stricture. This type of incontinence accounts for 10% to 15% of all incontinent clients.

Functional incontinence refers to involuntary urination because of the inability to reach a bathroom due to a specific disability, such as a physical or cognitive impairment, an inaccessible toilet, inattentive or inaccessible caregivers, or an unwillingness to move. This type of incontinence, which accounts for 25% of all incontinent clients, is common after admission to an acute care hospital.

D. Newman and D. A. Jakovac-Smith, *Geriatric Care Plans* (Springhouse Corp., 1991), p. 128. Figure 13-2 provides an illustrative guide to help you understand and remember the causes of incontinence.

It is important that the home health aide is aware of the potential for skin breakdown resulting from exposure to urine leakage. Figure 13-3 shows a sample nursing care plan that addresses the signs and symptoms, interventions, and rationales to reduce the potential for impaired skin integrity resulting from urinary incontinence.

Cystitis

Cystitis occurs when the membrane lining of the urinary bladder becomes inflamed. It can be caused by bacterial infection or a kidney inflammation that has spread to the bladder. This condition usually results in painful urination. It is generally treated with medication.

Kidney Stones

Kidney stones are usually caused by an excess of calcium. The urine becomes crystallized (hardened) and stones may block the ureters and cause painful urination. A new technique is available now for some clients, whereby the stones can be destroyed by sound waves rather than by surgery.

CLIENT CARE PROCEDURES

The remainder of this unit addresses commonly performed client care procedures that are related to the elimination system. In some states, home health aides are not allowed to do each of the procedures described. It is important that you check with your agency to clarify those procedures that will be your responsibility and those responsibilities that belong to other members of the team.

Measuring and Recording Fluids

Intake is a measure of all the fluids or semiliquids that a person drinks. Output is all the fluid that passes out of the body. The abbreviation for measuring fluid intake and output is I&O. This may be done for a person who has heart or kidney disease. Procedure 18 demonstrates the proper method for measuring and recording fluid intake and output.

Giving and Emptying the Bedpan or Urinal

The bedpan is used for clients who are confined to bed. The bedpan should be given whenever the client requests it. The client may be undergoing retraining to establish bowel and bladder continence. The aide should follow a regular schedule of offering the bedpan or urinal. If the client does

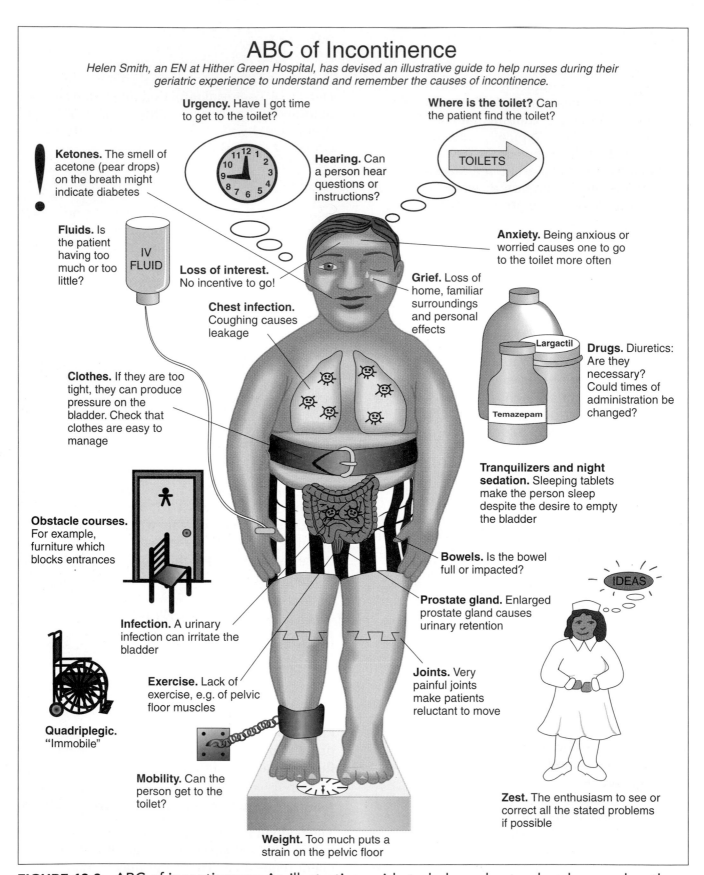

FIGURE 13-2 ABC of incontinence: An illustrative guide to help understand and remember the causes of incontinence. (Reproduced by kind permission of *Nursing Times* where this was first published on November 13, 1985.)

FIGURE 13-3   Sample care plan for impaired skin integrity

Nursing diagnosis: *Potential for impaired skin integrity related to urinary incontinence*

NURSING GOAL: To prevent skin breakdown caused by exposure to urine leakage

Signs and symptoms

- Frequent incontinence
- Itching and burning in the groin or on the upper thighs and buttocks
- Excoriated epidermis
- Pain over the entire affected area
- Ammonia body odor

Interventions	Rationales
1. Assess the client's perineum for signs of skin breakdown, rash, or infection.	1. Constant moisture in the perineal area can cause skin softening and infection.
2. Wash the affected area with mild soap and warm water whenever the client's clothing or pad is changed.	2. Cleaning the skin of urine prevents odor and the breakdown of the epidermal layer.
3. Apply a moisture barrier cream to the affected area.	3. Moisture barrier creams help protect sensitive skin from irritation and possible breakdown.
4. Apply vitamin E oil from capsules to reddened areas.	4. Vitamin E soothes rashes and excoriated (abraded) areas.
5. Instruct the client or caregiver to change saturated pads or diapers promptly.	5. Heavy, wet pads or diapers promote chafing and excoriation.
6. Dry the client's skin thoroughly and apply cornstarch to the affected area.	6. Thorough drying and cornstarch applications protect the skin from softening.
7. Inspect the client's skin frequently.	7. Frequent inspection is necessary to ensure early detection of skin breakdown, which can lead to pressure sores, urinary tract infections, and systemic sepsis.
8. Advise the female client to avoid using feminine hygiene deodorants on the affected area.	8. Certain ingredients, such as alcohol, in commercial products may cause an allergic response—for example, a rash, that can lead to skin breakdown.
9. Review incontinence management methods, such as condom catheters, external drainage systems, and behavioral interventions, with the client and caregiver.	9. Such methods may be necessary to ensure continence and prevent the possibility of skin breakdown.
10. Frequent toileting routine.	10. Helps maintain continence.

OUTCOME CRITERIA

- The client's skin will remain intact.
- The client and caregiver will perform necessary self-care measures to prevent skin breakdown.

(From Kashak-Neuman, D., Jakovac-Smith, D. A., *Geriatric Care Plans,* 1991, Springhouse Corporation. Reprinted with permission.)

not remember to ask, the home health aide should offer to bring the bedpan or urinal. The aide can politely remind the client by asking, "Do you need to use the bedpan or urinal?"

Procedures 19 and 20 demonstrate the proper way to give and empty a bedpan and urinal. A female client will use the bedpan for both urinating and defecating. A male client will

CLIENT CARE PROCEDURE

18

Measuring and Recording Fluid Intake and Output

PURPOSE

• To identify food items that need to be measured for fluid intake
• To measure and record fluid intake and output accurately

NOTE: Figure 13-4 shows the fluids that should be included in the measurement of intake and output.

Measure for Intake

ice	water
juices	pop
coffee	ice cream
yogurt	soup
jello	pudding
any other food that is liquid at room temperature	

Measure for Output

vomitus (emesis)	liquid stools
urine	
blood or drainage from wounds	

FIGURE 13-4 Various fluids and substances are measured and recorded as intake and output.

PROCEDURE

1. Assemble supplies:
   measuring cup or container for intake
   large measuring container for output
   disposable gloves
2. Wash hands and apply gloves if measuring output.
3. Measure and record all liquids taken by the client (Figure 13-5). This includes all fluids taken with meals and between meals: coffee, milk, fruit juices, beer, and water. Liquids are recorded in cubic centimeters, abbreviated cc (Figure 13-6). You need to remember that 30 cc equals 1 ounce. (One cc equals one mL.) Example:

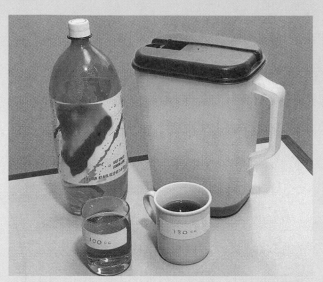

FIGURE 13-5   It is a good idea to measure the cubic centimeter (cc) capacity of commonly used glasses and cups. This will be helpful in recording the intake of a client.

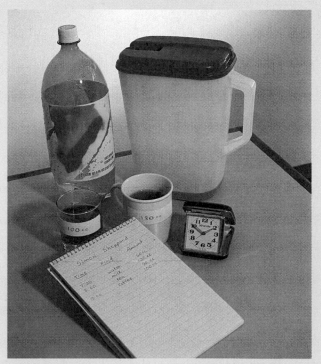

FIGURE 13-6   Intake is recorded in cubic centimeters (cc) after the client has drunk the liquid.   *(continues)*

CLIENT CARE PROCEDURE **Measuring and Recording Fluid Intake and Output** *(continued)*

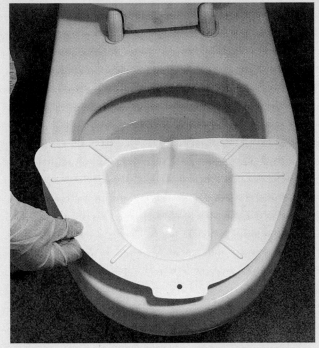

FIGURE 13-7 If a client's urine needs to be measured, a special toilet insert (potty hat) may be used to collect the urine.

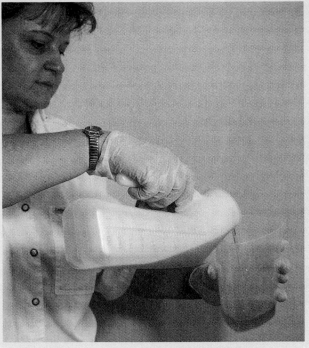

FIGURE 13-8 Urine can be measured with a special plastic container or a large measuring cup.

If a client drank a can of pop that is 12 ounces, you need to multiply 12 by 30, which equals 360 cc.

4. Ask the client to use a urinal or bedpan for all voiding. If the client can use the toilet, a special plastic hat can be placed in the toilet to collect the urine (Figure 13-7). All urine must be collected so that it can be measured.

5. Pour urine from bedpan or urinal into a measuring device (Figure 13-8). Record the amount. Always record output in cc.

6. Be sure to explain to the client how to keep exact records. The client will need to record the fluids at times when the aide is off duty.

7. Clean equipment after each use.

8. Remove gloves and wash hands.

need a urinal if he needs to urinate. If the client is very small or has a body cast, a smaller bedpan or fracture pan can be used.

Collecting a Urine Specimen

A **clean-catch specimen** is requested to obtain a urine sample that is as free of contamination as possible. This is required to provide a urine sample for a diagnostic test and to ensure that the test results are as accurate as possible. Procedure 21 demonstrates the correct way to collect a clean-catch urine specimen.

Caring for Catheters

A **urinary catheter** is a tube inserted into the bladder to drain urine. Germs can easily enter the bladder while the catheter is in place. Therefore, cleaning around the urinary opening is important. The catheter is inserted by the nurse. The catheter is replaced weekly or once a month. Procedure 22 demonstrates the proper way to care for a urinary catheter.

The leg urinary collection bag is smaller than the bedside urinary collection bag to provide a smaller collection bag for the client when out of

CLIENT CARE PROCEDURE

19

Giving and Emptying the Bedpan

PURPOSE

- To provide for routine elimination of bladder and bowels
- To observe or measure urinary or fecal output

PROCEDURE

1. Assemble equipment and supplies needed (Figures 13-9 and 13-10):
   disposable gloves
   bedpan and bedpan cover
   toilet tissue
   moistened washcloth
2. Wash hands and apply gloves.

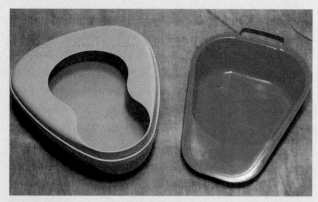

FIGURE 13-9 Regular bedpan (*left*) and fracture bedpan (*right*)

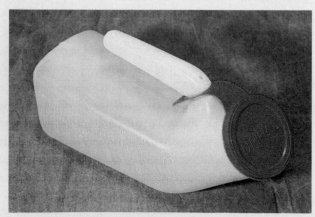

FIGURE 13-10 Male urinal

3. Tell client what you plan to do.
4. If a metal bedpan is used, first warm it by running hot water over the rim. Dry the rim and sprinkle it with powder if available. The powder prevents the client's buttocks from sticking to the bedpan.
5. Place bedpan near the bed. Put toilet tissue near the client's hand.
6. Fold top blanket and sheet at an angle. Remove the client's bottom clothing.
7. To raise the buttocks, have the client bend knees and push on the heels. As the client lifts, place your hand under the small of the client's back.
8. Lift gently and slowly with one hand. Slide the bedpan under the hips with the other hand. The client's buttocks should rest on the rounded shelf of the bedpan. The narrow end should face the foot of the bed. If the client cannot assist, turn the client to one side and position the bedpan over the buttocks (Figure 13-11). Roll the client onto the bedpan. The aide

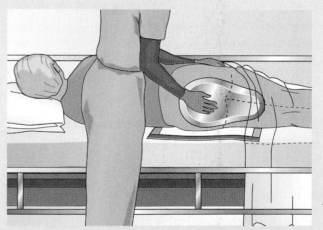

FIGURE 13-11 Roll client away from you while supporting client with one hand on client's hip and arm. Place bedpan with the other hand. Then roll client back onto bedpan. *(continues)*

CLIENT CARE PROCEDURE **Giving and Emptying the Bedpan** *(continued)*

holds the bedpan in place when the client is lying on his or her backside and then turns the client. Make sure the client's head is elevated.

9. Pull sheet over the client for added privacy. Make sure the client is as comfortable as possible. An extra pillow under the head may be used.

10. While client is using the bedpan, the aide can be moistening the washcloth.

11. Remove the bedpan when the client is finished using it. Do not leave the client sitting on the bedpan for longer than 15 minutes. Remove the bedpan by having the client bend the knees and push on the heels. Place one hand under small of client's back and lift. Remove the bedpan with the other hand.

12. If possible, have client wipe him or herself. If client is not able to do this, the aide must wipe the client. Discard tissues in the bedpan.

13. Replace the client's clothing. Give client washcloth to wipe hands.

14. Take bedpan to toilet, observe contents and measure if necessary. Empty contents into toilet. Flush. Fill bedpan with cold water and empty. Clean bedpan by using warm soapy water and the toilet brush. Empty water into toilet and rinse bedpan. Dry well.

15. Return bedpan to proper storage area.

16. Remove gloves and wash hands.

17. Record color and amount of urine; color, amount, and consistency of stool.

CLIENT CARE PROCEDURE

20

Giving and Emptying the Urinal

PURPOSE

- To provide for routine elimination of urine for a male client

PROCEDURE

1. Wash your hands and apply gloves.

2. Lift the top bedcovers and place the urinal under the covers so that the client can grasp the handle. If he cannot do this, you must place the urinal in position and ensure that the penis is placed in the opening of the urinal. If possible assist the client to stand when using the urinal.

3. Remove gloves and dispose of them properly. Leave client alone if possible. You may give the client a bell to ring when he is done.

4. Put on gloves and remove urinal once client is done using it.

5. Take the urinal to the bathroom and observe contents. Measure if required. Empty the urinal. Rinse with cold water and clean with soapy water. Rinse with disinfectant or water; dry, store properly.

6. Remove gloves and wash hands.

7. Record amount and color of urine, as required.

---

bed. The leg bag is attached to the client's thigh (upper leg). The leg bag allows for greater mobility for the client, but must be emptied more frequently. A client may use the leg bag while in the wheelchair or ambulating, and it can be connected to the bedside draining bag when in bed for the night. The leg bag must be rinsed according to agency policy and hung in the bathroom to drain (over bathtub towel bar). A clean cap or stopper must be used at the end of the

CLIENT CARE PROCEDURE

21

Collecting a Clean-Catch Urine Specimen

PROCEDURE

1. Assemble needed supplies:
   disposable gloves
   sterile urine specimen container with completed label
   plastic or resealable bag and paper bag
   clean bedpan or urinal
   antiseptic soaked wipes
2. Wash hands and apply gloves.
3. Inform client of what you plan to do.
4. Wash the client's genital area or have the client do so, if able. It is especially important for the urinary opening to be cleansed.
5. Give the client a labeled specimen container.
6. Explain the procedure to the client.
7. Have the client begin to void into the bedpan, urinal, or toilet. After a small amount of urine has been voided, have the client catch some of the urine in midstream in the sterile specimen container. You will only need 2 ounces, or 60 cc. After the specimen has been collected, the client can resume voiding into the bedpan, urinal, or toilet.
8. Immediately place the sterile cap on the specimen container (Figure 13-12) so the specimen will not become contaminated.
9. Remove bedpan and wipe client.

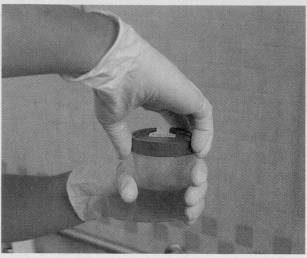

FIGURE 13-12 Screw top on securely. Wipe outside of container with paper towel.

10. Place labeled specimen container inside a plastic bag or resealable bag, then put this bag inside the paper bag with completed label.
11. Remove gloves and wash hands.
12. Store the specimen bag according to the nurse's instructions until time to take to local laboratory.
13. Document time of collection and type of specimen.

CLIENT CARE PROCEDURE

22

Caring for a Urinary Catheter

PURPOSE

- To clean the area around where the catheter enters the body
- To prevent infection of the urinary tract
- To decrease odors and make the client comfortable
- To maintain closed drainage system correctly

NOTE: The collection bag, tubing, and catheter are referred to as the *closed drainage system* (Figure 13-13). The system should

(continues)

CLIENT CARE PROCEDURE 22 Caring for a Urinary Catheter *(continued)*

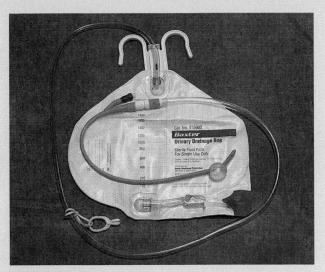

FIGURE 13-13 Closed drainage system. Note tubing, urine collection bag, and indwelling catheter with bulb inflated.

never be disconnected except to reconnect it to a leg bag. The reason the system should not be disconnected is to prevent germs from entering the system (Figure 13-14). You should never raise the collection bag higher than the client's bladder. Always check to see if the tubing is lying in correct position and not kinked. Never pull on a catheter. If possible, cover bag with a cloth to prevent embarrassment of your client.

PROCEDURE

1. Assemble supplies:
   disposable gloves
   antiseptic wipes
   basin of warm water
   plastic bag for waste
   cotton-tipped applicators
2. Wash your hands and apply gloves.
3. Tell client what you plan to do.
4. Position client on his or her back. Expose only the small area where the catheter enters the body. Using soap and warm water or antiseptic wipes, wash area surrounding the catheter. Observe for any skin breakdown, signs of infection, crusting, leakage or bleeding, which should be reported to the nurse immediately.
5. Using antiseptic wipes or gauze pads dipped in warm water, wipe the catheter

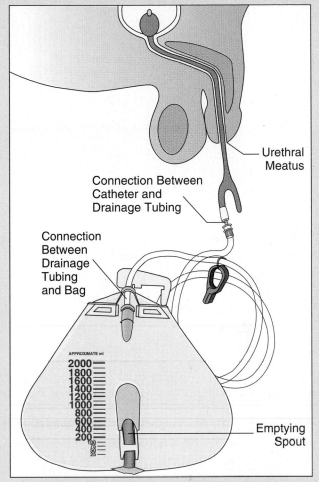

FIGURE 13-14 Special care must be taken to protect the possible sites of contamination in the closed urinary drainage system.

tube. Make only one stroke with each swab or pad. Discard each wipe after one stroke. Start at the urinary opening and wipe *away* from it. Be careful not to dislodge the catheter. Clean the catheter down to the connection of the drainage tubing.
6. Remove gloves and discard into plastic bag.
7. Check to be sure tubing is coiled on bed (Figure 13-15) and hanging straight down into the drainage container. Check level of urine in the collection bag. Tubing should not be below the collection bag (Figure 13-16). Do not raise collection bag above the level of the client's bladder.

(continues)

CLIENT CARE PROCEDURE ⟨22⟩ **Caring for a Urinary Catheter** *(continued)*

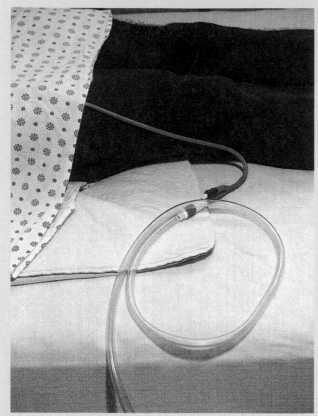

FIGURE 13-15 Tubing should be placed on top of the leg. The excess tubing should be coiled on the bed.

8. Cover client and discard wastes properly.
9. Wash hands.

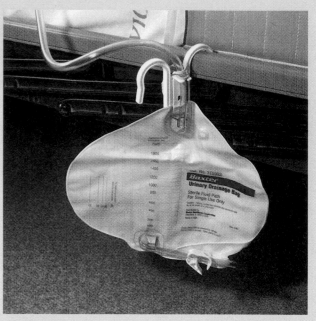

FIGURE 13-16 The urinary collection bag should be attached to the bed frame. Check to see that the tubing does not fall below the level of the collection bag. Never attach the bag onto the side rails because raising and lowering the rails can dislodge the catheter.

10. Document procedure and time, your observations, and client's reaction. Observe color, consistency, and odor of urine, and document.

tubing while the bedside urinary collection bag is not in use. Refer to Procedures 23 and 24 for the proper ways to connect a leg bag, and to empty a drainage unit.

Retraining the Bladder

A home health aide may need to keep a record for a few days of how often and how much the client voids throughout the day and night. Once the client's voiding pattern is known, the nurse supervisor can analyze the client's voiding record and formulate a schedule for the aide to follow. The schedule developed by the nurse

will include regularly scheduled times for the aide to have the client drink a measured amount of fluids, and then to toilet the client at regular intervals. Procedure 25 discusses the proper method to retrain the bladder.

Enemas and Rectal Suppositories

An **enema** is the technique of introducing fluid into the rectum to remove feces and flatus (gas) from the rectum and colon. A rectal **suppository** is a cone-shaped, easily melted, medicated mass that can readily be inserted into a client's rectum. The suppository contains ingredients

CLIENT CARE PROCEDURE

23

Connecting the Leg Bag

PURPOSE

- To connect a leg urinary collection bag

PROCEDURE

1. Assemble needed equipment:
   disposable gloves
   leg bag
   alcohol wipes
   paper towels
2. Wash your hands and apply gloves.
3. Tell client what you plan to do.
4. Place paper towel underneath catheter connection area.
5. Use alcohol to disinfect area to be disconnected.
6. Disconnect catheter from tubing. Wipe end of catheter with alcohol (Figure 13-17). Remove cap from end of leg bag and connect leg bag to catheter. Wipe end of bedside drainage bag tubing with alcohol wipe. Place cap on end of closed drainage system.
7. Attach leg straps and bag to leg of client (Figure 13-18). Check to see if the part marked "top of bag" is in the correct position.
8. Empty and measure urine from bedside collection bag.
9. Remove gloves and wash hands.
10. Document procedure completed.

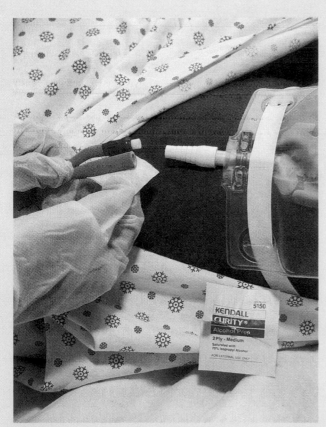

FIGURE 13-17 Wipe end of catheter with alcohol before connecting leg bag.

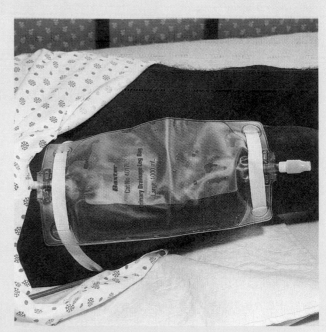

FIGURE 13-18 Apply leg bag to client's upper leg. Be sure the straps are smooth and not too tight.

CLIENT CARE PROCEDURE

24

Emptying a Drainage Unit

PURPOSE

• To empty urinary collection bag

PROCEDURE

1. Assemble equipment:
   disposable gloves
   alcohol wipes
   measuring device
   paper towel
2. Wash hands and apply gloves.
3. Tell client what you plan to do.
4. Place paper towel and measuring device on floor below drainage bag.
5. Open drain or spout and allow the urine to drain into measuring device (Figure 13-19A). Do not allow the tip of tubing to touch sides of the measuring device.
6. Close the drain and wipe it with the alcohol wipe. Replace it in the holder on the bag (Figure 13-19B).
7. Note the amount and color of urine. Empty urine into toilet. Wash and rinse measuring device.
8. Remove gloves and wash hands.
9. Document amount.

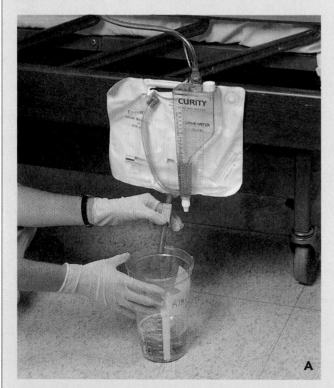
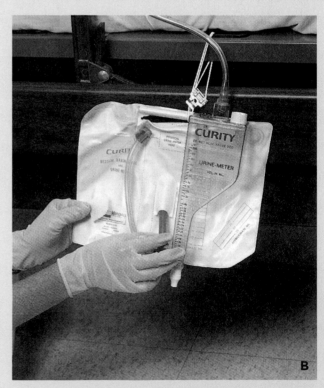

FIGURE 13-19 A. Open the drain on the bottom of the collection bag. B. Allow the urine to drain into the graduate. Note that the end of the drain is not touching the sides of the container. Wipe the drain off with alcohol before replacing. It is a good idea to place paper towels under the graduate, just in case some urine is spilled.

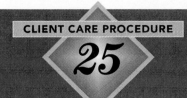

CLIENT CARE PROCEDURE
25

Retraining the Bladder

PURPOSE

• To regain bladder control

PROCEDURE

The schedule developed by the nurse will include regularly scheduled times for the aide to have the client drink a measured amount of fluid. After the client has drunk the liquid, the aide notes the time and then 30 minutes later the aide will toilet the client.

The aide will need to encourage the client to void each time the client is positioned on the commode or toilet. It is helpful at times to run water from the faucet to give the client an urge to void. Other methods of encouraging the client to void are to have the client apply light pressure to the bladder area to stimulate the urge to empty the bladder; to pour warm water over the genital area; or have the client lean forward on the toilet to stimulate emptying the bladder.

Remember that the client needs to be toileted at regular intervals to prevent accidents. The client will need consistent positive reinforcement to remain dry. At first it may be necessary to take the client to the bathroom every 2 hours; intervals may be lengthened as control is gained. A common cause of incontinence is delay in getting the client to the bathroom. It is of utmost importance to take the client to the bathroom on a *regular* time schedule.

The plan will also call for the aide to maintain the client's fluid intake at about 2500 cc/day, except for persons with fluid restriction, i.e., congestive heart failure or renal failure. The aide should encourage the client to wear regular underwear to enhance the client's self-esteem and to help the client from reverting back to the previous incontinence habit.

---

that once absorbed by the lining of the colon will give a stimulus to the colon to evacuate stool. Either of these techniques may be necessary to relieve the client of constipation, to make the client more comfortable, or to prepare the client for diagnostic tests. Procedures 26 and 27 demonstrate the proper way to give a commercial enema and a rectal suppository.

Bowel Retraining

Constipation can result from illness, poor eating habits, drug therapy, and lack of exercise. Constipation causes the client added discomfort when it occurs, in addition to other physical problems. An individualized bowel program is designed by the health care team for each client. For instance, one client can regulate the bowels

by adding prune juice to the diet twice a day. Another client may need to drink prune juice daily, but also take a daily laxative and stool softener by mouth. The frequency of bowel movements may range from three times a day for one person to only once every 2 or 3 days for another. Therefore, the term constipation should not be used to describe a missed movement or two, but only the unusual retention of fecal matter along with infrequent or difficult passage of stony, hard stool. Procedure 28 discusses retraining of bowels.

Adult Briefs

Although bed pads are used to keep the sheets from becoming wet or soiled, special supplies can be used for both men and women. The adult

CLIENT CARE PROCEDURE

26

Giving a Commercial Enema

PURPOSE

- To help cleanse the bowel

NOTE: Because enemas distend or dilate the rectum, the client may experience a feeling of urgency in the bowel, that is, a very strong need to empty the bowel as soon as possible.

Enemas can only be given on a doctor's orders.

The two commercially prepared enemas are the chemical (often referred to as Fleets) and oil-retention enemas. Oil-retention enemas are given to soften hard feces in the rectum and are usually followed by a soap solution enema.

PROCEDURE

1. Assemble supplies (Figure 13-20):
   disposable gloves
   commercial prepackaged enema
   protective pad
   bedpan (if client is bedridden)
   toilet paper
   lubrication jelly
   water, washcloth, soap, towel
2. Wash hands and put on gloves.
3. Tell client what you plan to do.
4. Provide for the client's comfort and privacy.
5. Place protective pad underneath the client's buttocks.
6. Have client turn to the left side. Turn covers back to expose only the buttocks.
7. Remove cover on the tip of enema. Apply extra lubricant to tip to ensure easy insertion.
8. Separate the buttocks and insert the tip into rectum for at least 3 inches. Tell client to take a deep breath and hold the solution as long as possible. Slowly squeeze the bottle (Figure 13-21). This

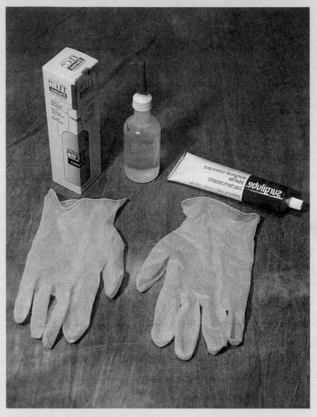

FIGURE 13-20 Equipment needed to give a commercial enema

forces the solution to flow evenly into the rectum.

9. Remove enema tip while holding the client's buttocks together.
10. Position client on bedpan, commode, or toilet.
11. After client has expelled feces and enema solution, assist the client in cleaning area around anus and buttocks.
12. Return client to comfortable position. It may be necessary to leave the protective pad in place until the effects of the enema are complete.

(continues)

CLIENT CARE PROCEDURE **26** **Giving a Commercial Enema** *(continued)*

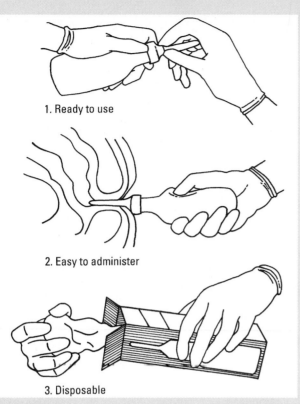

FIGURE 13-21 Administering a commercial enema. (Courtesy of C. B. Fleet Co., Inc.)

13. Remove gloves and wash hands.
14. Record results of enema—color, amount, consistency; for example: 10:00 AM, Fleets enema given, good results—large, brown, formed stool.

CLIENT CARE PROCEDURE
27
Giving a Rectal Suppository

PURPOSE

• To facilitate a bowel movement

NOTE: Suppositories are usually stored in the client's refrigerator and are wrapped in foil. The suppository will melt once inserted into the warm environment of the rectum and colon. It will take the suppository at least 5 to 10 minutes to melt. It is important that the aide inform the client to wait a few minutes after the suppository is inserted before trying to have a bowel movement.

PROCEDURE

1. Assemble supplies:
   disposable gloves
   rectal suppository
   lubricant, water soluble
   protective pad or paper towels
2. Wash hands and apply gloves.
3. Tell client what you plan to do.
4. Open foil-wrapped suppository. Turn client to one side.
5. Lubricate tip of suppository and gloved finger and insert suppository into rectum

(continues)

CLIENT CARE PROCEDURE **27** **Giving a Rectal Suppository** *(continued)*

(Figure 13-22). Push the suppository along the lining of the rectum with your index finger as far as your finger allows. Be careful not to insert suppository into the feces. The suppository needs to be next to the lining of the colon for it to be effective.

6. After 10 minutes have passed, assist the client to the toilet or commode.
7. After client has had a bowel movement, assist client back to bed or chair.
8. Observe results of elimination.
9. Remove gloves and wash hands.
10. Record results. It is important to note color, consistency, and amount of stool.

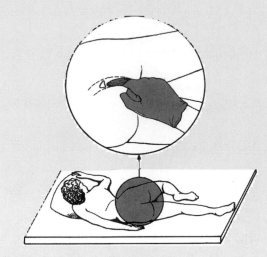

FIGURE 13-22   Carefully place the rectal suppository into the rectum about 3 inches for adults.

CLIENT CARE PROCEDURE

28

Retraining the Bowels

PURPOSE

- To retrain a client to be continent of bowel movement
- To regulate a client to have regular bowel movement

NOTE: Among the elderly, constipation is often encountered. If a client is unable to exercise and move about regularly, bowel action becomes sluggish. Sometimes medications, especially painkillers, can cause constipation. If a client has hemorrhoids, there may be a fear of pain and so the client avoids trying to have a bowel movement. If a client does not have a bowel movement for a few days, the client may develop an impaction. An **impaction** is a large amount of hard stool in the lower colon or rectum that cannot be expelled normally. This is a very painful condition. If a client does develop an impaction, the nurse will need to remove the stool manually.

PROCEDURE

1. The health care team assesses prior habits of client. If client always had a bowel movement early in the morning, this would be important to know in planning the client's retraining program.
2. A plan is designed and implemented. Important elements of the plan are:
   - High intake of fiber foods
   - Adequate intake of liquids

(continues)

CLIENT CARE PROCEDURE *28* **Retraining the Bowels** *(continued)*

- Regular exercise
- Toileting client at regular intervals
- Praise by aide of slightest progress of client
- Less reliance on laxatives and enemas
- Privacy for client for bowel movements
3. Follow bowel retraining program developed by the health care team. If plan does

appear to be working, note success of program. If plan does not work, report. It is also important to give some suggestions to the health care team of possible solutions for retraining of the client.

brief is used to keep the incontinent client dry and to minimize embarrassment to the client in the event of accidents. The adult brief will also reduce odor and the chance of developing urinary infections and pressure sores. Refer to Procedure 29.

Collecting a Stool Specimen

On occasion it may be necessary to collect a stool sample for a diagnostic test. Procedure 30 demonstrates the proper method to collect a stool specimen.

CLIENT CARE PROCEDURE

29

Applying Adult Briefs

The adult brief comes in various styles and sizes. One design may be an insert to go inside a specially designed brief. Another popular type is a "wrap-around brief" fastened with Velcro-like tabs (Figure 13-23). It is important to have the correct size for your client to ensure their effectiveness. It is also important to read the instructions on the package on how to apply each particular style of brief. Many briefs have a strip on them that changes color when the brief needs to be changed. The brief should be checked at regular intervals and changed as needed. Do not apply powder to the client's perineal area when adult briefs are used. Many of the briefs have specially treated wipes to use to clean the client's perineal area **(perineum)** when changing the briefs. They are very reasonable in cost and are recommended over soap and water. If a certain brief does not appear to be working, report this to

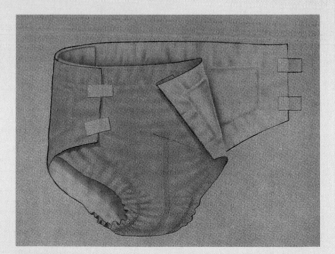

FIGURE 13-23 Disposable incontinence briefs

the nurse. There are many different types on the market, and some work better on some clients than others.

CLIENT CARE PROCEDURE

30

Collecting a Stool Specimen

PURPOSE

• To collect a stool sample for a diagnostic test

PROCEDURE

1. Assemble needed supplies:
   disposable gloves
   bedpan
   specimen container or hemoccult slide packet with label completed
2. Inform client of need for specimen. Certain foods, such as organ meats, can change the color of stool and test positive or false. Many of the tests on the market will indicate which foods should be avoided for several days before testing.

3. After client has defecated in bedpan, apply gloves and with wood applicator remove stool (Figure 13-24A). If specimen is to be collected in specimen container, place small amount (approximately 1 tablespoon) of stool in container (Figure 13-24B). If the test is for occult blood or guaiac, place small amount of stool on hemoccult blood card with the applicator stick included in the test (Figure 13-25).
4. Place specimen in proper storage place. Be sure the specimen is sent to laboratory as directed by your supervisor.
5. Remove gloves and wash hands.
6. Document stool specimen collection.

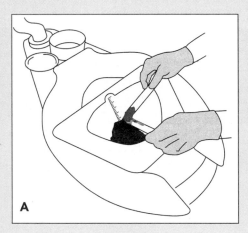
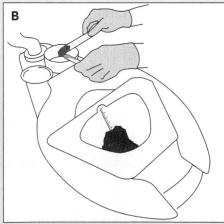

FIGURE 13-24 Use tongue blades to transfer the stool specimen from the collection container to the specimen container.

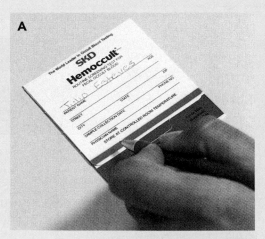
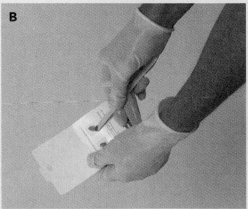

FIGURE 13-25 A. Fill in label on specimen card. B. Open card and apply a small sample of stool on the special area on the card for occult blood test.

Caring for an Ostomy Bag

An **ostomy bag** is sometimes called a stoma bag. It is used for clients who have had a sur-gical operation called a colostomy or an ile-ostomy. In these operations, the intestine is cut and brought to the outside of the body (Figure 13-26). Body wastes (feces) are expelled

A

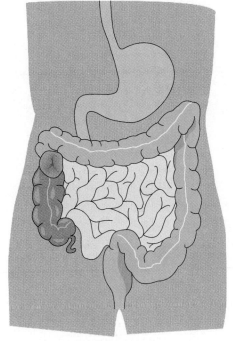

Ascending colostomy

B

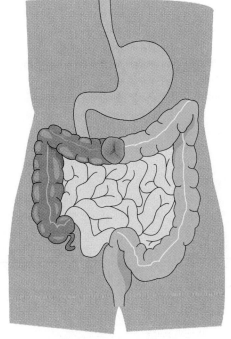

Transverse colostomy

C

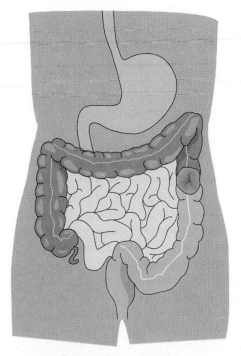

Descending colostomy

D

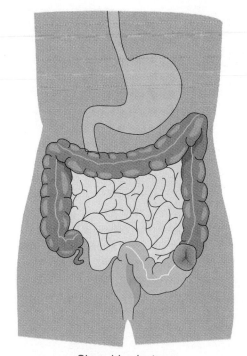

Sigmoid colostomy

FIGURE 13-26 Colostomy sites vary depending upon the part of the bowel that needs to be removed. A. Ascending colostomy. B. Transverse colostomy. C. Descending colostomy. D. Sigmoid colostomy.

through an opening in the abdomen instead of the rectum. This opening in the abdomen is called a **stoma**. The ostomy bag is placed over the opening to collect the wastes (Figure 13-27). Instructions for changing an ostomy bag are discussed in Procedure 31.

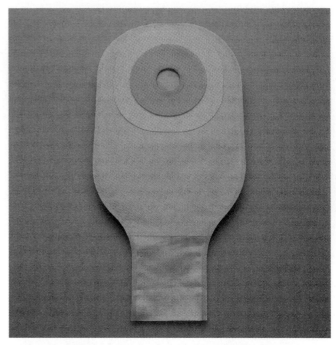

FIGURE 13-27 Stoma protector and drainage bag. (Permission to use this copyrighted material has been granted by the owner, Hollister Incorporated.)

CLIENT CARE PROCEDURE

31

Assisting With Changing an Ostomy Bag

PURPOSE

- To keep the client clean
- To prevent skin breakdown around the stoma
- To regulate and establish a daily routine for removing wastes

NOTE: An ostomy bag should be changed when it becomes one-third or one-half full. Once regulated the client can change it at about the same time each day. In some cases, the client may wear a gauze pad instead of a bag or pouch.

In addition to changing the bag, the client may need to wash out the intestines. If the client needs to do this, the client would have been taught at the hospital or by the nurse how to irrigate (wash out) the intestine. An aide may assist the client with this procedure. However, the aide may not do the procedure unless advanced training in the procedure has been learned and the agency requirements have been met.

Until a client has adjusted to using the ostomy bag there may be strong feelings of em-

(continues)

barrassment. The home health aide can help the client accept the inconvenience by being understanding. The aide should not show displeasure in assisting the client.

The bags and attachments come in many styles today. They are lighter, odor proof, and fit more tightly. Many types of bags and appliances are available; a few require a belt to attach the appliance, others do not require a belt. Colostomy bags can be in one-piece disposable pouches or two-piece disposable pouches. A popular method of attachment is with a synthetic preparation resembling real skin that is attached to the area around the stoma. On this artificial skin is a raised seal that the colostomy bag may attach to. This artificial skin protects the real skin from irritation and contamination with the client's feces and also serves as a place where the colostomy bag can be put on and taken off. Another popular method for attaching a colostomy bag is with a brown-colored, gum-type substance called Karaya, which does not irritate the client's skin and prevents skin breakdown. The nurse will give you special instructions on the type of skin attachment and bag the client is using.

PROCEDURE

1. Assemble supplies:
   disposable gloves
   basin of warm water and soap
   clean ostomy bag
   double bags
   skin ointment (if ordered)
   toilet tissue
2. Wash your hands and apply gloves.
3. Tell client what you plan to do.
4. Gently remove soiled colostomy bag from the stoma. Place in double-bagged receptacle. In a few instances, the colostomy bag can be washed and reused.
5. If there is stool on the skin remove with toilet tissue. Wash area around the stoma with mild soap and water. Pat the area dry. Occasionally a special substance may be applied to assist the new colostomy bag to adhere better.
6. Apply ointment if ordered. Observe area around the stoma for redness or open areas.
7. Apply client's pouch.
   * If one-piece pouch or bag is being used, remove self-stick backing from new ostomy appliance. Press the new bag to the area around the stoma, being sure to seal tightly.
   * If two-piece pouch is being used, be sure to cut opening to the correct size. (A few bags are premeasured and this step is not necessary.) Remove adhesive backing on face plate. Firmly apply face plate to client's skin around stoma, working from the stoma outward. Then apply the bag to this face plate. Let your client assist you as much as possible. Be sure to follow any special manufacturer's instruction in application of appliance.
8. Assist the client to connect belt to appliance, if client is using this type of appliance.
9. Remove wastes. Check skin and stoma for signs of irritation and breakdown. Observe stool for color, amount, and consistency. If necessary spray the room with deodorizer.
10. Remove gloves and wash hands.
11. Document procedure and time, your observations, and client's reaction. The aide should report to a supervisor any changes in the skin color of the stoma or changes noted in the way the stoma is emptying.

REVIEW

1. What is the medical term for inflammation of the bladder?

2. When measuring intake and output, 1 ounce is equal to how many cc?

3. Fill in the blank: _____ incontinence refers to the involuntary loss of small amounts of urine during activities such as coughing, running, laughing, or lifting heavy objects.

4. Fill in the blank: _____ incontinence refers to an involuntary loss of urine because of the inability to reach the bathroom in time.

5. T   F   A client should be given a bedpan two times a shift.

6. T   F   Once a client is offered a bedpan, it should be removed no longer than 5 minutes later.

7. When collecting a clean-catch midstream urine specimen, always:
   a. Do it in the morning.
   b. Take the first few drops of urine.
   c. Maintain a sterile collection container.

8. A surgically placed opening in the abdomen, such as a colostomy, is called:
   a. Scar
   b. Stoma
   c. Wound

9. T   F   Clients with bowel or bladder problems are never helped with a toileting schedule.

10. T   F   Clients are always constipated if they do not move bowels daily.

11. Mr. Jones is on a bladder retraining program, and the nurse has developed a schedule that requires you to toilet him every 2 hours. When it is time for Mr. Jones to be toileted, he tells you that he does not need to go. What steps could you take to encourage him to cooperate with this procedure? What methods could you suggest that may stimulate his bladder to release urine?

12. You have been assigned to change Mrs. Smith's ostomy bag. In doing so, you notice that the color of the stoma has changed significantly since the last time. What should you do?

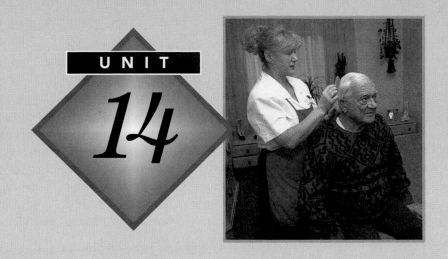

UNIT
14

Integumentary System

KEY TERMS

bony prominence   hyperthermia   pressure sore
dermis   hypothermia
epidermis   perineum

LEARNING OBJECTIVES

After studying this unit, you should be able to:

- Identify one function of the integumentary system.
- List the symptoms of pressure sore development.
- Describe good skin care.
- Describe treatment of heatstroke.
- Demonstrate the following:

PROCEDURE 32	Applying Clean Dressing and Ointment to Broken Skin
PROCEDURE 33	Assisting with Tub Bath or Shower
PROCEDURE 34	Giving a Bed Bath
PROCEDURE 35	Giving a Back Rub
PROCEDURE 36	Giving Female Perineal Care
PROCEDURE 37	Giving Male Perineal Care
PROCEDURE 38	Assisting with Routine Oral Hygiene
PROCEDURE 39	Caring for Dentures
PROCEDURE 40	Shaving the Male Client
PROCEDURE 41	Performing a Warm Foot Soak
PROCEDURE 42	Giving Nail Care
PROCEDURE 43	Shampooing the Client's Hair in Bed
PROCEDURE 44	Caring for an Artificial Eye

INTEGUMENTARY SYSTEM

The skin, hair, and nails make up the integumentary system. The skin is the largest organ of the body. It covers the entire outer surface of the body. Skin is made up of two layers of tissue. The outer layer is the **epidermis** and the inner layer is the **dermis** (Figure 14-1). Other parts of the integumentary system are the nails, hair, oil and sweat glands, and mucous membranes.

The integumentary system protects the body but also has other functions. It regulates body temperature and works with the nervous system to sense touch, pressure, pain, heat, and cold.

The pores or natural openings in the skin surface are protected by oil glands and sweat glands. As the body perspires (sweats) through the skin pores, the air evaporates the perspiration and the body feels cooler. Secretions from these glands are helpful in keeping germs from entering the pores. When the skin is cut or there is an open sore, germs can enter the body easily. Once germs get beyond the skin, the other body defenses start to work. White blood cells surround the germs and try to stop them from going deeper into the body. The pus that forms on a skin wound is made up of dead white blood cells that have fought off the germs.

Hair protects the body in several ways. The eyebrows keep sweat from falling into the eyes. The tiny hairs inside the nose and ears stop small particles from entering and causing damage. The eyelashes keep small objects from getting into the eyes. These hairs all act very much like a screen door on a house in keeping out unwanted organisms. The skin itself is a protective covering that helps to maintain body temperature and excretes waste products through perspiration.

COMMON DISORDERS OF THE INTEGUMENTARY SYSTEM

Pressure Areas (Bedsores)

The care given to the skin of a person confined to bed or a wheelchair is extremely important. When the body gets little exercise, the skin is one of the first areas to break down. Breakdown most often occurs where the skin covers the bones. These places are called **bony prominences** (Figure 14-2).

The back of the head, buttocks, coccyx, elbow, knees, and heels are common places to watch for signs of skin breakdown. A **pressure sore** is a

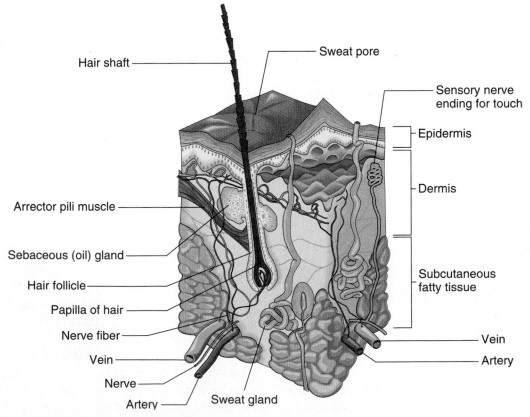

Hair shaft

Sweat pore

Sensory nerve ending for touch

Epidermis

Dermis

Arrector pili muscle

Sebaceous (oil) gland

Hair follicle

Papilla of hair

Nerve fiber

Vein

Subcutaneous fatty tissue

Vein

Artery

Nerve

Artery

Sweat gland

FIGURE 14-1 Cross-section of the skin

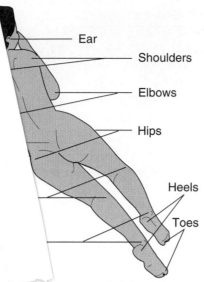

Ear

Shoulders

Elbows

Hips

Heels

Toes

...ssure sores most often form ...ences.

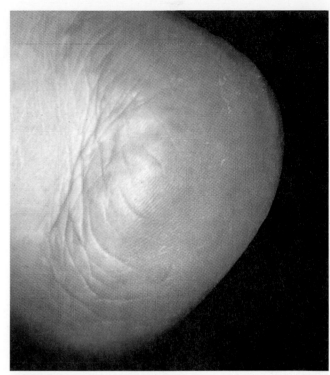

FIGURE 14-3A First indication of tissue ischemia (stage 1) is redness and heat over a pressure point such as this heel. (Courtesy of Emory University Hospital, Atlanta, GA)

...kin that covers a bony area. ...s of pressure sore develop- ...skin due to leaving a client ...ong, friction and shearing ...tioning a client, poor skin ..., and incontinence.

of Bedsores. Pres- ...ized by stages, depend- ...rity.

...ng reddened area. ...4 hours the reddened ...e an open sore. If ...ill soon develop ...Figure 14-3A).

...n and there will be ...le on the client's ...it will soon pro- ...(Figure 14-3B).

...pen and there ...e visible (Fig-

...ls to the mus- ...ying struc- ...ese sores ...places ...sily and

Pre... ...alth aide's
role ... ...develop-
ment... ...velops a

reddened area, the aide should notify a nurse or supervisor. The aide will need to reposition the client every 2 hours. The client's bed linens should be kept clean and dry at all times. If the client is left in a urine-saturated bed, the skin may begin to break down quickly. The client should be exercised as his or her condition

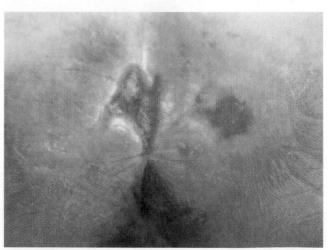

FIGURE 14-3B Stage 2 is marked by destruction of the epidermis and partial destruction of the dermis. (Courtesy of Emory University Hospital, Atlanta, GA)

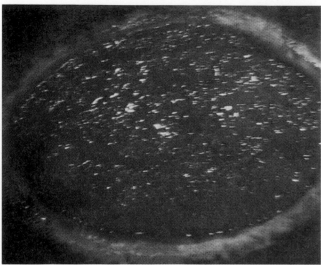

FIGURE 14-4 In stage 3, all layers of skin have been destroyed. A deep crater has been formed. (Courtesy of Emory University Hospital, Atlanta, GA)

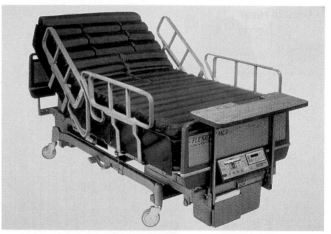

FIGURE 14-6 Alternating air pressure mattress overlay. Alternating air pressure in mattress cells constantly changes pressure points against the client's skin and gently massages the skin. (Courtesy of Hill Rom, Charleston, SC)

allows. The aide can assist the client with exercises. When bathing a client be sure to use soap sparingly because soap dries the skin and makes it susceptible to breakdown. Many special devices are available to place on the bed or on the specific part of the body to aid in the prevention of pressure sores. Examples of these are air mattress, water mattress, gel foam pad, egg crate mattress or cushion, lamb's wool or sheepskin pads, and elbow and heel pads.

An alternating pressure air mattress is a mattress filled with air (Figure 14-6). This works by

continuously changing the pressure areas on the client's back. One can improvise an air mattress designed for camping instead of buying a medical air mattress. A water mattress is also effective in reducing pressure on the skin, but causes problems when transferring clients in and out of bed, because it is not as firm as a regular mattress.

An egg crate mattress is a mattress made of foam rubber that is molded like an egg crate (Figure 14-7). They are inexpensive but effective

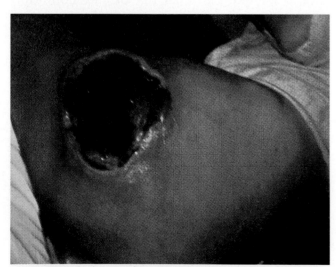

FIGURE 14-5 In stage 4, tissue destruction can involve muscle, bone, and other vital structures. (Courtesy of Emory University Hospital, Atlanta, GA)

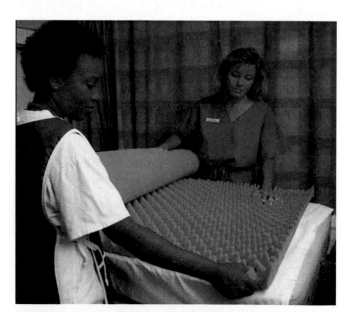

FIGURE 14-7 Egg crate mattress provides cushioning and mild redistribution of pressure beneath the client.

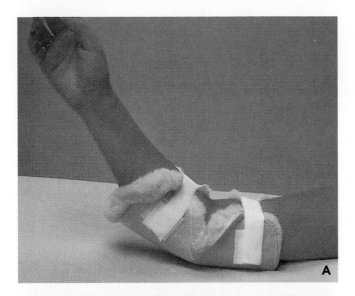

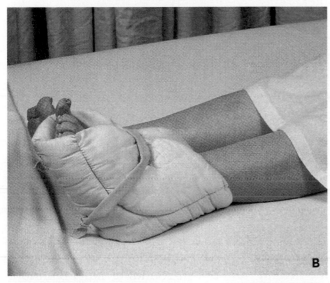

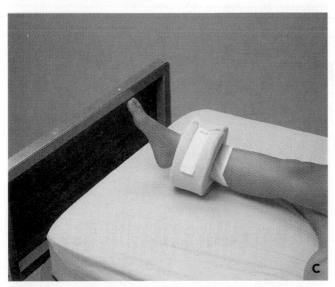

FIGURE 14-8 Pads reduce skin irritation and help prevent pressure sores. (14-8A and 14-8C, Courtesy of J. T. Posey Company, Arcadia, California)

in reducing pressure on the skin. You can also purchase one the size of a seat for the client to sit on during the day when up in a chair. A gel foam cushion is a special cushion filled with a solution or gel. This style of cushion is effective in the prevention of pressure sores for a client who sits in a wheelchair for long periods of time.

Sheepskin or lamb's wool pads or elbow or heel pads prevent pressure sores by acting as a barrier between the client's skin and the sheets (Figures 14-8 and 14-9). A bed cradle is another device to keep linens off the client's legs and feet. In the home a client may substitute a box or other device to keep linens off the legs and feet.

These special devices can prevent the skin from rubbing against the bedclothes, but do not take the place of good skin care.

Good skin care includes changing the client's position at least every 2 hours, quickly removing feces or moisture from the skin, encouraging clients in wheelchairs to reposition themselves every 15 minutes, promoting good nutrition and plenty of fluids, keeping bed linens dry, using moisturizing lotion, and avoiding soaps that dry the skin. The home health aide should watch for skin irritation when applying braces and splints, and report the first sign of a reddened area to the nurse supervisor. Some other common skin disorders and their treatments are described in Figure 14-10.

Applying Skin Dressings. Occasionally it may be necessary to apply a dressing for minor cuts and scrapes. Applying a clean dressing and ointment to broken skin helps to protect the area from contamination and irritation. Although

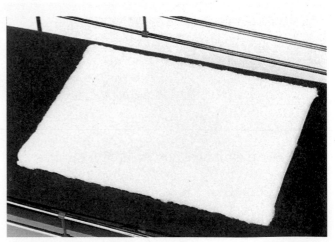

FIGURE 14-9 Pad of synthetic sheepskin. (Courtesy of J. T. Posey Company, Arcadia, California)

FIGURE 14-10 Common skin disorders and their treatments

Disorder	Description	Treatment
Acne	Chronic inflammatory disease of the sebaceous (oil) glands and hair follicles. Characterized by eruptions, cysts, nodules, or pustules that may lead to scarring and pitting of the skin. Often appears at puberty when major body changes commence. Usually appears on the face, neck, and shoulders.	Diet modification Topical medication Cleansing of the skin Surgical skin peeling and removal
Psoriasis	Scaly, itchy skin eruptions that appear at any age.	No cure, but can be controlled by topical medication to relieve itching
Dermatitis	Skin inflammation that causes itching, redness, and skin lesions (sores). May be caused by skin irritants such a poison ivy, allergies, sunburn, or adverse reaction to heat or cold.	Topical medication and avoidance of causal factors.
Scabies	Skin lesions caused by mites that burrow into the skin. Transmitted by direct contact, clothing, and linen. Itching may persist several days after treatment. Noticed around fingers, wrists, axilla, waist, under the breasts, abdomen, buttocks, and genitalia. Infection of the lesions is common.	(ordered by physician) Topical medication Antibiotics if infection occurs Antihistamines to relieve the itching

most dressings will be changed as indicated by the nurse, occasionally the dressing change is done by the home health aide, with the approval of the nurse supervisor. In these cases, the aide should observe and record the color, amount, and consistency of the drainage, the progress of the healing, and the surrounding skin condition. Refer to Procedure 32.

CLIENT CARE PROCEDURE

32

Applying Clean Dressing and Ointment to Broken Skin

PURPOSE

• To help skin heal and avoid infection.

PROCEDURE

1. Assemble supplies:
   disposable gloves
   two or more 4 × 4 gauze pads prepackaged
   over-the-counter ointment (if ordered)

   receptacle for wastes (e.g., plastic bag) tape and scissors
2. Wash your hands and apply gloves.
3. Tell client what you plan to do.
4. Position client so area with dressing is accessible while maintaining client comfort (Figure 14-11).
5. Remove old dressing. If the dressing does not lift off easily, pour warm water over it

(continues)

CLIENT CARE PROCEDURE **Applying Clean Dressing and Ointment to Broken Skin** *(continued)*

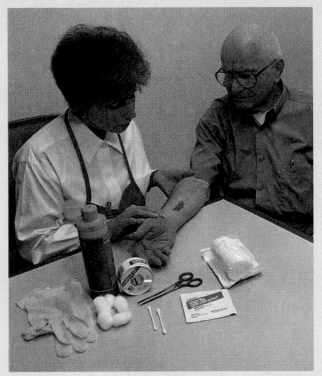

FIGURE 14-11 Assemble supplies and position client so area of dressing is accessible.

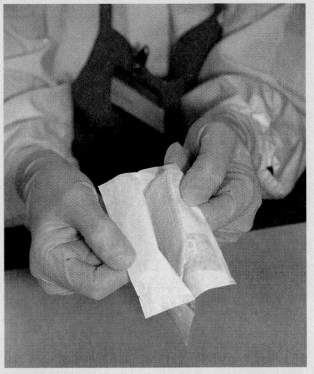

FIGURE 14-12 Correct method of opening dressing

to loosen it. Discard used dressing in open waste receptacle (plastic bag). Note color, amount of drainage, and condition of surrounding skin.

6. Open the package of gauze pads without touching the pads (Figure 14-12). Be careful not to have dressing touch bed linens or client's clothing. Cut tape. Apply ointment if ordered. Apply dressing. Do not touch center of dressing. Hold all dressings on the corners only. Apply tape correctly (Figures 14-13 and 14-14).

7. Position client comfortably.

8. Discard wastes and return supplies to storage. Be sure to follow standard precautions throughout this procedure.

9. Remove gloves and wash hands.

10. Record observations of the wound and skin condition. Report signs of redness, swelling, heat, foul odor, or amount of drainage. Document that dressing was changed. In addition, report client complaints of pain around the wound.

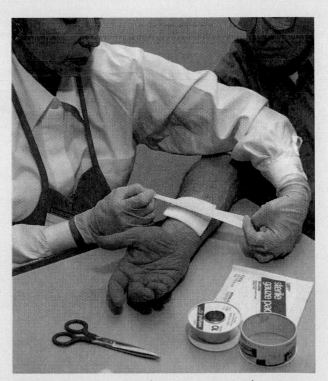

FIGURE 14-13 Apply tape correctly over dressing. *(continues)*

CLIENT CARE PROCEDURE ⟨32⟩ **Applying Clean Dressing and Ointment to Broken Skin** (continued)

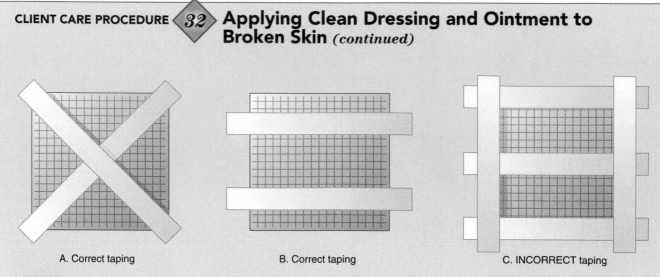

A. Correct taping B. Correct taping C. INCORRECT taping

FIGURE 14-14 Correct taping allows for air circulation. Ends of gauze should never be taped down.

Topical Applications to Unbroken Skin

1. Obtain correct topical medication. Check label of medication with nursing care plan.
2. Position client so area is accessible, while maintaining client comfort.
3. Wash hands and apply gloves.
4. Apply medication in a thin layer to affected area only. Note color and appearance of skin.
5. Remove gloves and reposition client.
6. Wash hands.
7. Return medication to correct storage area.
8. Chart treatment and appearance of skin.

DANGERS OF EXTREME BODY TEMPERATURE

Hyperthermia (heatstroke) and **hypothermia** (abnormally low internal body temperature) are two conditions that may occur when the environmental conditions are extreme and the person's skin is unable to regulate body temperature, a situation not uncommon among the elderly and children.

The home health aide may be the only member of the health care team to see an older person in his or her home on a regular basis. It is important to know the signs of hyperthermia or hypothermia and to report your concerns to a supervisor or family member.

Hyperthermia

Older people are more likely to die from heat-related causes than younger persons. Chances of experiencing heatstroke are increased by a weak or damaged heart, hypertension, circulatory problems, diabetes, being overweight, infection or fever, drinking alcohol, or a previous stroke.

Hyperthermia Signs and Symptoms.

1. Lack of energy
2. Mild discomfort
3. Lack of appetite
4. Dizziness
5. Muscle cramps
6. Diarrhea, nausea
7. Chest pain
8. Excessive weakness
9. Severe mental changes
10. Breathing problems
11. Vomiting
12. Dry skin (no sweating)

An older person may be reluctant to run an air conditioner or a fan because of the cost. He or she may not want to keep open a window due to fear of crime, or may be unable to manage opening a window that is stuck or painted shut. For the client's and your own safety try to gently convince the client to open a window while you are there. If the client is afraid, be sure to close it again before you leave. Be sure to encourage your client to drink plenty of fluids on very hot days.

If any client, older or younger, shows many of the above symptoms and has an elevated body temperature due to heat, take the following steps:

1. Loosen clothing.
2. Place the client in a semi-sitting position, the head slightly elevated to the body.
3. Bathe the head and body in cool water to lower the body temperature.
4. Give drinks of cool water or ice chips to suck on.
5. Call for medical assistance whenever you suspect a person is suffering from hyperthermia.

Hypothermia Cold

Hypothermia is a condition marked by an abnormally low internal body temperature, usually 95°F (35°C) or under. This decrease in body temperature is due to exposure to a cold environment. Infants are at risk because of immature temperature control. The risk factors to the elderly are increased due to chronic illness, poverty, and some medications. Antidepressants, sedatives, tranquilizers, and cardiovascular medications can increase the risk of hypothermia.

Hypothermia Signs and Symptoms.

1. A change in appearance or behavior during cold weather
2. Uncontrollable shivering or lack of shivering
3. Slow and sometimes irregular heartbeat, shallow or very slow breathing
4. Weak pulse, low blood pressure
5. Confusion, disorientation, or drowsiness
6. Pain in the extremities
7. Slurred speech
8. Lack of coordination, sluggishness
9. Stiff muscles
10. Low indoor temperatures and other signs that the person has been in a cool or cold room

You may visit a home that has little or no heat due to a lack of money for gas or oil, a lack of wood for a wood-burning stove, or no heating appliances in the home. If the client is experiencing money problems that have caused the heat to be turned off be sure to let your supervisor know. Most states have emergency money available for utilities that can be given to individuals or families in need.

If your client's primary source of heat is a wood-burning, oil, or kerosene stove, you may find that bringing in the wood or filling the stove with oil is a part of the care plan.

Be cautious about the use and placement of electric space heaters. Never place a space heater near loose bed covers, clothing, or tablecloths. **NEVER** turn on an oven with the door open to heat a room. The danger of breathing in gas fumes or starting a fire is too great.

To warm a person whom you suspect of having hypothermia take the following steps:

1. Take the person's temperature. If it is below 95°F (35°C) call a doctor or ambulance.
2. Wrap the person in a warm blanket, quilt, towels, or extra clothes. Make sure that you cover the head and neck.
3. Use hot water bottles or electric heating pads on the person's abdomen (never on a high setting or with water too hot). Do not place hot water bottles on the feet. Do not rewarm extremities and the core (trunk of body) at the same time.
4. If the person is alert give small quantities of warm (not hot) food or a sweet, warm drink—but nothing alcoholic.
5. Do not rub the person's limbs.
6. Call for medical assistance whenever you suspect the person is suffering from hypothermia.

HYGIENE

Good hygiene is an important part of the care a home health aide provides to a client. Practicing good hygiene is important to maintain skin integrity, prevent infection, as well as to refresh and clean the client. The home health aide may be responsible for providing bathing, oral care, and personal care to the client. It is important for the aide to be sensitive to cultural reactions of clients with regard to providing this type of care. A client's cultural ideas about health, illness, hygiene, and rules for behavior may be different from your own. It will be helpful for you to understand your client's customs, practices, and beliefs so you can provide the best care and be respectful of individual differences. If you are unsure of your client's cultural patterns with regard to personal hygiene, it is a good idea to talk with your supervisor.

Bathing a Client

A tub bath or shower will clean and refresh the client, as well as stimulate the circulation in the skin. While bathing a client, the aide should check the client's skin for any signs of irritation. Procedure 33 demonstrates the proper procedure for assisting with a tub bath or shower.

CLIENT CARE PROCEDURE

33 Assisting with Tub Bath or Shower

PURPOSE

- To clean and refresh the client
- To check client's skin for signs of irritation
- To stimulate circulation in the skin

PROCEDURE

1. If possible, plan the tub bath or shower for a time convenient for the client. A tub bath or shower should not take more than 15 minutes unless there is a special reason for a longer bath.
2. Assemble needed supplies and place in bathroom (Figure 14-15):
   clean clothing
   bath seat or stool
   2 washcloths and towels
   shampoo (if needed)
   plastic pitcher (if shampooing client's hair)
   hose attachment
   comb and brush
   skidproof bath mat
   soap
3. Wash hands.
4. Tell client what you plan to do.
5. Fill tub one-third full with warm water. **CAUTION:** Test the temperature with a thermometer or inside the wrist to be sure it will not burn the client. The water should be about 115°F (46°C°). Place a skidproof bath mat in the bottom of the tub. If client is taking a shower, regulate the flow and be sure the temperature is correct.

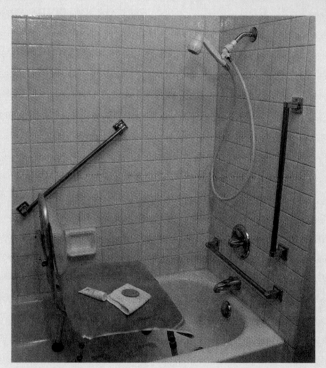

FIGURE 14-15 Gather equipment needed for bath.

6. Assist the client to sit on a chair or on the closed toilet seat. Help the client undress. Place soiled clothing in the hamper. Close the bathroom door so the client will not be chilled.
7. For a tub bath, help client to sit on the edge of the tub. If there is a safety bar, have client hold onto it. When client has gained balance, help the client to turn and lift both legs into the tub. Give assis-

(continues)

CLIENT CARE PROCEDURE ◆*33*◆ **Assisting with Tub Bath or Shower** *(continued)*

tance by supporting the client under the arms and helping the client to slowly sit down in the tub facing the faucets. If the client cannot sit in the tub, place a bath stool in the water. Help the client to sit on the stool (Figures 14-16 and 14-17).

8. If the client needs a shampoo, wet the hair, rub in shampoo, lather, and massage head. If possible, have the client tilt head back. Pour water over the head using the pitcher, or attach the hose to the faucet and use it to rinse the head. Repeat shampoo, massage, and rinse. Client may hold a washcloth over the eyes during the shampoo to prevent soap from entering the eyes.

9. Give the client a washcloth and soap. Allow the client to do as much bathing or washing possible. Assist as necessary (Figure 14-18). If shower is running, make sure the flow is not too heavy; check water temperature often.

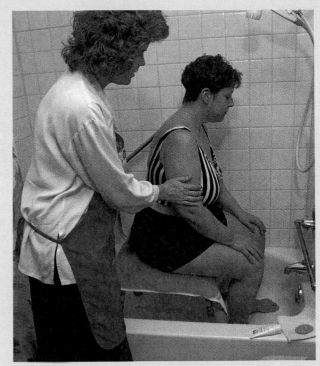

FIGURE 14-17 Have client sit on tub chair.

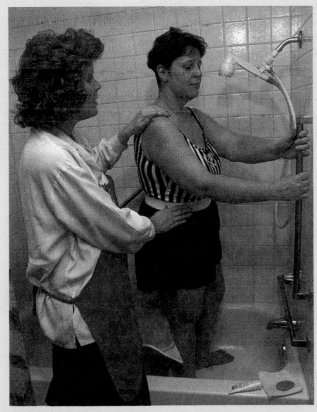

FIGURE 14-16 Instruct client to hold onto grab bars.

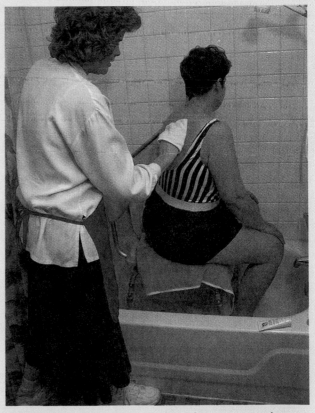

FIGURE 14-18 Assist the client in washing her back. *(continues)*

CLIENT CARE PROCEDURE **33** ▶ **Assisting with Tub Bath or Shower** *(continued)*

10. Remain beside the tub at all times during the bath or shower. **CAUTION:** Be ready to help the client at any moment. If the client should feel faint, empty water from the tub, cover the client with a towel to avoid unnecessary chilling, and lower the client's head between the client's knees.

11. For a tub bath, help the client raise out of the water. Assist the client out of the water. Assist the client to sit on the edge of the tub. Bring client's legs over to outside and assist the client to stand. Allow the client to sit on the closed toilet seat or the chair.

12. Make certain that the client's body is thoroughly dry. Help dry difficult areas such as the back and shoulders (Figure 14-19). Be sure underarms and area under breasts are completely dry. Pay special attention to the feet. Dry soles of feet and between toes. Apply lotion to the client's skin as required (Figure 14-20).

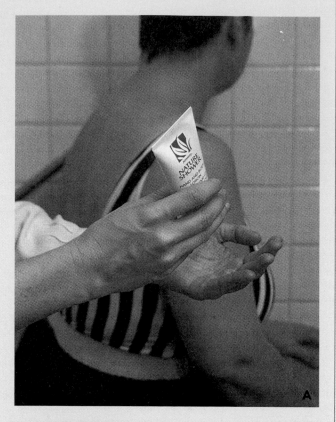

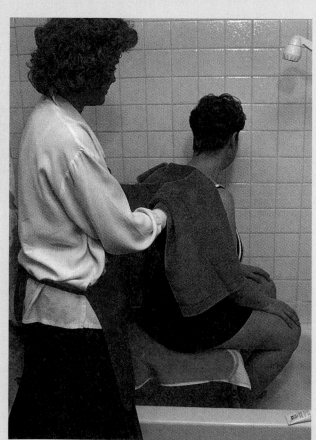

FIGURE 14-19 Dry client's back.

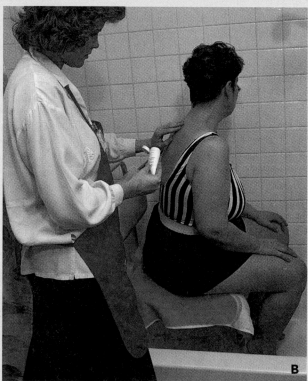

FIGURE 14-20 A. Place lotion in your hands to warm. B. Apply lotion to client's back.

(continues)

CLIENT CARE PROCEDURE **Assisting with Tub Bath or Shower** *(continued)*

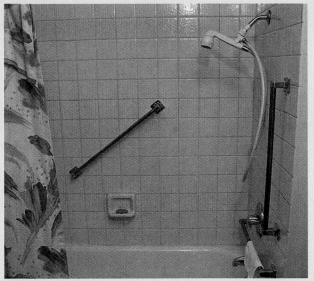

FIGURE 14-21 Be sure to clean tub after the bath.

13. For a shower, make sure the client is completely washed and rinsed and then turn off the shower. Towel dry and assist client out of the shower area.
14. Assist client to dress in clean clothes.
15. Help client back to bed, to a wheelchair, or to a lounge chair.
16. Return to the bathroom and drain and clean tub or shower stall (Figure 14-21). Place dirty clothes and towels in the hamper. Put supplies away.
17. Wash hands.
18. Document procedure, any observations, and client's reaction.

Giving a Bed Bath

If the client is bedbound, the bath will need to be given in bed. Procedure 34 demonstrates the proper way to give a bed bath. A partial bath is given on days a complete bed bath is not given. A partial bath is given the same as a bed bath, except that the legs and feet are not washed. If the client is able, this type of bath can be given by the bathroom sink.

CLIENT CARE PROCEDURE

34

Giving a Bed Bath

PURPOSE

* To clean and refresh the client
* To stimulate circulation
* To observe the client's skin for signs of irritation
  NOTE: The bed bath is usually given in the morning. This procedure is one of a series of procedures performed in the same time period. This will require the home health aide to organize and plan ahead. All materials and supplies needed can be gathered and placed conveniently so that each separate procedure can be completed easily.

* If client needs to use the bedpan, offer it before the bath.
* Gather supplies needed for making the bed and put them near at hand.
* Organize materials needed for oral hygiene, denture care, and nail care to move easily from one procedure to another as needed.

PROCEDURE

1. Gather supplies for the complete series of procedures including:

(continues)

CLIENT CARE PROCEDURE **Giving a Bed Bath** *(continued)*

soap and disposable gloves
washcloths and towels
fresh clothes
body lotion
orange stick
change of bed linens
bath basin, two-thirds filled with water
adult brief if needed

2. Close windows to prevent a draft from blowing on the client. If there are other people in the home, ask not to be disturbed. Close the door for privacy.
3. Wash your hands.
4. Tell client what you plan to do.
5. Remove blankets, leaving the top sheet covering the client. Place one pillow under client's head.
6. Pull out bottom part of top sheet so it covers client loosely. Remove client's clothing.
7. Place a basin of water on the chair or dresser at the bedside.
8. Assist client in moving to side of bed nearest you.
9. Moisten washcloth, squeeze out excess water. Form a mitt by folding a washcloth around one hand (Figure 14-22).

10. Using clear water only, wash the client's eyes first. Wipe from the inner corner to the outer corner of the eye. Using a mild soap, wash the face, ears, and neck. Pat dry with the face towel.
11. Lift client's farthest arm and lay a bath towel under the area to keep bed dry. Wash with soap, rinse, and pat dry, making sure the arm, underarm, and hand are cleaned and thoroughly dry. Repeat for other arm. Apply underarm deodorant or bath powder if client desires.
12. Give nail care using an orange stick to clean nails. Trim nails *if allowed.* Refer to Procedure 42 for a description of the proper method to give nail care.
13. Place towel over client's chest, then pull sheet down to waist. Working under the towel, wash with soap, rinse, and dry chest. Rinse and dry area under a woman's breasts carefully to prevent skin irritation and redness. Replace sheet over chest.
14. Have client bend one knee. Fold sheet up from the foot of the bed. Expose the thigh, leg, and foot. Place a towel under

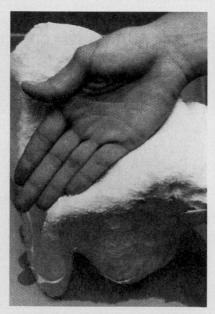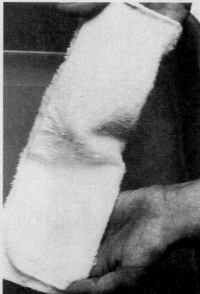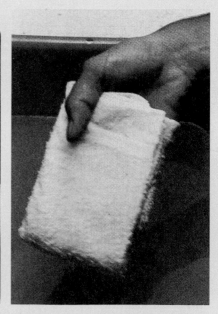

FIGURE 14-22 To make a bath mitt, wrap the washcloth around one hand, bringing free end over palm, and bringing the free-hanging end up over palm and tucking in the end.

(continues)

CLIENT CARE PROCEDURE **34** **Giving a Bed Bath** *(continued)*

the area, and put the basin on the towel, placing client's foot in basin. Wash and rinse foot. Remove the foot from the basin and dry it well.

15. Remove the basin from the bed. Follow the same procedure for the other leg and foot.
16. Lightly apply lotion on legs and feet if skin is dry (never massage legs).
17. Change the water in the basin before proceeding with the bath. If at any time during the bath the water becomes dirty or cool, change it.
18. Place bath towel lengthwise by the client's back and buttocks. Starting at the hairline use long, firm strokes while washing the back.

19. Prepare washcloth with soap and have client wash the genital area, if able. Rinse the cloth and have client wipe and dry the genitals, if capable.
20. Spread the towel under client's head and comb or brush hair.
21. Assist the client into clean clothes.
22. Remove the basin, dirty linens, and the other equipment away from the bed.
23. Change the bed linens using the procedure for making an occupied bed.
24. Leave the client in a comfortable position. After all the activities, the client may require a rest period.
25. Wash your hands.
26. Document procedure and time, observations, and client's reaction.

Back Rub

A back rub is helpful to increase the blood circulation to the back area, and to provide comfort and relaxation to the client. It is also a good opportunity for the aide to observe the skin for signs of skin breakdown. Procedure 35 demonstrates the proper way to give a back rub.

CLIENT CARE PROCEDURE
35 **Giving a Back Rub**

PURPOSE

- To increase the blood circulation to the back area
- To give comfort to the client and provide relaxation
- To observe the skin for signs of skin breakdown

PROCEDURE

1. Wash hands
2. Assemble supplies:
   small towel
   lotion
3. Provide privacy for the client.
4. Position client on back or side.

5. Place small amount of lotion on your hands. Rub together to warm the lotion.
6. Begin by starting at the base of the spine; rub toward the neck in the center of the back. Use both hands in one long stroke (Figure 14-23).
7. When reaching the neck, continue back down the sides of the back. When reaching the base of the spine, rub up the center again. Repeat several times (Figure 14-24).
8. If necessary, add more lotion and use a spiral motion for several minutes.
9. Remove excess lotion with small towel. Reposition client.
10. Wash hands and return supplies to proper place. *(continues)*

CLIENT CARE PROCEDURE **35** **Giving a Back Rub** *(continued)*

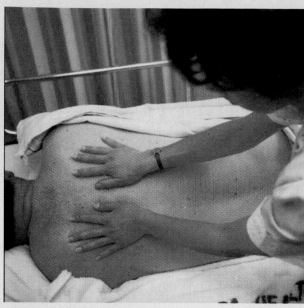

FIGURE 14-23 Use long, smooth strokes as you apply the lotion.

11. Record and report any sign of skin irritation.

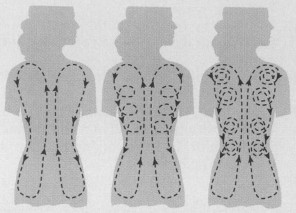

FIGURE 14-24 Place a small amount of lotion on your hands and rub together to warm the lotion. Give the patient a gentle back rub using strokes as shown.

Perineal Care

Part of good skin care includes keeping the **perineum** clean, which is the area from the genitals to the anus. Keeping the perineum clean is important to prevent infections, to prevent skin breakdown, and to reduce odor. Procedures 36 and 37 demonstrate the proper way to give female and male perineal care.

CLIENT CARE PROCEDURE
36
Giving Female Perineal Care

PURPOSE

- To prevent infections
- To clean the genital and anal area
- To prevent skin breakdown
- To prevent odors

PROCEDURE

1. Assemble supplies:
   disposable gloves
   soap
   basin
   water
   washcloths and towel
2. Wash your hands and apply gloves.
3. Tell client what you plan to do.
4. Position client on back and place sheet or thin cotton blanket over client.
5. Position towel under client's buttocks.
6. Wet washcloth with soap and water. Help the client flex her knees and spread her legs if able.

(continues)

CLIENT CARE PROCEDURE **Giving Female Perineal Care** *(continued)*

7. Separate the vulva. Clean downward from front to back with one stroke, first the inner labia, and then rinse. Repeat with outer labia. Repeat on other side. Dry with the towel.
8. Help the client lower her legs and turn onto her side away from you.
9. Apply soap to washcloth.
10. Clean the rectal area by cleaning from the vagina to the anus with one stroke.

Rinse washcloth and repeat until area is clean.
11. Pat the area dry with towel.
12. Cover client with sheet or blanket and make her comfortable.
13. Remove basin and supplies from bedside.
14. Remove your gloves and wash your hands.
15. Document procedure completed, observations, time, and client's reactions.

CLIENT CARE PROCEDURE

37

Giving Male Perineal Care

PURPOSE

- To prevent spread of infection
- To promote comfort
- To prevent odors

PROCEDURE

1. Repeat steps 1 through 6 as for female perineal care.
2. Grasp penis gently with gloved hand. Clean the tip of the penis using gentle circular motion. You will need to pull

back the foreskin if the man is uncircumcised. Start at the urinary meatus and work outward. Rinse the area well and dry. Return the foreskin to its original position.
3. Clean the remaining portion of the penis with firm downward strokes. Rinse well.
4. Wash the scrotum and pat dry.
5. Turn client to side and clean rectal area in the same way as for the female.
6. Follow steps 11 through 15 as for female perineal care.

Oral Care

Some clients will be unable to give themselves oral care. In these instances, the aide must assist the client with oral hygiene, including brushing teeth and caring for dentures. Good oral hygiene is important to keep the client's teeth and gums healthy, to observe the gums for irritation, to refresh the client's mouth, and stimulate the client's appetite. Procedures 38 and 39 demonstrate the proper ways to assist with routine oral hygiene and to care for dentures.

CLIENT CARE PROCEDURE

38

Assisting with Routine Oral Hygiene

PURPOSE

- To keep client's teeth and gums healthy
- To refresh client's mouth and improve appetite

  NOTE: Clients who are helpless are unable to give themselves oral care. In these cases the aide must give special mouth care:
- Wash hands and apply gloves.
- Place small towel under client's head and turn head to one side.
- Dip padded tongue blade (toothette) into mouthwash solution or other special solution.
- Clean teeth, tongue, and inside surfaces of the mouth. Hold an emesis basin under the client's chin to collect secretions.
- Apply pleasant-tasting lubricant to lips. Repeat procedure as ordered.
- Clean and replace equipment. Remove gloves. Wash hands.
- Document procedure and time, observations, and client's reaction.

PROCEDURE

1. Assemble needed equipment and supplies (Figure 14-25A):

   disposable gloves
   toothbrush
   toothpaste
   glass of water
   towel
   small bowl or basin or emesis basin
   mouthwash if available
   tissues or damp washcloth
2. Wash your hands and apply gloves.
3. Tell client what you plan to do and position the client in a sitting position (if allowed).
4. Place a towel over the client's chest and under the chin.
5. Moisten toothbrush and apply toothpaste.
6. Let client brush teeth, if able. If not, carefully brush the client's teeth (Figures 14-25B through E.)

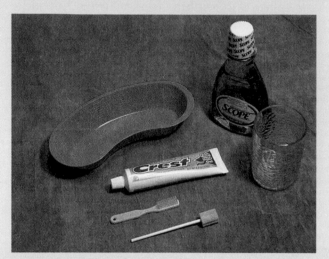

FIGURE 14-25A Supplies needed for oral hygiene

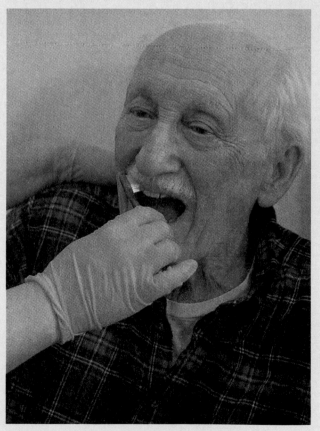

FIGURE 14-25B Hold soft, wet toothbrush at a 45° angle and brush back teeth.

(continues)

CLIENT CARE PROCEDURE **Assisting with Routine Oral Hygiene** *(continued)*

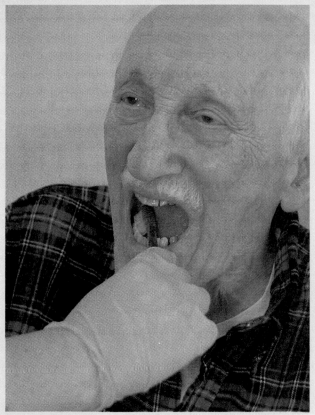

FIGURE 14-25C   Brush top and bottom teeth thoroughly.

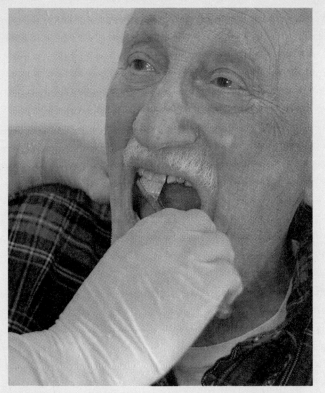

FIGURE 14-25D   Be sure to brush behind the front teeth.

7. Give the client a glass of water; be sure client rinses mouth well. Hold the basin underneath the client's chin and have client return the fluid. If mouthwash is available, have client rinse mouth with the mouthwash.
8. Give the client a moistened washcloth to wipe mouth.
9. Reposition client.
10. Clean and replace equipment.
11. Remove gloves and wash hands.
12. Document procedure completed and time, any observations and client's reaction.

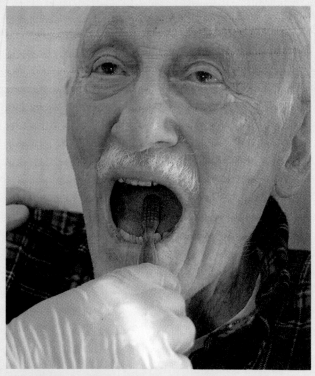

FIGURE 14-25E   Brush tongue.

39

Caring for Dentures

PURPOSE

- To clean dentures and refresh client's mouth
- To provide opportunity to observe client's gums for irritation or soreness
- To stimulate client's appetite

PROCEDURE

1. Assemble the needed supplies (Figure 14-26A):

   disposable gloves
   denture cup or two small containers lined with gauze or washcloth
   toothbrush and toothpaste
   mouthwash with small cup
   small towel and dampened washcloth

2. Wash your hands and apply gloves.

3. Tell client what you plan to do.

4. Ask client to remove dentures (Figure 14-26B), helping if needed. Place dentures in padded container or denture cup (Figure 14-26C). Be very careful in handling client's dentures. They may become slippery to hold.

5. Place approximately 2 to 3 inches of water and a small paper towel or washcloth in bottom of sink (Figure 14-26D). This will protect the dentures in case they are dropped. Turn on cold water and brush all surfaces of the upper and lower plate (Figure 14-26E). Rinse denture cup

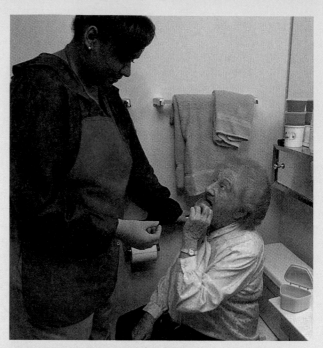

FIGURE 14-26B Ask client to remove dentures.

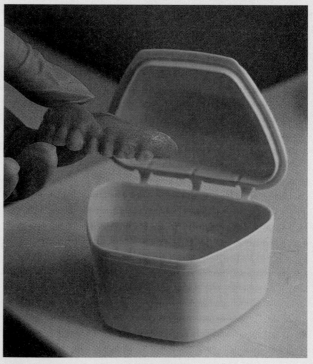

FIGURE 14-26C Place dentures into container.

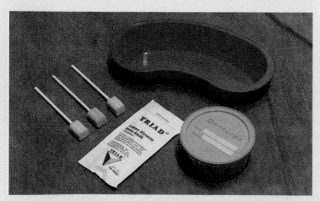

FIGURE 14-26A Assemble needed supplies.

(continues)

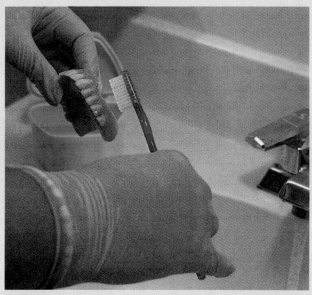

FIGURE 14-26D   When cleaning dentures under cool running water, protect the dentures by placing a paper towel or washcloth in the bottom of the sink.

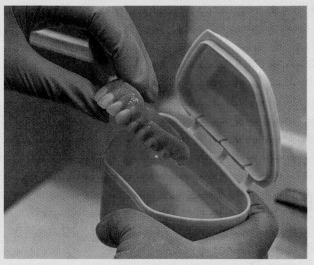

FIGURE 14-26F   Place clean dentures in clean denture cap.

and place fresh gauze squares into bottom. Place dentures in cup (Figure 14-26F) and take to client's bedside.

6. Assist client to rinse mouth with mouthwash.
7. A soft toothbrush or other type of applicator may be used to clean the mouth while dentures are out (Figure 14-26G). This is a good time to observe the inside of the client's mouth for signs of irritation or soreness.
8. Have client, if capable, insert clean dentures into mouth.
9. Clean and replace equipment.
10. Remove gloves and wash hands.
11. Document procedure completed and time, observations, and client's reaction.

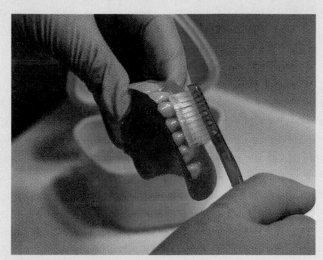

FIGURE 14-26E   Be sure to brush all surfaces of dentures.

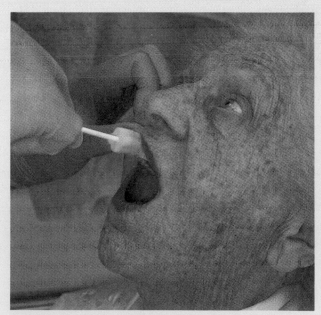

FIGURE 14-26G   Use toothette and clean inside of mouth. Remember to clean the tongue.

Personal Care and Grooming

The home health aide will be responsible for providing personal care to clients to keep clients well-groomed so that they look and feel good about themselves. Personal care will include shaving, nail care, and shampooing. Depending on the needs of your client, personal care may also include performing a warm foot soak or caring for an artificial eye. Procedures 40, 41, 42, and 43 demonstrate the proper ways to shave a male client, perform a warm foot soak, give nail care, and shampoo the client's hair in bed. Procedure 44 demonstrates how to care for an artificial eye.

CLIENT CARE PROCEDURE

40

Shaving the Male Client

PURPOSE

* To remove unwanted hair
  NOTE: Shaving can be planned for the same time that other daily hygiene tasks are done. For shaving, the electric razor is usually the easiest to use. However, it may be necessary to use a safety razor or disposable razor. In some instances, older women also may request to have facial hair shaved to improve cosmetic appearance. Remember standard precautions; wear gloves. If you accidentally cut the client while shaving him or her, report the cut to your supervisor.

PROCEDURE

1. Wash hands and apply gloves.
2. Ask client if he wants a shave.
3. Assemble needed supplies. If possible, have client shave in bathroom by the mirror.
     disposable gloves
     razor and shaving cream
     basin of hot water
     washcloth and towel
     aftershave lotion (optional)
4. Position client in sitting position and place towel under chin and across his chest.
5. Apply shaving cream (Figure 14-27A). With one hand, pull the skin tight above area to be shaved. With razor in other hand, gently take short, even strokes. Shave in the direction the hair grows

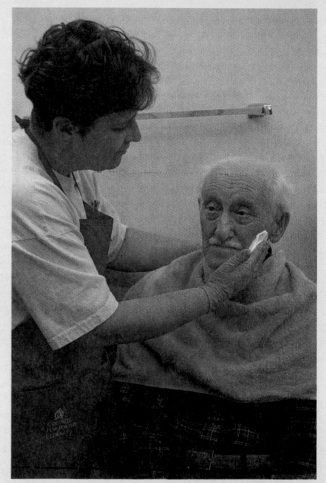

FIGURE 14-27A Apply shaving cream to face.

(Figures 14-27B through D). If client is capable, let him do as much as possible.

6. Rinse the razor frequently. After shave is completed, place used uncapped razor in "sharps" container. *(continues)*

CLIENT CARE PROCEDURE **Shaving the Male Client** *(continued)*

7. Change water in basin when shave is completed. Rinse the client's face in clear warm water and pat dry.
8. If desired, apply aftershave lotion. Remove gloves.
9. Return equipment and supplies, clean and rinse basin, dry and store.
10. Reposition client.
11. Wash hands.
12. Document completion of procedure and time, observations, and client's reaction.

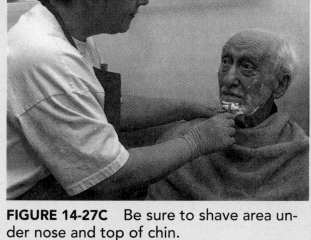

FIGURE 14-27C   Be sure to shave area under nose and top of chin.

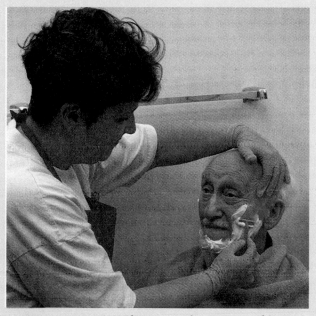

FIGURE 14-27B   Shave in direction of hair growth.

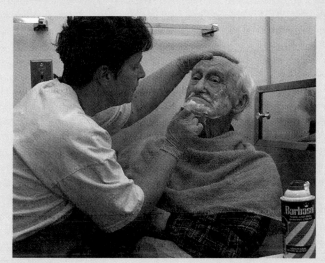

FIGURE 14-27D   Shave area under the client's chin.

CLIENT CARE PROCEDURE

41

Performing a Warm Foot Soak

PURPOSE

- To stimulate circulation in a client's feet
- To relieve pain or discomfort

- To soften the toenails to make them easier to cut
  NOTE: Never cut toenails unless directed by supervisor and follow agency policies.

(continues)

CLIENT CARE PROCEDURE **Performing a Warm Foot Soak** *(continued)*

PROCEDURE

1. Assemble equipment:
   disposable gloves
   large basin—plastic oblong dishpan
   warm water—100° to 110°F
   large plastic garbage bag or sheet
     of plastic
   small thin blanket
   2 towels
2. Wash hands and apply gloves.
3. Tell client what you plan to do.
4. Have client sit in comfortable chair if possible.
5. Place plastic bag on floor and place basin of water on top of plastic covering.
6. Remove client's shoes and socks and slowly place client's feet in basin of warm water (Figure 14-28). Be sure to follow any special instructions for special soaps or solutions that might be ordered.
7. Place thin blanket over the client's legs and feet.
8. Replenish water as necessary to maintain proper temperature.
9. Discontinue treatment in 20 to 30 minutes.
10. Remove feet from the basin and pat dry. Be sure to dry the skin well in between toes. When feet are dry, massage lotion on both feet. Put socks and shoes on client's feet.
11. Clean up equipment and return to storage area.
12. Remove gloves and wash hands.
13. Document completion of procedure, your observations, and client's reaction.

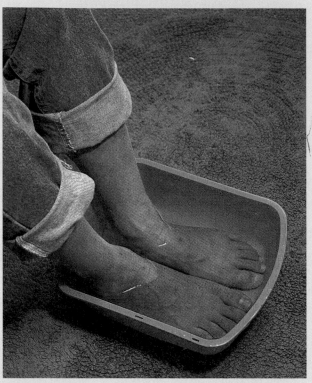

FIGURE 14-28   Client is sitting in a comfortable chair while she soaks her feet.

CLIENT CARE PROCEDURE

42

Giving Nail Care

PURPOSE

- To keep the client's nails clean and well groomed
- To observe for signs of irritation

NOTE: You never cut a diabetic client's toenails or fingernails. Nail care is usually given at bath time or when there is a need because of a broken nail or hangnail. A manicure may be done to make the client feel more attractive. In the elderly, you might note very thick toenails, which require special clippers to cut; this usually is done by a podiatrist (foot doctor).   *(continues)*

CLIENT CARE PROCEDURE **Giving Nail Care** *(continued)*

PROCEDURE

1. Assemble supplies:
   soap, water, and basin
   nail brush
   towel and lotion, preferably lanolin lotion
   small scissors or clippers
   emery board or nail file and orange stick
2. Wash your hands.
3. Tell client what you plan to do.
4. Soak toenails or fingernails in soap and water for 10 minutes.
5. Brush nails with nail brush. Clean under nails. Rinse well. Dry hands and nails.
6. Wear gloves if clipping nails/toenails.
7. If nails are too long, make a straight cut for toenails and a curve cut for fingernails. Check to make sure that you are allowed to cut nails. If you accidentally cut a client's skin while cutting nails, remember to use standard precautions. Report the cut to your supervisor.
8. Use file or emery board and smooth edges of nails (Figure 14-29).
9. Massage lotion on the hands or feet.
10. Clean the basin, brush, and scissors or clippers. Return equipment to proper place.
11. Wash your hands.
12. Document procedure, any observations, and client's reaction.

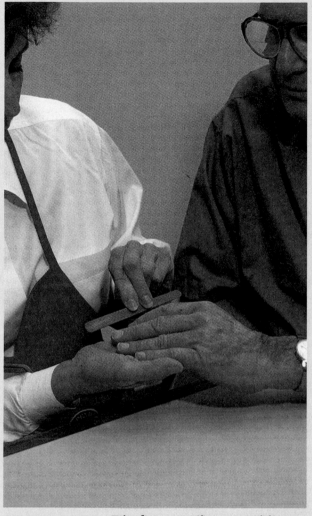

FIGURE 14-29   File fingernails smoothly.

CLIENT CARE PROCEDURE

43

Shampooing the Client's Hair in Bed

PURPOSE

- To clean the hair and scalp
- To stimulate circulation in the scalp
- To make the client feel and look better
- To prevent accumulation of dandruff or formation of scalp crusts

NOTE: A plastic shampoo tray may be used in a client's home, if available. Occasionally your agency may supply you with this shampoo tray. The shampoo tray is used in place of a rubber sheet or plastic bag and is easy to use.

(continues)

CLIENT CARE PROCEDURE **43 Shampooing the Client's Hair in Bed** *(continued)*

PROCEDURE

1. Assemble equipment:
   shampoo and hair conditioner or rinse (optional)
   3 to 4 towels
   large plastic garbage bags or rubber sheet
   large empty container or large waste-paper basket or bucket
   large pitcher for warm water
   comb and brush
   disposable gloves
   newspapers
2. Wash your hands. If client has sores or lesions of the scalp, wear gloves.
3. Tell client what you plan to do.
4. Position client so that the head rests over the edge of the bed. The back and shoulders should rest on the edge. (Your instructor will demonstrate this procedure.)
5. Loosen clothing from around client's neck. Roll a towel to be placed around neck (Figures 14-30A and B).

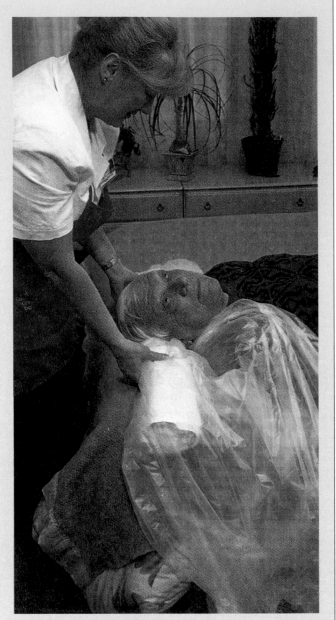

FIGURE 14-30B Place towel on large piece of plastic and roll to form a trough at the top and both sides.

6. Spread a newspaper on a chair or on the floor and set large empty bucket or container on the newspaper. Move the chair with the basin to a position beneath the head of the client.
7. Slide a plastic bag or sheet under the client's shoulders. Let the other end of the plastic fall into the basin. This allows the water to go from the head into the catch basin or bucket. *(continues)*

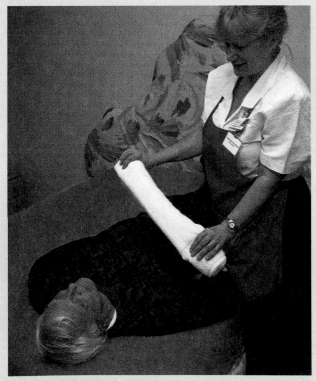

FIGURE 14-30A Fold large towel into a roll lengthwise.

CLIENT CARE PROCEDURE **Shampooing the Client's Hair in Bed** *(continued)*

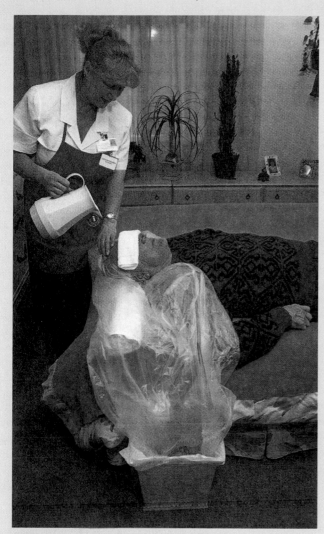

FIGURE 14-30C Position client on side of bed and moisten hair with a pitcher of water. Be sure to cover client's eyes. Note placement of bucket.

8. With pitcher full of warm water, wet the client's hair (Figure 14-30C). The client can use a washcloth to cover the eyes for protection.
9. Apply shampoo to the head, lather well, and massage scalp with your knuckles. If nonprescription medicated shampoo is ordered, follow any special instructions on label.
10. Rinse hair with water thoroughly, making sure to remove all traces of shampoo.
11. If necessary, reapply shampoo, lather well, and rinse thoroughly.

12. Apply hair conditioner or rinse. Follow directions on the bottle because some need to be diluted and others do not.
13. Dry client's hair with large towel. Comb and brush hair (Figure 14-31). If female, you may need to set hair on rollers. If hair dryer is available, blow-dry hair gently.
14. Return equipment to proper storage area.
15. Wash hands.
16. Document procedure completed, your observations, and client's reaction.

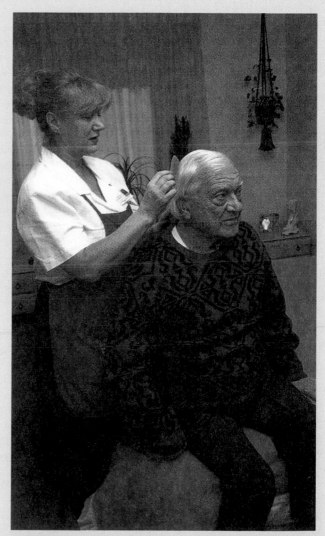

FIGURE 14-31 Comb and dry hair after shampoo. Before combing, be sure to place towel on shoulders to collect fallen hair.

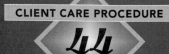

CLIENT CARE PROCEDURE 44

Caring for an Artificial Eye

PURPOSE

- To ensure proper care of client's artificial eye
- To prevent infection or irritation of the eye socket

PROCEDURE

1. Assemble equipment:
   disposable gloves
   eyecup with gauze square (not cotton filled)
   cleansing solution, if ordered
   washcloth and basin of lukewarm water
   cotton balls
   small plastic bag for wastes
2. Wash hands and apply gloves.
3. Tell client what you plan to do.
4. Have client lie down if possible. Position yourself and equipment to be on the same side as the client's artificial eye.
5. With moistened cotton balls clean the outside of the eye from the nose to the outside of the face. Stroke once only with each cotton ball.
6. Remove artificial eye by depressing lower eyelid with your thumb while lifting upper lid with your index finger. If client can remove artificial eye, let the client do it. Carefully take eye and place in gauze lined eyecup. Place eyecup in a safe place nearby while you clean the outside of the eye socket.
7. Clean eye socket using warm water and cotton balls. Pat area around eye dry. Observe area for signs of irritation or infection.
8. Carry eyecup to bathroom. Place washcloth in bottom of sink, as a precaution against breakage. Remove eye from eyecup and gently wash in sink. Remove all secretions on outside of the eye. Do not use any cleaner on eye unless specifically ordered.
9. Place clean gauze in bottom of eyecup and return to client. Assist the client to insert eye into socket. If eye is moist, it will slide in easier. You may need to depress the lower eyelid and replace the lid gently over the eye as it slips into the socket.
10. If client does not wish to have eye inserted into socket right away, the eye needs to be stored in water in the eyecup.
11. Return equipment and wastes to correct areas.
12. If client wears glasses, clean the glasses with a cleaning solution, rinse with clear water, and dry with tissues. Handle the glasses only by the frame. Return glasses to client or place in case.
13. Remove gloves and wash hands.
14. Document procedure completion, your observations, and client's reaction.

REVIEW

1. What is the largest organ of the body? *The Skin*
2. What might be suspected if a red, warm-looking spot appears on a bony prominence? *Brack down of skin*
3. List the elements of the integumentary system.
4. You notice an open sore over the elbow of a new client when you give her a bath. What stage of bedsore is this?
   a. Stage 1
   b. Stage 2
   c. Stage 3
   d. Stage 4

REVIEW

5. At what stage should you notify a nurse about a bed sore?
   a. Stage 1
   b. Stage 2
   c. Stage 3
   d. Stage 4

6. Which of the following are aspects of good skin care?
   a. Nutrition and hydration
   b. Clean bedclothes and clean skin
   c. Repositioning every 2 hours
   d. All of the above

7. Fill in the blank: Another word for hyperthermia is _____ .

8. Fill in the blank: Two conditions that may occur when the environmental conditions are extreme and the person's skin is unable to regulate body temperature are _____ and _____ .

9. Fill in the blank: _____ is a condition marked by abnormally low internal body temperature, usually 95°F (35°C) or under.

10. On a cold day in January you visit a client whom you see twice a week for postpartum care. You notice that the apartment feels cold when you walk in. The mother is lethargic, cannot concentrate on a conversation with you, and her speech is slurred. The baby's skin is cool to the touch, and she is stiff and has a weak pulse. What do you suspect the mother and child are suffering from? List the steps you would take to help the mother and baby.

11. It is a hot, summer day when you visit your elderly client Mr. Banks, who lives in a large, public housing complex. The housing complex he lives in is known for having a high crime rate, where the elderly are particularly vulnerable. He rarely leaves his apartment and refuses to open a window.

    When you arrive for today's visit you notice that his face is flushed and his skin is warm and dry to the touch. He is feeling weak and complains of chest pains when he greets you. His pulse is irregular, and his temperature is elevated to 101°F. What are the signs and symptoms present? Would you call for medical assistance? Why or why not?

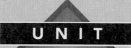

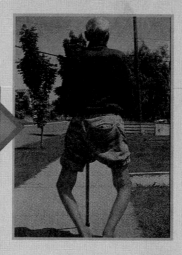

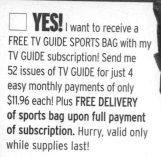
al System: Arthritis,
and Restorative Care

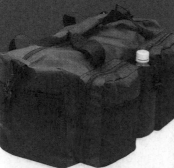

rheumatoid arthritis
steroids
tophi

...s
...hritis
...ism

...NG OBJECTIVES

...s unit, you should be able to:

...itis.

...,

...bed

...a

Name two joints that can be replaced by surgery.
- Demonstrate the following:

PROCEDURE 45	Turning the Client Toward You
PROCEDURE 46	Moving the Client up in Bed Using the Drawsheet
PROCEDURE 47	Making an Occupied Bed
PROCEDURE 48	Log Rolling the Client
PROCEDURE 49	Positioning the Client in Supine Position
PROCEDURE 50	Positioning the Client in Lateral/Side-lying Position
PROCEDURE 51	Positioning the Client in Prone Position
PROCEDURE 52	Positioning the Client in Fowler's Position
PROCEDURE 53	Assisting the Client from Bed to Wheelchair
PROCEDURE 54	Assisting the Client from Wheelchair to Bed
PROCEDURE 55	Transferring the Client from Wheelchair to Toilet/Commode
PROCEDURE 56	Lifting the Client Using a Mechanical Lift
PROCEDURE 57	Caring for Casts
PROCEDURE 58	Applying an Ice Bag, Cap, or Collar
PROCEDURE 59	Dressing and Undressing the Client

MUSCULOSKELETAL SYSTEM ·············

The musculoskeletal system is made up of bones and muscles. It protects the internal body organs and makes body movement possible. The skull, for instance, forms a protective covering for the brain. The spinal column surrounds the spinal nerves leading from the brain.

There are more than 200 bones in the body (Figure 15-1A and B). Bones are joined together by tough elastic fibers called **ligaments.**

Joints allow the bones to be moved in certain ways (Figure 15-2). The elbows and knees have hinge joints, which move in only two directions like hinges on a door. The joints at the shoulder and pelvis are ball and socket joints. They provide circular movements. The wrist,

ankles, and spinal column have gliding joints connecting the various bones. These allow only a limited sliding movement.

Skeletal muscles are attached to the bones by tendons and are stretched over joints. Certain muscles produce motion by pulling on the bone when they receive messages from the nervous system. These muscles are called voluntary muscles because their movement is controlled by the brain. For example, the eye sees a $5.00 bill on the floor. The picture is relayed to the brain. The brain, through the nervous system, tells the body to bend over and pick up the bill. This is an example of voluntary muscle action or one that the body chooses to perform.

Other muscles, called involuntary muscles, form the walls of organs. They, too, receive messages through the nervous system but they

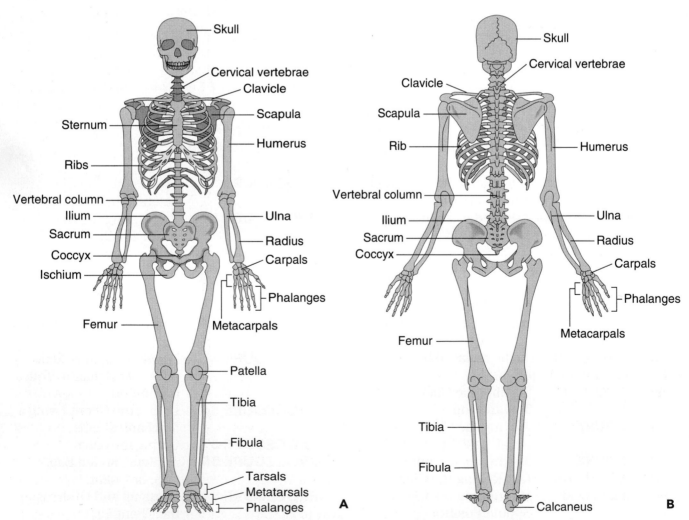

FIGURE 15-1 Bones of the skeleton. A. Anterior view B. Posterior view

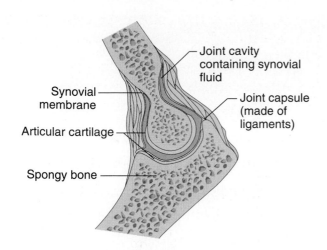 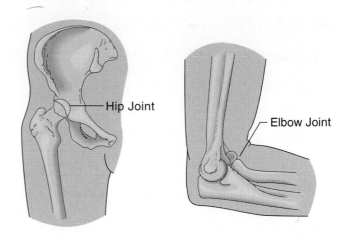

FIGURE 15-2   Diarthrotic joints

work automatically, or without any conscious effort by the individual. The heart is an example of an involuntary muscle because it pumps blood throughout the body without any conscious effort.

The musculoskeletal system constantly interacts with other systems. The interior of the bone produces new blood cells for the circulatory system. Muscles move in response to messages from the nervous system. It is not necessary to understand these complex interrelationships. However, it is interesting to note how one system depends on another.

Common Disorders of the Musculoskeletal System

The musculoskeletal system can be invaded by disease-causing microorganisms. However, the most common problems are fractures that are caused by falls.

Fractures.   A **fracture** is a break in a bone. Fractures are treated by immobilizing the bone or fixing it into position. Often the bone is immobilized by the application of a cast. Healing of bones may take several weeks; older people require a healing period similar to all individuals. This is about 6 weeks, providing there are no underlying illnesses. Procedure 57, presented later in this unit, demonstrates the proper method of caring for casts.

Arthritis.   A musculoskeletal problem the home health aide will probably encounter is arthritis. Although arthritis affects people of all ages, it more commonly occurs in the elderly.

Arthritis is an inflammation of the joints. It is usually painful and causes the joints to swell and become enlarged. Sometimes the bones of the hands and feet curl inward and become deformed.

There is no specific cure for arthritis, but there are treatments to relieve some of the symptoms. Pain, muscle spasms, and cramps can be relieved by heat from hot baths, heat lamps, paraffin baths, or hot packs. Aspirin, or aspirin substitutes such as nonsteroidal **anti-inflammatory** drugs are considered the safest medication for long-term use. However, the doctor should determine the amount of aspirin the client is allowed to take. Other drugs are also used in the treatment of arthritis, but these drugs must be prescribed by a physician. A client with arthritis may need physical therapy or may be treated with a special diet.

DEFINITION OF ARTHRITIS ···············

Arthritis means inflammation of a joint. Many people complain of **rheumatism** in relationship to their many aches and pains. The Arthritis Foundation states that arthritis is the number one crippler in the United States, affecting one in seven people. There are several types of arthritis. The two main ones are rheumatoid arthritis and osteoarthritis. A comparison of the two types is shown in Figure 15-3. Other types of arthritis are gout and ankylosing spondylitis. Arthritis affects 50% of persons over 65 years of

FIGURE 15-3 Comparison of rheumatoid arthritis and osteoarthritis

Rheumatoid Arthritis	Osteoarthritis
Affects the lubricating fluid in the joints	Affects cartilage-connective tissue
Inflammation	Wearing down condition
System disease (total body)	Health not generally affected
Good and bad periods of pain	No particular good periods without pain
Results in deformity	Limits motion only
Affects any joint	Affects weight-bearing joints
Affects all ages—even young people	Affects older age group

age. Twice as many women as men are afflicted with the disease. The major warning signs of inflammatory arthritis are:

• Swelling in one or more joints
• Early morning stiffness
• Recurring pain or tenderness in any joint
• Inability to move a joint normally
• Obvious redness and warmth in a joint
• Unexplained weight loss, fever, or weakness
• Symptoms and signs of the above persisting for 2 weeks

Other infections such as gonorrhea, tuberculosis, syphilis, Lyme disease, and streptococcal infections can also cause arthritis. There is no cure for the disease. It can be managed with diet, medication, surgery, and exercise.

Rheumatoid Arthritis

Rheumatoid arthritis affects individuals of all ages, the very young to the very old. The cause of this condition is that the immune system that normally protects the body works the opposite way and fights against the body. However, the joints are generally affected the most. It is a disease that affects the whole body, not only the joints. It can occasionally cause problems with the muscles, skin, blood vessels, nerves, and eyes. Additional signs besides joint enlargement that accompany the disease are weight loss and fatigue. A client may have a very mild case, which might cause mild discomfort, or a severe case where widespread joint deformities are present. The morning is usually the most difficult part of the day for clients with this type of arthri-

tis; at this time, stiffness and fatigue are more evident. As the disease progresses, joint problems increase in severity. These deformities of the joints are usually seen in the hips, knees, wrists, fingers, and ankles (Figure 15-4A to D).

Osteoarthritis

Another term for **osteoarthritis** is "wear and tear" arthritis. This type of arthritis affects the weight-bearing joints, such as the spine, hip, and knee. It is most often seen in clients over 65 years of age. The cause of this type of arthritis is not clearly understood. A few of the possible causes might be attributed to the aging process, obesity, heredity, stress, trauma, unbalanced hormone levels, or overuse of the joint. The affected joint or joints become enlarged and painful. Osteoarthritis is the most common type of arthritis.

Gout is a form of arthritis that affects mainly men over the age of 40. This type of arthritis is due to the presence of too much uric acid in the client's system. The first sign of this disease is a painful big toe. It can also affect other joints such as the foot, ankle, and wrist. These areas of the body have little outpouches or protruding lesions called **tophi** that contain abnormal amounts of uric acid. The affected joint becomes extremely painful.

MANAGEMENT OF ARTHRITIS

Arthritis is a chronic **degenerative** (weakens and becomes abnormal) **disease.** It is generally

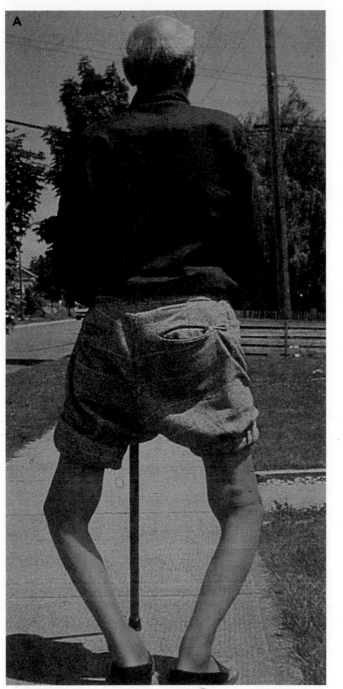
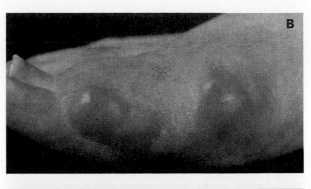
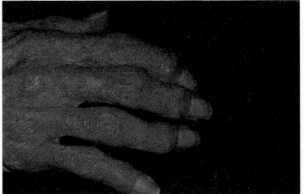
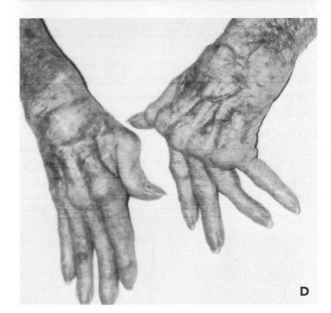

FIGURE 15-4   Joint deformities caused by arthritis

managed with diet therapy, an exercise program, medication and surgery. In some cases assistive devices can also be helpful.

Diet Therapy

The diet is individualized to meet the person's needs. If the client is overweight, the diet will need to be low in calories; if the client is underweight, the diet will need to be high in calories and protein. If the client has the gout form of arthritis, the client is placed on a low-purine diet prescribed and explained by a dietitian. Individuals crippled with arthritis may have a few of the following problems that interfere with their nutritional status.

- Pain may be a factor in lack of appetite.
- Decreased activity can cause weight gain, immobility, and pressure sore development.

- Impaired movement (Figure 15-5) may cause lack of energy for preparing foods and grocery shopping.

As a home health aide, you will most likely be employed to work in the home to assist the client with cooking, cleaning, and laundry duties. The client will be able to assist you to do a few of these tasks but will tire easily. You need to encourage the client to do as much as possible. Be sure you do not overtire or rush the client. The client will need a longer time to accomplish a task.

Exercise

Another form of treatment for arthritis is exercise. Exercise can be passive (you do it for the client) or active (the client performs the exercise without assistance). The goals of the exercise program are to maintain complete joint movement and in some cases strengthen the muscles around the specific joint. The physical therapist will develop a care plan for your client. If the joints are very painful and swollen, the exercises should be done gently but consistently. The exercises are usually ordered three (tid) to four times (qid) a day. It is helpful to have the client take pain medication a half-hour before the exercises are started. With his or her pain reduced, the client might be more willing to do the exercises. If the client does not exercise these joints, they will quickly become frozen or immobile.

Medication

The third method of treatment is through drug therapy. The specific drug used by clients will depend on many factors, such as:

- Severity of the arthritis
- Tolerance to the drug (aspirin is the drug of choice, but many individuals with stomach problems cannot tolerate aspirin)
- Cost
- Type of arthritis (gout responds to certain drugs only)
- Client's response (some clients respond positively to a drug and others do not respond at all)
- Presence of other chronic diseases (if a client has a stomach ulcer, certain drugs cannot be prescribed)

The largest class of drugs used to treat arthritis are called anti-inflammatories, which decrease pain and swelling in the joints and muscles. Some drug names are ibuprofen, ketoprofen, and naproxen; many are now available over the counter. They have significant side effects, such as black stools, bloody urine, ringing in the ears, and skin bruises. It is important that your client not self-medicate with these over-the-counter drugs. He or she should be encouraged to discuss treatment options with a doctor.

Other drugs used to treat arthritis are a group called **steroids.** These powerful drugs can cause edema, weight gain, susceptibility to infections, and elevated blood pressure.

Your nurse supervisor will inform you of the side effects to watch for in your client. More than 100 drugs are used to treat arthritis; all have different side effects.

Surgery

In the last 20 years, surgery has become successful in helping the arthritic client maintain independence. Doctors can now replace arthritic knees and hips. Surgery can also be done on the client's spine, jaw, wrist, fingers, and shoulder. An aide may be employed to care for these clients on a temporary basis after they

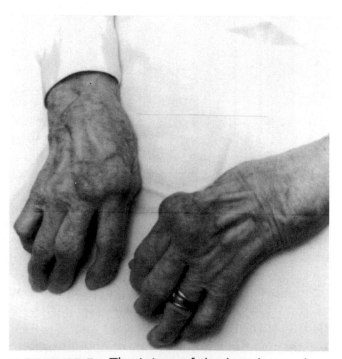

FIGURE 15-5 The joints of the hands are deformed because of arthritis.

return home from the hospital. Clients will have their own individualized plan of care designed by a team consisting of the doctor, nurse, physical therapist, occupational therapist, and case manager. You need to be fully informed of your responsibilities and what you are allowed and not allowed to do.

Assistive Devices

An aide employed in a home with a client with arthritis will need to take special care when moving or transferring a client. It is normal for the client to be able to do everything one day but the next day very little. Encourage the client to function at the highest level of wellness possible and to be as independent as possible. Try to assist the client in making tasks as simple as possible. A suggestion might be to have Velcro closures rather than buttons on clothes. Have elastic waist slacks rather than zipper and button closures. Bars may need to be placed by the bathroom and in the tub area to assist the client to get up and down. Portable whirlpool attachments can be placed in the client's tub to help soothe the client's pain. Another effective therapy is exercising or swimming in warm-water pools.

Assistive devices are often used in caring for clients with arthritis (Figure 15-6). Assistive devices are used mainly to maintain or increase independence, simplify tasks, reduce pain, and minimize stress on joints. Clients are more likely to use and accept simple devices over complicated devices (Figure 15-7). Your nurse supervisor will explain how to use these devices for your client (Figure 15-8).

In some cases the physical therapist will come directly to the home and do specialized treatments such as ultrasound or hot and cold treatments for your client (Figure 15-9). In other instances you might need to take your client to see the physical therapist for specialized therapy.

POSITIONING

Often a home health aide will need to position a client with mobility impairments. Positioning can make the client more comfortable and assist the body to function more efficiently. The

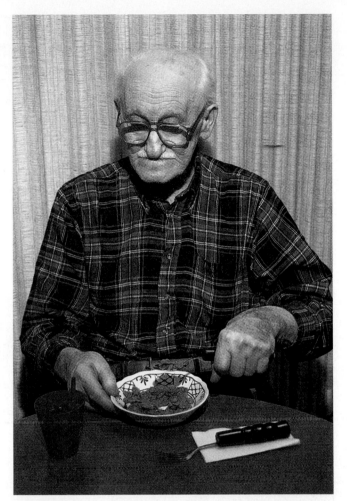

FIGURE 15-6 Client feeding himself using special cup, foam-handled fork and spoon

correct positioning can relieve pressure on body parts, aid in breathing, as well as preventing injury to the client. Some clients may need your assistance in positioning so that they can engage in activities such as eating, reading, watching television, or visiting. If the client is in the sitting position, you should check to make sure that the head is erect and the spine is in straight alignment (Figure 15-10). Body weight should be evenly distributed on the buttocks and thighs. Feet should be supported by the floor with ankles comfortably flexed. Forearms should be supported on an armrest, on the lap, or on a table positioned in front of the chair. For a side-lying position, pillows and other positioning supports should be correctly placed (Figure 15-11). The spinal column should be in correct alignment. Procedures 45 through 52 address many different positioning techniques and the proper procedures for each position.

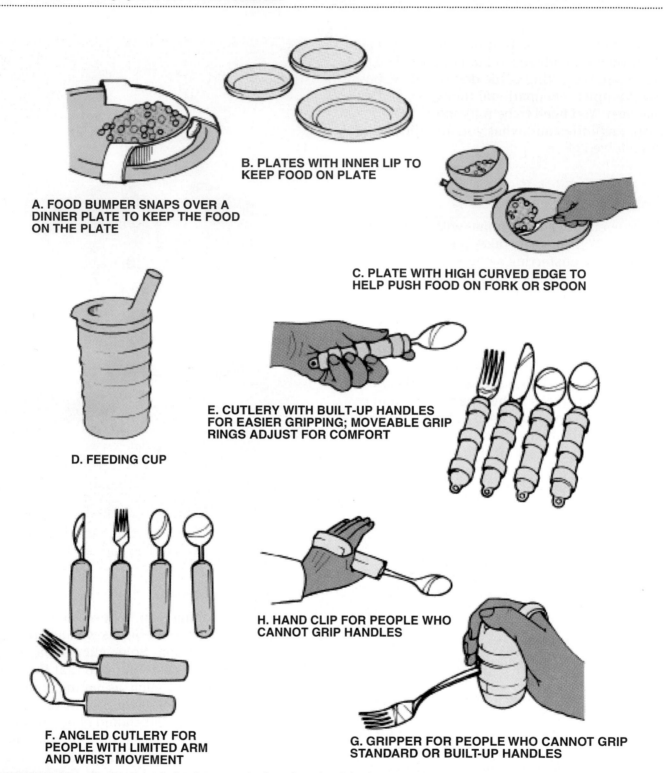

A. FOOD BUMPER SNAPS OVER A DINNER PLATE TO KEEP THE FOOD ON THE PLATE

B. PLATES WITH INNER LIP TO KEEP FOOD ON PLATE

C. PLATE WITH HIGH CURVED EDGE TO HELP PUSH FOOD ON FORK OR SPOON

D. FEEDING CUP

E. CUTLERY WITH BUILT-UP HANDLES FOR EASIER GRIPPING; MOVEABLE GRIP RINGS ADJUST FOR COMFORT

F. ANGLED CUTLERY FOR PEOPLE WITH LIMITED ARM AND WRIST MOVEMENT

H. HAND CLIP FOR PEOPLE WHO CANNOT GRIP HANDLES

G. GRIPPER FOR PEOPLE WHO CANNOT GRIP STANDARD OR BUILT-UP HANDLES

FIGURE 15-7 Eating and drinking aids for the disabled

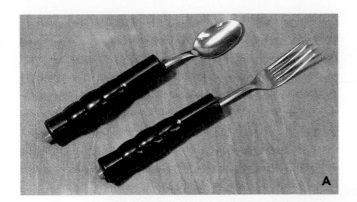

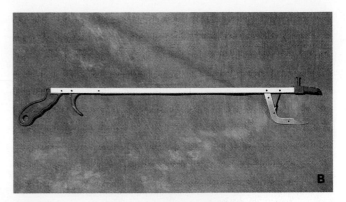

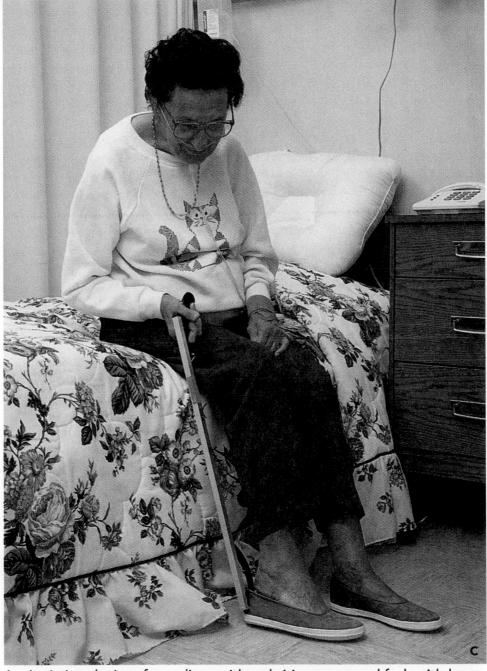

FIGURE 15-8   A. Assistive devices for a client with arthritis: spoon and fork with large, easy-to-hold foam handles   B. Assistive device used to pick up items from the floor or to reach for items on shelves   C. Using an assistive device to put on shoes

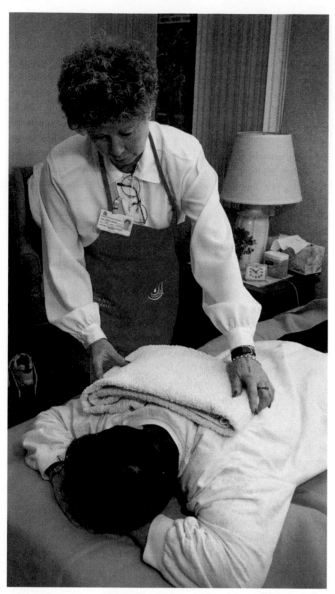

FIGURE 15-9 Physical therapist doing specialized treatment to client's shoulder

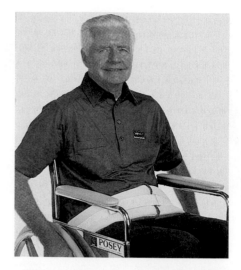

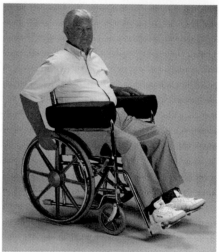

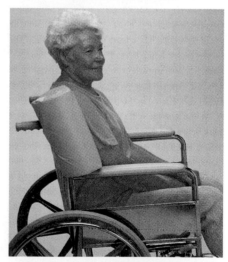

FIGURE 15-10 Supports help position patients and maintain body alignment without restricting movement. Clients are supported and protected without being restrained. (Courtesy of J. T. Posey Company, Arcadia, California)

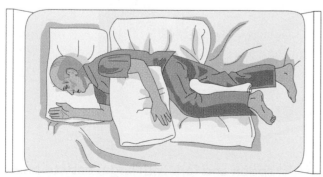

FIGURE 15-11 Check to see if the hips and legs are in correct alignment.

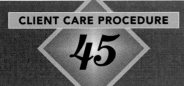

CLIENT CARE PROCEDURE

45

Turning the Client Toward You

PURPOSE

- To make the client more comfortable
- To change the client's position
- To improve circulation and reduce skin pressure

PROCEDURE

1. Wash your hands.
2. Tell client what you are going to do.
3. Lift client's far leg and cross it over the leg that is nearest you.
4. Lift the far arm over the chest, bend the elbow, and bring the hand toward the client's shoulder. Position the nearest arm so you will not roll client on it when you turn him.
5. Place the hand nearest the head of the bed on the far shoulder and place your other hand on the client's hip on the far side.
6. Brace your one thigh against the side of the bed and smoothly roll client toward you. Make sure that the client's upper leg comes over and bend it at the knee to ensure that the new position is stable.
7. Go to opposite side of bed and place your hands over the client's shoulder and pull upper body to the center of the bed. Place your hands over client's hips and pull the rest of the client's body to the center of the bed and into good body alignment.
8. Place a pillow against the client's back and secure it by pushing part under the client's back. The client's upper arm also should be supported with a pillow.
9. Support the knee, ankle, and foot of the upper leg with a pillow, which also prevents the knees and ankles from rubbing against each other and causing skin irritation. Cover client.
10. Wash your hands.
11. Document procedure completion, time, and client's reaction.

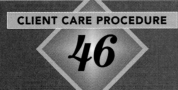

CLIENT CARE PROCEDURE

46

Moving the Client up in Bed Using the Drawsheet

PURPOSE

- To move client up in bed with minimum discomfort
- To relieve pressure on body parts
  NOTE: Very often a client will slide down in the bed away from the headboard. This is uncomfortable for the client. The sheets become wrinkled and undue pressure may be placed on the bony prominences, allowing the formation of pressure sores. You will need a partner to accomplish moving the client.

PROCEDURE

1. Wash your hands.   *(continues)*

CLIENT CARE PROCEDURE **Moving the Client up in Bed Using the Drawsheet** *(continued)*

2. Tell client what you plan to do. Have your partner stand on the opposite side of the bed to assist you.
3. Place pillow at the head of the bed to protect the client's head. Roll both sides of the drawsheet or flat sheet folded in fours toward the client. Place the client's feet 12 inches apart, so that they will not bump together as you move the client. Bend the client's knees, if possible.
4. With the hand nearest the client's feet, firmly grasp the rolled drawsheet or folded sheet. With the other hand, both of you cradle the client's head and shoulders and firmly grasp the top of the rolled drawsheet or folded sheet.
5. Turn your body and feet toward the head of the bed. Keep your feet about 12 inches apart and bend your knees slightly to achieve good body mechanics as you lift the client.
6. Coordinate your lift—on the count of three, together lift the drawsheet and the client up toward the head of the bed without dragging the client (Figure 15-12A). Align the client's body and limbs so that the client is straight and comfortable.
7. Place the pillow back under the client's head (Figure 15-12B), and tighten the drawsheet. Replace the covers and make the client comfortable.
8. Wash your hands.

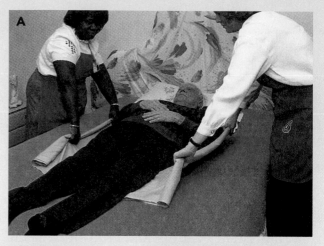

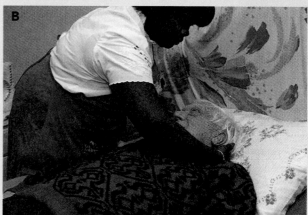

FIGURE 15-12 A. Lifting a client up in bed using a drawsheet B. Be sure to position client's head comfortably.

9. Document completion of the procedure, time, and client's reaction.

CLIENT CARE PROCEDURE

47

Making an Occupied Bed

PURPOSE

• To apply clean linens while the client remains in the bed

• To add to the client's comfort by removing soiled and wrinkled sheets *(continues)*

CLIENT CARE PROCEDURE **Making an Occupied Bed** *(continued)*

PROCEDURE

1. Wash your hands.
2. Assemble clean linens.
   flat sheet and fitted bottom (if available)
   extra flat sheet or drawsheet if used by client
   pillow cases
   large plastic bag (for soiled linens)
3. Tell client what you plan to do and provide for the client's privacy by closing the bedroom door.
4. Place clean linens on a clean chair or table in room in the order you plan to use them.
5. Loosen bedding from under mattress by lifting the mattress with one hand as you pull out bedding with the other hand.
6. Remove top covers one at a time, folding each to the foot of the bed.
7. Leave top sheet covering the client to prevent chilling and afford privacy.
8. Place two straight chairs against one side of the bed. This helps protect the client from falling out of bed. If the bed has side rails this is not necessary. Simply raise the side rail on the opposite side of the bed.
9. Assist the client to turn on the side facing the chairs or side rail. Assist the client to move near the edge of the bed by the chairs. Stand at the other side of the bed.
10. Roll or fanfold (fold in pleats) the soiled bottom sheet to the center of the bed beside the client's back.
11. Fold the clean bottom sheet lengthwise and place the fold at the center of the bed. Fanfold half the clean sheet next to the soiled sheet. Tuck the other half under the mattress. Make a mitered corner at the top. Tuck from the top or head of bed and move toward the foot of the bed.
12. Help client turn toward you onto the clean sheet. Bring the chairs to the other side of the bed for the client's protection (or raise the side rail).
13. Go to the other side and remove soiled sheet. Place dirty linens into large plastic bag.
14. Pull clean sheet across bed and tuck under mattress. Miter corner at top and tuck along side from head to foot of bed. Make certain the sheet is tight and wrinkle free.
15. Turn client onto the back in center of the bed. Place clean top sheet over the soiled top sheet. Slide the soiled sheet out from under the clean sheet. Have client hold fresh top sheet in place.
16. Place soiled sheet in large plastic bag.
17. Unfold blanket and bedspread and place over top sheet.
18. Tuck in the bottoms of the sheet, blanket, and bedspread at the foot of the bed. Miter the two corners; leave extra room for foot and toe movement.
19. Change the pillow cases and replace pillows under client's head. Put soiled cases in large plastic bag.
20. Be sure client is comfortable and that the room is neat. Remove soiled linens from room.
21. Wash your hands.
22. Document procedure completed.

CLIENT CARE PROCEDURE

Log Rolling the Client

PURPOSE

- To ensure the spinal column is kept straight because of special medical conditions

NOTE: You will need help to perform this procedure. *(continues)*

CLIENT CARE PROCEDURE ◆48◆ **Log Rolling the Client** *(continued)*

PROCEDURE

1. Wash your hands.
2. Tell the client what you plan to do.
3. With both you and your helper on the same side of the bed, remove the top covers.
4. Place your hand and arm under the client's head and shoulder to stabilize the neck. Your helper places his arms under the client's body and legs. On the count of three, lift the client toward you as a single unit.
5. Do not allow the client to bend and use good body mechanics yourselves by bending your knees and keeping your backs straight.
6. Place a pillow lengthwise between the client's thighs and legs and fold the client's arms over the chest.
7. Go over to the other side of the bed. You are in a position to keep the shoulders and upper body straight and your helper is positioned to keep the client's lower body, hips, and legs straight. Reach over the client and roll the drawsheet firmly against the client. On the count of three, the client is rolled toward you in a single movement, keeping the client's head, spine, and legs in a straight position.
8. To maintain the client's new position and alignment, place pillows against the spine and leave the pillow between the client's legs. Other small pillows or folded towels can be placed under the client's head and neck and under the arms for support.
9. Fold the drawsheet back over the pillows supporting the spine. Make sure the client's alignment is straight and that the client is comfortable. Arrange covers for the client.
10. Wash your hands (Figure 15-13).
11. Record this repositioning, time, and any observation you made.

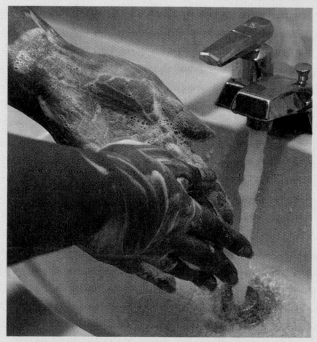

FIGURE 15-13 Wash your hands.

CLIENT CARE PROCEDURE

49

Positioning the Client in Supine Position

PURPOSE

- To make client more comfortable
- To assist the body to function more efficiently

PROCEDURE

1. Wash your hands.
2. Tell client what you plan to do.

(continues)

CLIENT CARE PROCEDURE **Positioning the Client in Supine Position**
(continued)

3. Place pillow under the client's head, so that the client's head is about 2 inches above the level of the bed. The pillow should extend slightly under the shoulders (Figure 15-14).
4. Have client's arms extended straight out with palms of the hands flat on the bed. The arms can be supported by pillows or covered foam pads placed under the forearms and extending from just above the elbows to the ends of the fingers.
5. Place a small pillow or rolled towel along the side of the client's thighs and tuck part of the support under the thigh, ensuring that the part under the thighs is smooth. This maintains alignment of the hips and thighs and helps prevent the hips from rotating outward or externally.
6. Place a pillow under the back of the ankle to relieve pressure on the heels.
7. Wash your hands.

8. Document the time, position change, and the client's reaction.

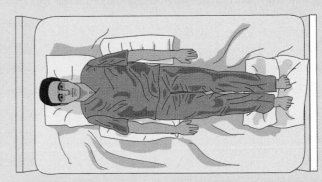

FIGURE 15-14   A client in supine position. The head may be elevated slightly with a pillow and the arms may be elevated slightly with a pillow and the arms may also be supported with pillows. A trocanter roll may be placed along the side of the client's thighs to keep legs in good alignment.

CLIENT CARE PROCEDURE
50
Positioning the Client in Lateral/ Side-lying Position

PURPOSE

- To provide for client comfort
- To relieve pressure on body parts

PROCEDURE

1. Wash your hands.
2. Tell client what you plan to do.
3. Go to opposite side of bed from the direction you are planning to turn the client toward.
4. Cross the client's arms over the chest. Place your arm under the client's neck and shoulders. Place your other arm under the client's midback. Move the upper part of the client's body toward you.
5. Place one arm under the client's waist and the other under the thighs. Move the lower part of the client's body toward you.
6. Turn client to opposite side. Pull shoulder that is touching the bed slightly toward you. Pull buttock that is touching the bed slightly toward you. Place pillow under back and buttocks. Place bottom leg in extension and flex upper leg. Place small folded blanket or pillow between the upper and lower leg.
7. Place pillow under client's head. Rotate the arm up to bring it up to the pillow with the palm facing up. Place the other arm

(continues)

CLIENT CARE PROCEDURE 50 **Positioning the Client in Lateral/ Side-lying Position** (*continued*)

on a pillow that extends from above the elbow to the fingers. Extend the fingers.

8. Check the client's position to see if the body is in good vertical alignment (Figure 15-15).
9. Wash your hands.
10. Document time, change of position, and client's reaction.

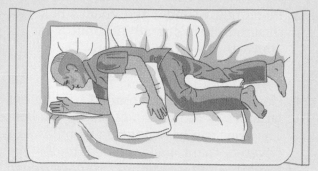

FIGURE 15-15 Lateral/side-lying position

CLIENT CARE PROCEDURE

 51 **Positioning the Client in Prone Position**

PURPOSE

- To relieve pressure on body parts
- To provide for client comfort
  NOTE: Most elderly clients are not able or do not like to be in this position for long because it is uncomfortable. In fact, it would be preferable to use frequent position changes from side to back (if possible), to side again, to increase client comfort and to reduce pressure points.

  Before turning a dependent client prone, make sure client's arms are straight down at sides to avoid injury while turning. Never leave an older client in this position more than 15 to 20 minutes.

PROCEDURE

1. Wash your hands.
2. Tell client what you plan to do.
3. Turn client on abdomen. Check to see if spine is straight and face is turned to either side.

4. Client's legs are extended. Arms are flexed and brought up to either side of head.
5. A small pillow can be placed under the abdomen. (For women, this will reduce pressure against their breasts.) An alternate method is to roll a small towel and place it under shoulders to reduce pressure.
6. Place another pillow under lower legs to prevent pressure on toes (Figure 15-16).

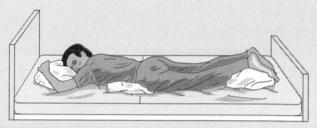

FIGURE 15-16 Prone position

CLIENT CARE PROCEDURE

52

Positioning the Client in Fowler's Position

PURPOSE

- To provide client comfort
- To aid in breathing
- To position client so the client can engage in activities such as eating, reading, watching television, visiting

   NOTE: If the client is weak or frail, the sitting position may be hard for the client to maintain. Supporting the client with pillows may help the client maintain the sitting position.

PROCEDURE

1. Wash your hands.
2. Tell the client what you plan to do.
3. Check to see if the client's spine and legs are straight and in the middle of the bed.
4. Support client's head and neck with one, two, or three pillows. If client has a hospital bed, raise bed to 45° angle.
5. Knees may be flexed and supported with small pillows (Figure 15-17).
6. Pillows may be placed under each arm from elbows to fingertips to support shoulders.
7. Place pillow or padded footboard against feet.
8. Wash your hands.
9. Document time, position change, and client's reaction.

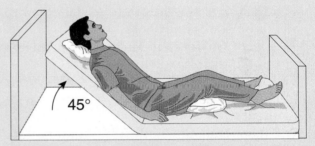

FIGURE 15-17   Fowler's position

TRANSFERS

Often an aide will be asked to transfer a client who is wheelchair bound. Using the proper transfer techniques will ensure that the client is moved safely from one location to another. Procedures 53 through 56 address various transfer techniques and the proper method for each.

CLIENT CARE PROCEDURE

53

Assisting the Client from Bed to Wheelchair

PURPOSE

- To move client from one location to another safely and without discomfort

NOTE: There should be a specific transfer procedure for each client who is not an independent, self-transfer.   *(continues)*

CLIENT CARE PROCEDURE ◆53◆ **Assisting the Client from Bed to Wheelchair**
(continued)

PROCEDURE

1. Wash your hands.
2. Tell the client what you plan to do.
3. Assemble needed equipment.
   wheelchair
   transfer belt
   client's shoes and socks
4. Place chair so client moves toward client's strongest side. Set chair at 45° angle to bed. Lock wheels. Move footrests out of the way.
5. Assist client to sit at edge of bed (Figure 15-18A).
6. Wait a few seconds to allow the client to adjust to sitting position. Assist client to put on socks and shoes.
7. Apply transfer belt. Make sure the belt is not too tight or too loose.
8. Spread your feet apart and flex your hips and knees, aligning your knees with client's.
9. Grasp transfer belt from underneath. Rock the client up to standing on the count of three (Figure 15-18B), while straightening your hips and legs, keeping knees slightly flexed.
10. If client has a weak leg, press your knee against it or block client's foot with yours to prevent weaker leg from sliding out from under the client.
11. Instruct client to use armrest on chair for support and be sure to flex your hips and knees while lowering client into chair. Remove transfer belt.
12. Check alignment of client in chair and make adjustments accordingly (Figure 15-18C).
13. Wash your hands.
14. Document time, position change, and client's reaction.

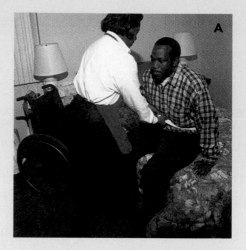

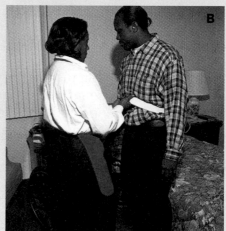

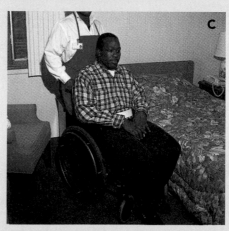

FIGURE 15-18 A. Lift belt is applied to client. An aide holds onto belt to assist the client to stand. B. Client stands and pivots on his good leg. C. Client is positioned comfortably in chair.

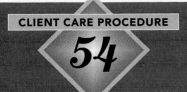

Assisting the Client from Wheelchair to Bed

PURPOSE

- To change client's position
- To transfer client safely from one location to another

PROCEDURE

1. Wash your hands.
2. Tell client what you plan to do.
3. Position client with strong side toward bed with wheelchair at 45° angle. Lock wheels.
4. Apply transfer belt and place both hands on back of the belt. Instruct client, if able, to put feet flat on the floor and hands on the chair. On the count of three, have client push up to standing position. While standing, have the client pivot (turn) on strong leg toward the bed. Have the client lower himself or herself to the bed to a sitting position.
5. Assist the client to lying position. Position client in comfortable position and in good alignment. Remove shoes, socks, and transfer belt.
6. Wash hands.
7. Document time, change of position, and client's reaction.

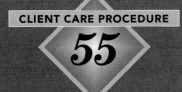

Transferring the Client from Wheelchair to Toilet/Commode

PURPOSE

- To enable client to sit on toilet for normal excretion of body wastes
  NOTE: It is essential to have grab bars, preferably secured to the wall, but they can be attached to the toilet seat.

PROCEDURE

1. Wash hands.
2. Tell client what you plan to do.
3. Have client in wheelchair with strong side nearer to the toilet or commode.
4. Lock the wheelchair. Apply transfer belt. Lift foot pieces out of way.
5. Loosen clothing on the client, but not too loose that the slacks fall while transferring.
6. Have client slide forward in chair and place feet apart. Place your hand on the back of the transfer belt. Have client place hands on armpiece and on the count of three push up.
7. Stand client up and have client place strong arm on grab bars (Figure 15-19).

(continues)

CLIENT CARE PROCEDURE ⟨55⟩ **Transferring the Client from Wheelchair to Toilet/Commode** (*continued*)

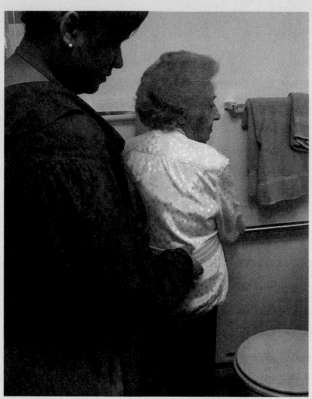

FIGURE 15-19 Assist the client to the toilet with client holding onto grab bars.

You continue to hold onto the transfer belt and slowly lower client onto the toilet or commode. Have client hold onto grab bar while you lower the client's pants.

8. Remove belt and move wheelchair out of way.
9. Provide privacy for client. Check often to see if client is all right. Give client toilet paper.
10. Assist the client as needed, return to wheelchair, and assist back to prior activity.
11. Wash client's hands and your hands.
12. Document bowel movement or urination.

CLIENT CARE PROCEDURE

56

Lifting the Client Using a Mechanical Lift

PURPOSE

- To transfer client from one place to another, usually from bed to chair
- To safely transfer a client who is heavy or has no weight-bearing ability
  NOTE: Check slings, chains, and straps for frayed areas or defective hooks. Two types

of slings are supplied with the Hoyer lift: hammock style and two-piece canvas strips. The hammock type can be made out of mesh or canvas. This type of sling is better for clients who are weak and need support (Figure 15-20). The canvas strips can be used for clients with normal muscle tone.

(continues)

CLIENT CARE PROCEDURE ◆*56*◆ **Lifting the Client Using a Mechanical Lift**
(continued)

PROCEDURE

1. Wash your hands and assemble equipment.
2. Tell client what you plan to do.
3. Position chair near bed and allow adequate room to maneuver the lift.
4. Roll client away from you.
5. Place hammock sling or canvas strips under client to form seat; with two canvas pieces, lower edge fits under client's knees (wide piece); upper edge goes under client's shoulders (narrow piece).
6. Go to opposite side of bed, roll client away from you and straighten hammock or strips through.
7. Roll client supine into canvas seat.
8. Place lift's horseshoe bar under side of bed (on side with chair). Have base of lift in maximum open position and lock.
9. Lower horizontal bar to sling level by releasing hydraulic valve. Lock valve.
10. Attach hooks or strap (chain) to holes in sling. Short chains/straps hook to top holes of sling; lower chains to bottom of sling. Point hooks to the outside when attaching.
11. Fold client's arm over the chest.
12. Pump handle until client is raised free of bed, but no higher than necessary.
13. Use steering handle to pull lift from bed and maneuver to chair.
14. Roll base around chair. Slowly release check valve and lower client into chair.
15. Check to see if client is positioned correctly. Unhook chains or straps and remove lift.

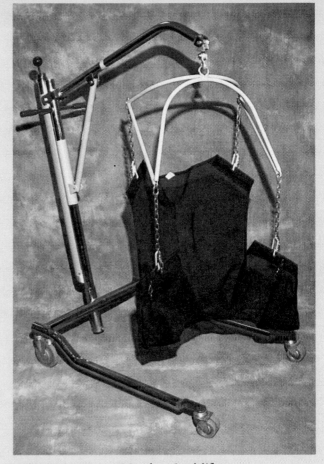

FIGURE 15-20   Mechanical lift

16. If straps are used, they can be removed. If the hammock sling is used, sling will remain underneath client so it is in position for transfer back to bed.
17. Wash your hands.
18. Document transfer, time completed, and client's reaction.

CAST CARE ⋯⋯⋯⋯⋯⋯⋯⋯⋯

Casts are used to immobilize extremities or joints following trauma or fractures, or to correct a body bone/joint defect. Casts may be applied to an extremity or to the entire body. Casts may be made of plaster of Paris, fiberglass, or polyester. Casts promote healing of the injured area, while providing comfort to the client. Procedure 57 demonstrates the proper method to care for casts.

CLIENT CARE PROCEDURE

57

Caring for Casts

PROCEDURE

1. Observe the new cast every 2 to 3 hours for the first 2 days and then four times daily. Check the skin for signs of irritation such as redness or swelling. Skin areas below the cast must be observed for signs of cyanosis (blue color), unusual coldness, or any unusual odor, which may indicate a serious problem. These signs and any complaints of numbness should be reported to the supervisor.
   - Note the color of the skin at the farthest end of cast—normal pink, warm to touch, and movable toes or fingers (Figure 15-21).
   - Look for edema at both ends of the cast; report and record this information.
   - Observe for response to touch (that is, the response of the nerves to stimulation); report and record this information. Report *any* numbness or tingling that persists.
2. Observe the cast daily for roughness around the edges. This may cause skin irritation and may be filed or covered with soft padding. These rough edges can be covered with plain white tape. This is called petaling and can be done by the nurse.
3. Observe the cast itself, noting any redness that may indicate bleeding or drainage from under the cast. Circle the area with a magic marker, noting the date and time that you first noticed the redness. Also note any unusual odor. Record and report immediately.
4. Observe the cast constantly for any cracks. Cracks are unsafe and you should notify your nurse supervisor of the crack. You must state the exact location and length of the crack as well as the depth of it.
5. When the cast is near the perineal area, protect it from moisture. Ask your case manager for special instruction on which

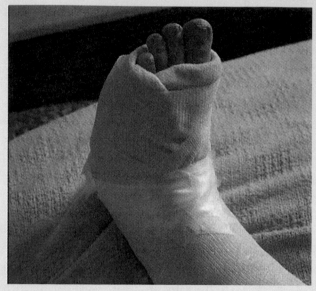

FIGURE 15-21 Frequently check the client's toes for warmth, color, and response to touch.

waterproof or protective device to use. Protect the cast and skin by preventing any dirt, sand, or small articles from getting inside the cast, which could cause an infection under the cast. Note that plaster of Paris tends to crumble and become soft when moist; therefore, this type of cast must always be kept dry.

6. Ask the client if he or she has pain in any particular area under the cast. This may indicate a pressure point and skin breakdown under the cast. Note this area. *Report and record immediately*. Be sure to position your client correctly. Figure 15-22 shows several types of casts commonly applied.

Safety for Client with a Cast

1. Check the house for throw rugs or objects on the floor. Remove any hazard that may cause the client to fall. Remind client to leave a nightlight on to prevent a fall in the middle of the night.

(continues)

CLIENT CARE PROCEDURE **Caring for Casts** *(continued)*

2. Remember that at first the client may not have a good sense of balance and may be unsteady in walking. Arrange the furniture so that the client may hold on to furniture or handrails while walking.

3. Assist the client in making changes in eating, dressing, writing, toileting, and walking.

4. Ask the case manager for specific orders for passive range of motion exercises. A physical therapist or occupational therapist may come to assist the client with specific exercises. A home health aide may not perform these exercises without orders and direct supervision.

5. Determine the composition of the cast by asking the case manager. Plaster of Paris casts take at least 24 hours to dry; polyester or fiberglass casting tape takes 5 to 15 minutes to dry. Be sure you do not touch the wet cast with the fingers because this may leave dents in the cast. Use the palm of the hand to move the cast. Do not allow the cast to dry on a hard surface because this will flatten the cast. Place the entire new cast on pillows and expose to air. Do not allow client to put anything between the cast and the skin if the skin under the cast starts to itch. If itching becomes unbearable, air can be blown in by use of a hair dryer, if the nurse supervisor gives you permission to do this. When positioning a client with an extremity cast, elevate the cast on pillows. Generally it is not allowed to have the client lie on the injured side. Instruct the client to wiggle toes or fingers frequently on cast extremity. Do not cover casted extremity because air needs to be allowed to circulate inside the cast.

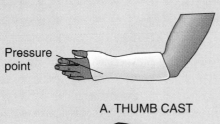

A. THUMB CAST

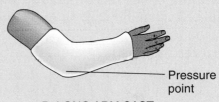

B. LONG ARM CAST

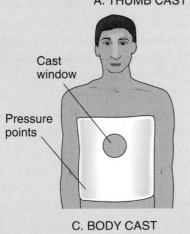

C. BODY CAST

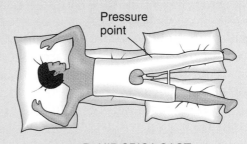

D. HIP SPICA CAST

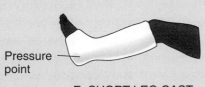

E. SHORT LEG CAST

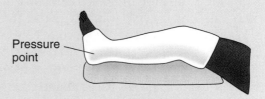

F. LONG LEG CAST

FIGURE 15-22 Casts that are frequently applied

APPLICATION OF COLD ·····················

Heat and cold applications are ordered by a physician to promote comfort and healing. Cold applications can ease pain or decrease swelling of localized areas. Heat applications can increase circulation to a body part, relax tension, and relieve pain. Because the application of heat and cold can cause injury and changes in bodily functions, some states and home care agencies do not allow home health aides to carry out these procedures. It is important to follow your employer's policies and procedures. Procedure 58 addresses the proper method to apply an ice bag, cap, or collar.

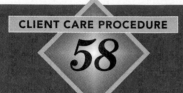
CLIENT CARE PROCEDURE

58 Applying an Ice Bag, Cap, or Collar

PURPOSE

• To ease pain
• To decrease swelling of localized area
  NOTE: Cold applications such as an ice bag, ice cap, or collar should **NOT** be applied without a doctor's order. The supervisor will tell the aide when to apply ice and how to do it.

  All ice applications must be covered with a cloth. Never apply ice or the cap, bag, or collar directly to the skin. A towel, face cloth, or fitted cover should be used against the skin.

PROCEDURE

1. Wash your hands before beginning the procedure.
2. Fill an ice bag, cap, or collar with ice cubes or crushed ice. Use a spoon to transfer the ice. Fill the container half full so that its weight will not be uncomfortable for the client (Figure 15-23).
3. Place the bag on a flat surface with the top in place but not tightened. Hold the neck of the bag upright. Gently press the bag from the bottom to the opening to expel the air.
4. Secure lid firmly and wipe dry with paper towels. Periodically test for leakage.
5. Wrap ice bag in towel or soft cloth. Covering it protects the client's skin from di-

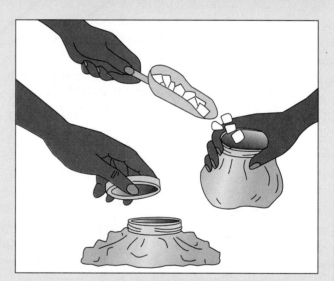

FIGURE 15-23 An ice bag should be half filled so it can lie flat against the client's body and not cause discomfort due to its weight.

rect contact. A disposable cold pack can also be used (Figure 15-24).
6. Apply to affected body area. Make sure that any metal parts face away from the skin. Place an extra towel around the bag if the skin appears sensitive to the cold.
7. Check the client's skin every 5 minutes. Look for signs of redness, whiteness, or cyanosis (blue color). If these signs appear, call the nurse or supervisor for instructions.

(continues)

CLIENT CARE PROCEDURE **58** **Applying an Ice Bag, Cap, or Collar** *(continued)*

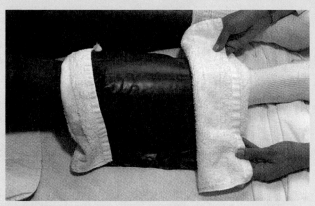

FIGURE 15-24 A disposable ice pack can be applied readily to a client's swollen ankle.

8. If ice melts, replace with fresh ice and continue treatment.
9. Remove ice bag after 20 minutes.
10. Empty bag, allow it to dry, and store properly.
11. Return client to a comfortable position.
12. Wash your hands after the procedure.

PERSONAL CARE

Some clients with functional or cognitive impairments may need assistance with personal care, such as dressing and undressing. Procedure 59 demonstrates the proper technique to dress and undress the client.

CLIENT CARE PROCEDURE

59 **Dressing and Undressing the Client**

PURPOSE

- To keep the client clean and comfortable
- To increase client's self-image and well-being
- To reduce client's discomfort and reduce client's risk of strain or injury

NOTE: Do not allow client to remain in nightclothes during the day (unless case manager states it is all right). The client needs to know that it is daytime and needs to dress accordingly.

PROCEDURE

1. Wash your hands and tell client what you plan to do.

2. Assemble clean items:
   undergarments
   clothing—let client select if possible
   stockings and shoes
3. If client is able, help the client to sit at the edge of the bed and dangle his or her legs. If the client is too weak to sit up, have client lie flat on the bed. Place a sheet or robe over client to avoid embarrassing or chilling the client.
4. Assist the client to put on undergarments. (A front closing bra is very convenient for women with limited movement in their arms.) If client has a weak leg,

(continues)

CLIENT CARE PROCEDURE ◇ 59 ◇ **Dressing and Undressing the Client** *(continued)*

place the weak leg in first, then the other leg. Then put on clothing in the same manner. If the client can stand, pull the pants or slacks up to the waist. If the client must remain on the bed, ask the client to press the heels into the bed and raise the buttocks. While the client is in this position, quickly slide the pants or slacks up to the waist. Assist the client as necessary. If the client is unable to lift buttocks up, roll the client from side-to-side as you raise the slacks over the hips. Slacks with elastic waist are preferred, as they are put on more easily than pants with zippers and buttons. Cotton jogging suits are becoming a popular option for the disabled or elderly clients. They are warm, easy to get off and on, and attractive. They also launder easily.

5. Assist the client to put on a shirt by placing the weaker arm in the sleeve first. Pull the shirt around for the client to place the other arm in the sleeve.

6. When removing a shirt, remove the sleeve of the strongest arm first, followed by the weaker arm. Encourage the client to do as much as he or she is able.

REVIEW

1. Fill in the blanks: Two common disorders of the musculo-skeletal system are _____ and _____ .

2. List three types of arthritis.

3. List two types of diets that can be prescribed for clients with arthritis.

4. List three side effects of steroids.

5. List two goals of an exercise program for a client with arthritis.

6. List two joints that can be replaced by surgery for a client with arthritis.

7. Describe special care that you as a home health aide would do for a client with arthritis.

8. A client has arthritis. Care will include all the following except:
   a. Assistance with activities of daily living
   b. Range of motion exercises
   c. Use of braces or prosthesis to prevent contractures
   d. Exercising painful joints gently and consistently

9. T F Osteoarthritis is often seen in women over 65 years of age.

10. T F Clients with rheumatoid arthritis experience more discomfort and pain in the evening than in the morning.

11. Signs of an osteoarthritis flare-up are:
    a. Swelling of one or more joints
    b. Inability to move a joint normally
    c. Obvious redness and warmth in a joint
    d. All are correct

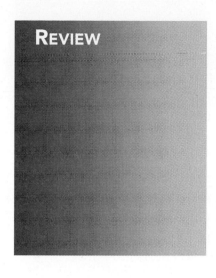

REVIEW

12. Arthritis can be treated by:
    a. Drug therapy
    b. Exercise program
    c. Surgery
    d. All are correct

13. Your client has a severe form of arthritis. The physical therapist has developed a care plan for your client; however, when you ask the client about it she tells you "it hurts too much to exercise." What three steps could you take to ensure that your client completes her exercises?

14. What are the advantages of having a wheelchair-bound person positioned properly? Describe in detail the proper body position for a person sitting in a wheelchair.

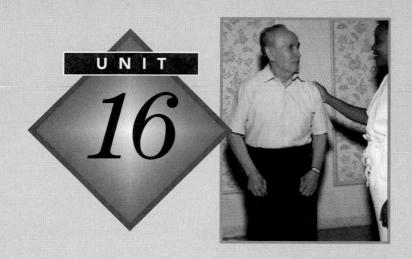

Nervous System

KEY TERMS

amyotrophic lateral
    sclerosis (ALS)
auditory
cerebral vascular
    accident (CVA)

hemiplegia
multiple sclerosis (MS)
muscular dystrophy
otosclerosis
paraplegia

Parkinson's disease
quadriplegia
seizure
sensory deficits

LEARNING OBJECTIVES

After studying this unit, you should be able to:

- Define paraplegia, quadriplegia, and hemiplegia.
- Identify three common sensory losses in older adults.
- Name and describe four common sensory disorders.

- Demonstrate the following:
  PROCEDURE 60   Caring for a Client
                  Having a Seizure

NERVOUS SYSTEM

The brain, spinal cord, and nerves make up the nervous system. This system is the communication center that sends messages to all parts of the body. It is the system that enables the body to see, hear, smell, taste, and touch. Sight, sound, taste, smell, and touch are known as the five body senses. The brain (Figure 16-1) is the master control or main switch of the nervous system. Messages are relayed to the brain from all parts of the body. The brain decides how to respond to each message (or stimulus) sent by the nerves. Each area of the brain performs a specialized duty. The brain alerts other control centers in the body so that the body correctly responds to a message.

The spinal cord can be compared to the electrical wiring system in a house. All the major nerves of the body are bound together in the spinal cord and lead into the brain. The spinal cord is protected by the spinal column. If the spinal column is damaged or diseased, the spinal nerves may be affected. For example, if a person suffers a broken back and the spinal cord is cut or damaged, the **nerves** below the cut could no longer send messages up to the brain. The parts of the body below the cut could no longer feel pain and the muscles would no longer move.

Paraplegia refers to paralysis of the lower part of the body and both legs. **Quadriplegia** refers to paralysis of both arms and both legs. Both paraplegia and quadriplegia can result from disease or injury to the brain or spinal cord. **Hemiplegia** is a paralysis of one side of the body. It is frequently the result of a **cerebrovascular accident (CVA)** or "stroke."

The nerves radiate from the spinal cord to all parts of the body, forming a network. The nerve endings might be compared to the electrical outlets in the house. In the body, the nerves are usually ready to receive stimuli. For instance, the hand touches a hot surface, the nerve sends the message to the spinal cord, and it goes to the brain. The brain sends back the message to move the hand off the hot surface. This entire process takes place in an instant so that one is only aware of the result. The time it takes to respond to a stimulus is known as reaction time. As the human body ages, reaction time often slows down a great deal. It also is affected when part of the brain has been damaged as with a stroke.

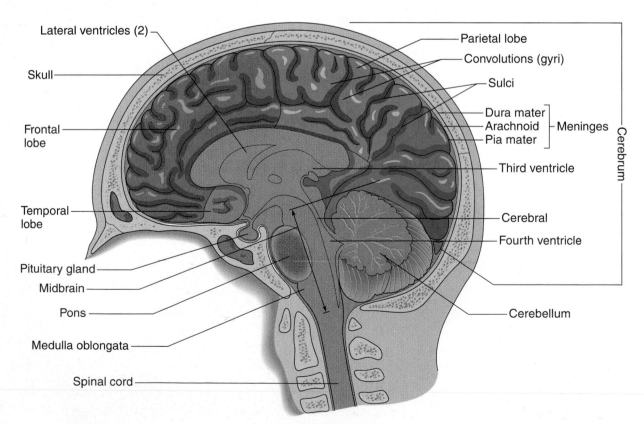

FIGURE 16-1 The central nervous system—brain and spinal cord

DISORDERS OF THE NERVOUS SYSTEM····························

Disorders of the nervous system can be the result of disease or injury to the brain or spinal cord. Many of these disorders cause mobility and cognitive problems. For example, shakiness in the extremities (tremors), difficulty walking, and mental changes are common symptoms of nervous system disorders. The home health aide can assist the client who has a nervous system disorder by being aware of the client's limitations, encouraging the client to complete the assigned exercises, and by observing and reporting changes in the client's health status and functioning levels to the health care team.

Parkinson's Disease

Parkinson's disease, first documented by James Parkinson in 1817, is a progressive degeneration of nerve cells in the area of the brain that controls muscle movements. The disease results from the inability of these nerve cells to produce dopamine, which is necessary for the transmission of signals within the brain. The cause of Parkinson's is not yet known.

Parkinson's disease often starts in middle or late life and is progressive in nature, with symptoms worsening over time. Characteristic symptoms of Parkinson's disease include shakiness of the body at rest (tremors), fixated or reduced facial expressions, slowness of movement, shuffling walking pattern (gait), stiffness or rigidity of limbs, and stooped posture (Figure 16-2). In its most severe form, the individual becomes incapacitated by rigidity and tremors. Depression is common among individuals diagnosed with this disease.

Treatment for Parkinson's disease involves drug therapy to restore the brain's supply of dopamine to reverse problems of the disease involving walking, movement, and tremors. Close medical supervision of the drug treatment is necessary. Patients should be monitored for serious side effects such as involuntary

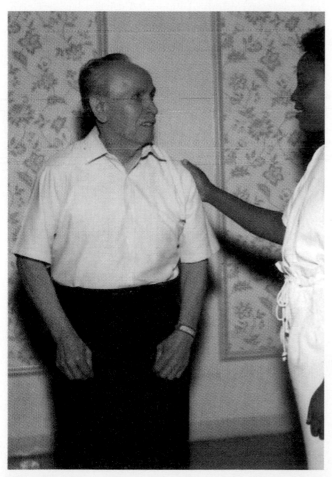
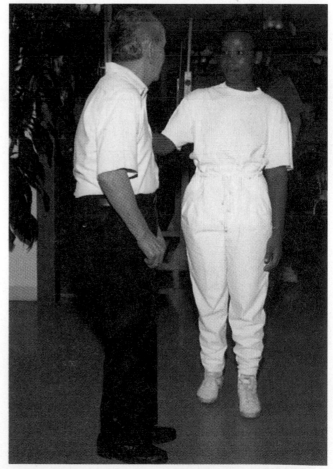

FIGURE 16-2 Characteristics of Parkinson's disease include fixated or reduced facial expression.

movements, nausea, dizziness, and mental changes so that medications can be adjusted to suit the patient. Regular exercise is another critical part of treatment. However, clients with Parkinson's disease will require many rest periods because their energy levels may go up and down throughout the day. Participation in support groups and physical therapy programs can play an important role in helping the client maintain a positive mental attitude and avoid depression.

Multiple Sclerosis

Multiple sclerosis (MS) is a disease affecting the central nervous system. In most cases, the disease begins with episodes that last only weeks or months that are separated by periods of remission (absence of symptoms). The cause of MS is not clearly understood. Multiple sclerosis produces a wide variety of symptoms, including movement or coordination problems; sensory problems involving brief pain, tingling, or electric shock sensations; vision problems, such as blurred or double vision; problems with bowel and bladder control; and problems with mental functions. Individuals with MS also suffer from a lack of energy and fatigue easily.

There is no current cure for MS. Treatment for MS involves the use of steroid drugs. Physical and occupational therapy are also an important part of a MS treatment plan. Most persons with MS live productive lives and are able to work. Although people with MS are capable of walking, occasionally they may need an assistive device such as a walker or cane. The average life expectancy is 35 years after the onset of the disease.

Amyotrophic Lateral Sclerosis

Amyotrophic lateral sclerosis (ALS) is more commonly known as Lou Gehrig's disease, after the famous baseball player who died from ALS. ALS is a progressive degeneration of the nerve cells in the brain and spinal cord that control the voluntary muscles. Its cause in unknown. A common misconception of ALS is that it is contagious; however, this is not true.

The signs and symptoms of ALS include slow loss of strength and coordination in one or more limbs, muscle twitches and cramps; increasingly stiff, clumsy gait; and difficulty with swallowing, speaking, or breathing. The onset of ALS is gradual, with weakness appearing first in one limb. Twitching and cramping follow. Additional muscle areas then become affected and complete paralysis may result. Following diagnosis, a person generally lives only 2 to 10 years.

Seizures

A **seizure** (or convulsion) is an involuntary episode of alternating muscular contractions and relaxations accompanied with a loss of consciousness. Under normal conditions, the brain cells produce coordinated electrical discharges. However, when a seizure occurs the electrical discharges of the brain cells become disorganized. There are several disorders that cause seizures. Seizures are caused by kidney failure; meningitis; high fever; toxemia of pregnancy; withdrawal from drugs such as Valium, barbiturates, or alcohol; intake of certain poisons or street drugs; and, in rare cases, are the first manifestation of a brain tumor. Procedure 60 identifies the proper method for caring for a client having a seizure.

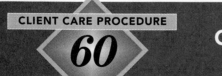

CLIENT CARE PROCEDURE

60 Caring for a Client Having a Seizure

DURING THE SEIZURE

1. Do not try to limit the movements of the person.

2. Keep the person from injuring himself or herself. Loosen the clothing, if possible, and place a pillow under the head.

(continues)

CLIENT CARE PROCEDURE *60* **Caring for a Client Having a Seizure** *(continued)*

3. Clear the areas around the person of furniture or other objects.
4. If vomiting occurs, try to turn the head so that the vomitus is not aspirated into the lungs or windpipe.
5. If poisoning is suspected, attempt to determine the poison consumed. Call for immediate medical assistance.

AFTER THE SEIZURE

1. If the person has never had a seizure before, has hurt him or herself, if the episode lasts more than a few minutes, or if the seizure recurs, call for an ambulance.

2. Once the seizure is over, position the person on his or her side. This will allow for normal breathing and for any vomitus, saliva, or blood to drain from the mouth.
3. Confusion may be present for a period of time. Watch the person until there is a complete return of mental function. A client may feel very tired after a seizure.
4. Treat any bumps, bruises, or cuts that may have resulted from the seizure. The client may have become incontinent during the seizure and will want to clean up.
5. Record details of the seizure for the physician. Important things to note are duration of the seizure, extremities involved, apparent precipitating factors, nature of the seizure, and any other characteristics noted.

Muscular Dystrophy

Muscular dystrophy is a progressive disease caused from insufficient nourishment of the muscles. The lack of a key protein essential to muscle function causes the muscles to decrease in size and grow weaker. Muscular dystrophy is a rare disease that is inherited in more than half of all cases. The disease usually strikes at an early age, usually before 5, and affects only boys. Muscular dystrophy ultimately cripples the person entirely.

Symptoms of the disease are muscle weakness, lack of coordination, clumsy gait, inability to lift the arms over the head, and progressive crippling resulting in a loss of mobility. By the teenage years, most patients require a wheelchair. Many persons with muscular dystrophy die before adulthood. There is no cure. The best treatment regimen involves physical therapy to help minimize deformities.

Spinal Cord Injuries

When a person has an injury to the spinal cord, loss of sensation and function in body parts below the level of that injury often results. Most spinal cord injuries are the result of traffic or industrial accidents, falls, gunshot wounds, and sports injuries. Clients who are paralyzed as a result of a spinal cord injury are often prone to the development of pressure sores and contractures, the abnormal shortening of muscle tissue.

Sensory Deficits

Sensory deficits (decreases in sensory ability such as hearing or vision) commonly affect elderly people, but they may also affect others as a result of disease. The home health aide is likely to encounter clients whose vision or hearing are impaired. Such conditions as glaucoma (an eye disorder caused by increased pressure of the fluid within the eye) and cataracts (a cloudy area in the lens of the eye) may severely limit the vision of a client. Elderly persons who are hard of hearing (HOH) may have nerve damage affecting the **auditory** (hearing) nerve, or a disorder called **otosclerosis**. This condition occurs when the bones of

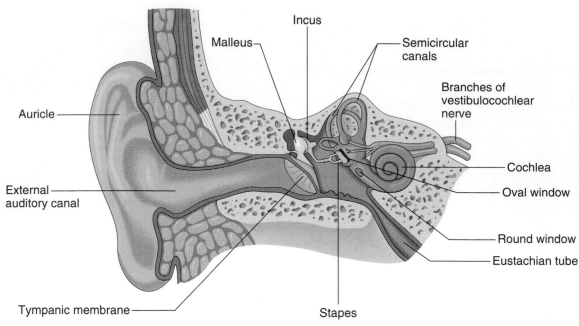

Incus

Malleus

Semicircular canals

Branches of vestibulocochlear nerve

Auricle

Cochlea

External auditory canal

Oval window

Round window

Eustachian tube

Tympanic membrane

Stapes

FIGURE 16-3 Internal view of the ear

the inner ear (Figure 16-3) harden and sound waves are no longer carried in the usual fashion. Hearing ability gradually diminishes. Aged persons also may experience a loss of taste sensation, which may have a negative effect on their appetite. The home health aide should be aware of any sensory deficits a client might have and accordingly adjust the care given. In Unit 3 you can find Procedure 1, Inserting a Hearing Aid.

REVIEW

Fill in the blanks for the following three questions:

1. Paralysis of the lower part of the body and both legs is called

    _____ .

2. Paralysis of both arms and both legs is referred to as _____ .

3. Paralysis of one side of the body is known as _____ .

Answer true or false to the following questions:

4. T F Parkinson's disease is marked by body tremors and a fixed facial expression.

5. T F Multiple sclerosis can be cured using a combination of drugs and therapy.

6. T F Amyotrophic lateral sclerosis (ALS) is a fatal disease.

7. T F Muscular dystrophy strikes only males.

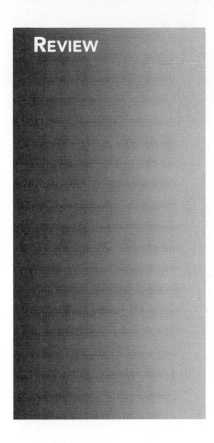

REVIEW

8. Match Column I with Column II.

Column I

_____ 1. amyotrophic lateral sclerosis

_____ 2. multiple sclerosis

_____ 3. Parkinson's disease

_____ 4. muscular dystrophy

_____ 5. seizures

Column II

a. inability of nerve cells to produce dopamine

b. electrical discharges of the brain cells disorganized

c. Lou Gehrig's disease

d. Disease that has no cure and for which the average life expectancy is 35 years after disease onset

e. a rare disease that is inherited in many cases

9. While you are visiting Ms. Jones at her home, she has a seizure. What steps should be taken to ensure that she does not hurt herself during the seizure? When should you call an ambulance? What steps should you take after the seizure has subsided?

10. What sensory deficits commonly affect the elderly? What are some of the causes of vision and hearing deficits in the elderly? What might be the result if a client experiences a loss in taste sensation? What steps would you take if you were assigned to care for a client with severe sensory deficits?

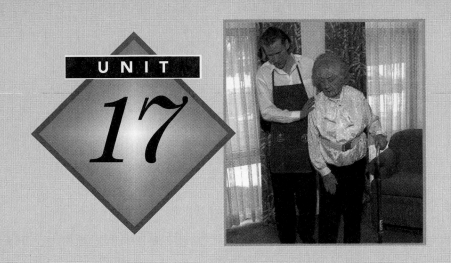

Circulatory System —Read

KEY TERMS

activities of daily
  living (ADL)
anemia
aneurysm
angina pectoris
anticoagulants
aphasia
arterial insufficiency
arteriogram
arteriosclerosis
artery
atherosclerosis
cardiac arrest
catheterization
cerebral hemorrhage
cerebral infarction

cerebral vascular
  accident (CVA)
collateral circulation
congestive heart failure
cyanosis
edema
embolus
expressive aphasia
gangrene
hemophilia
hypertension
hypotension
intermittent claudication
ischemia
leukemia
multi-infarct dementia

myocardial infarction
myocardium
nitroglycerin
occupational therapist
phlebitis
pulmonary embolus
receptive aphasia
sickle cell anemia
sublingually
thrombophlebitis
thrombus
transient ischemic
  attack (TIA)
venous insufficiency

LEARNING OBJECTIVES

After studying this unit, you should be able to:

- Identify symptoms of four heart conditions.
- Describe care given for clients with heart conditions.
- Explain the effect nitroglycerin has on the blood vessels.
- Give two other names for a CVA.

- List six risk factors for heart attacks and strokes.
- List three signs a client might display if suffering from a heart attack.
- List four warning signs of stroke.
- List three causes of stroke.

LEARNING OBJECTIVES

- List two types of aphasia.
- List three physical defects a client may have after a stroke.
- Explain the role of the aide in assisting a client recovering from a stroke.
- List three blood disorders.

- List three symptoms of arterial insufficiency.
- Describe three ways the aide can assist in the care of a client with thrombophlebitis.
- Demonstrate the following:
  PROCEDURE 61   Applying Elasticized Stockings

The organ that provides power to the body system is the heart. The heart is a hollow muscular organ about the size of a closed fist (Figure 17-1). Although it is one of the most important organs in the body, it has only one job—to pump blood throughout the body. From the time the fetus is 3½ months old, the heart continues to pump until death.

CIRCULATORY SYSTEM

The heart has four chambers, the right and left atria and the right and left ventricles. The right atrium receives oxygen-poor blood from the tissues. This blood is pumped to the lungs by the right ventricle, where carbon dioxide is exchanged for oxygen from the lungs. The oxy-

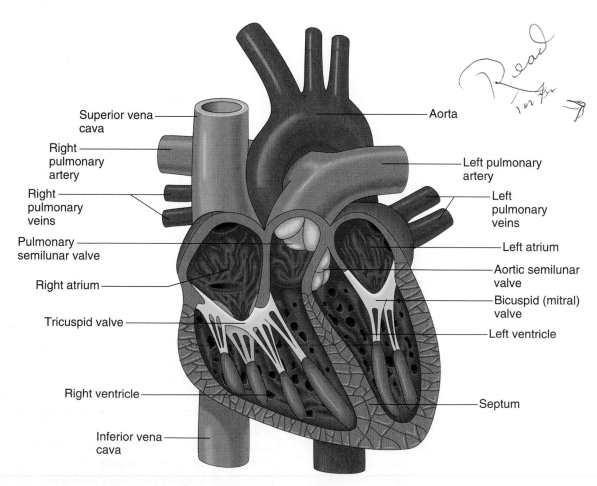

Superior vena cava — Aorta
Right pulmonary artery — Left pulmonary artery
Right pulmonary veins — Left pulmonary veins
Pulmonary semilunar valve — Left atrium
Right atrium — Aortic semilunar valve
Tricuspid valve — Bicuspid (mitral) valve
— Left ventricle
Right ventricle — Septum
Inferior vena cava

FIGURE 17-1 The heart is a hollow muscular organ about the size of a closed fist.

genated blood is received by the left atrium, which then pumps it to the left ventricle; it is then pumped out to all parts of the body.

Connected to these chambers are the largest blood vessels in the circulatory system. There are three kinds of blood vessels. The arteries carry blood away from the heart to the body cells. The arteries join the tiny blood vessels, called capillaries. The capillaries meet the veins. The veins carry the blood back to the heart. It takes 1 minute for blood to leave the heart, travel through the arteries, capillaries, and veins and return to the heart. This is a cycle that continues each minute of the day.

As the heart contracts (squeezes together) and expands (relaxes), it pushes the blood into the arteries. The arteries contract and expand in the same rhythm as the heart. The pulse measured at the wrist is the expansion of the radial artery. The blood carried in the arteries is a rich, bright red color. Venous blood is a darker red because it is low in oxygen. There are many disorders of the circulatory system that will be discussed. There are many age-related changes that affect the cardiovascular system. Heart muscle fibers become calcified and thick. The valves of the heart stiffen and become more rigid. The blood vessels become less flexible. These changes can increase the risk for older individuals to develop heart disease.

RISK FACTORS

Because of the many deaths due to heart problems, many research studies have been conducted on individuals with heart problems. Research has documented the following as major risk factors in heart disease.

- Heredity—Children of parents with heart problems have a greater risk of developing heart conditions.
- Male sex—Men have greater risk than premenopausal women and have heart attacks earlier in life.
- Increasing age—Fifty-five percent of all heart attacks occur in individuals who are 64 or older.
- Cigarette smoking—Smokers have twice as many heart attacks as nonsmokers.

- High blood pressure—High blood pressure increases the heart's workload and weakens the heart and also the blood vessels in the brain, which eventually can cause either a heart attack or stroke.
- High cholesterol levels—As cholesterol levels increase, the risk of having a heart attack increases.
- Diabetes—People with diabetes have a greater incidence of heart attacks and strokes.
- Obesity—Individuals who are 30% overweight have a greater incidence of strokes and heart attacks.
- Physical inactivity—Lack of exercise combined with obesity and high cholesterol levels will definitely increase the person's chances of having a heart attack or stroke.
- Stress—There is an increased risk of heart problems in people who are under continuous stress in their lives.
- Postmenopausal women not on hormone replacement therapy have increased risk.

DISORDERS OF THE HEART AND CIRCULATORY SYSTEM

The number one killer of individuals in the United States is cardiovascular disease. In 1990, more than 1 million Americans died as a result of some form of cardiovascular (heart) disease. Circulatory problems affect people of all ages. If an infant is born with a heart defect, it is called a congenital heart problem. Five percent of heart attacks occur in people under age 40, and 45% occur in people over age 65. The majority of individuals who survive after a heart attack or stroke will need some type of medical care and also assistance with **activities of daily living (ADL)**. A home health aide has an important role to play in the recovery of these clients. Some of these clients will need assistance with ADL for the rest of their lives.

In many cases, disorders of the heart and circulatory system force people to change their lifestyles. Many people become very frightened when a heart or circulatory condition is diagnosed. The psychological effects can be almost as crippling as the illness itself. People may think they will be permanently disabled or wonder how they can support themselves and their families. People who have had one heart attack may be afraid of having another heart attack. As a result, they often avoid moving about or doing any exercise. Inactivity usually leads to boredom, irritability, and depression.

The aide may be assigned to help clients with heart problems. Certain conditions require clients to reduce their activity. Clients may need assistance with household duties or child care. The aide may need to remind clients to avoid vigorous exercise or heavy lifting. The physician's orders explain a safe range of activity. Helping the client adjust to the necessary changes may be the focus of the aide's care plan.

Angina Pectoris

Angina pectoris is a symptom of a condition called myocardial ischemia, which occurs when the heart muscle (**myocardium**) does not get an adequate supply of blood and oxygen to do its work. Lack of blood supply is called **ischemia. Angina pectoris** is a mild pain in the chest radiating to the left arm and up through the neck area. This condition results from lack of oxygen in the heart muscle due to constricted blood vessels. An attack can last from a few seconds to several minutes. It may occur after physical exertion or during times of stress and anxiety. The person becomes pale and ashen and the body stiffens. Blood pressure increases dramatically (hypertension). The client becomes flushed and perspires heavily.

Immediate treatment for angina is physical rest. If this is not the first angina attack, the client is likely to have medication on hand. A common emergency medication used for angina is **nitroglycerin.** Nitroglycerin may be taken **sublingually,** in which case the tablet is placed under the tongue. It can also be applied topically in the form of a nitro-patch placed on the skin (Figure 17-2). The nitroglycerin is absorbed through the skin; a patch provides 24 hours of medication. Old nitroglycerin patches should be removed and the area of skin under the patch cleansed before a new patch is applied by the client. This is to prevent a buildup effect from residual nitroglycerin. Application sites should be alternated daily to prevent skin irritation.

Nitroglycerin opens the blood vessels to increase the blood flow. The effects of the drug occur within 2 to 3 minutes. The pain from angina is usually relieved in 5 to 10 minutes.

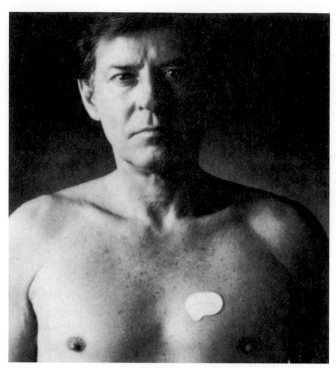

FIGURE 17-2 The client may receive nitroglycerin through the skin by means of a transdermal patch. (Courtesy of CIBA Pharmaceutical Co., Division of CIBA GEIGY, Summit, NJ)

Nitroglycerin is one of the medications that can only be used for a specified period of time because it loses its potency and effectiveness. The aide should check the expiration date carefully to be sure the medicine is still effective. This drug must be kept in the original bottle to maintain its potency.

When angina pectoris has been diagnosed, the client should avoid emotional stress, exercise after heavy meals, exposure to sudden cold, and overexertion. Medication should be placed near the client for immediate use in case of an attack. The medication often causes headaches. Frequent periods of rest with restricted activities, no smoking, medications such as a nitro-patch, and a special diet are commonly ordered by the physician. If three tablets taken over a time span of 15 minutes do not provide relief, emergency care is required. Call an ambulance, physician, family members, and case manager.

Myocardial Infarction

Myocardial infarction is more commonly known as a coronary, or a heart attack. A myocardial infarction is a condition in which a blood vessel of the heart muscle closes or is blocked by a blood clot. The size and location of the incident determines the seriousness of the attack. There can be permanent damage to the heart. In the case of permanent damage, parts of the heart muscle die and **collateral circulation** may develop. This means that other small blood vessels take over the job of bringing blood to the heart muscle. These smaller vessels actually become enlarged so they can carry the required amount of fresh, oxygenated blood to the heart muscle. The symptoms of a heart attack are shown in Figure 17-3.

The person may go into shock and collapse. Prompt emergency treatment is needed and is begun in the ambulance and continued in the hospital. In the hospital the client will be treated for a heart attack. The need for specialized treatment or surgery will be determined. A **catheterization** is often done to assist in diagnosing the client's problem. During cardiac catheterization, a catheter (thin tube) is introduced into a vein or **artery** and passed through the heart so that any abnormalities of the heart can be detected. One common operation is called coronary artery bypass grafting, or CABG. After release from the hospital, treatment at home may include increased activity with continuing periods of rest and a special diet.

Anticoagulants and other drugs may be part of the treatment when a person has had a coronary attack. **Anticoagulants** are drugs that reduce the ability of the blood to clot. A home health aide should observe and report any signs of side effects from the use of anticoagulants. These may include bleeding from the gums or bruising of the skin. To reduce the risk of bleeding, use of an electric razor instead of a blade razor is recommended for clients receiving anticoagulants. The home health aide *never* massages the legs. This could loosen a blood clot and send it directly to the lungs, causing pain and severe breathing problems or cardiac arrest. If a person's heart does stop beating, it is called **cardiac arrest.**

Congestive Heart Failure

Congestive heart failure is a condition in which the heart does not pump effectively. This condition can affect the right or left side of the heart, or even both sides at the same time. This is most often caused by heart muscle damage. Thus, the heart's pumping action is weakened. A client with congestive heart failure may have one acute attack and then develop a chronic condition. The symptoms include a cough, shortness of breath (dyspnea), bluish tinged skin and nails (**cyanosis**), and retention of fluid (**edema**). Fluid (frothy pink sputum) may accumulate in the lungs, causing pneumonia. Congestive heart failure can lead to chronic disability and death.

Treatment for congestive heart failure usually includes two types of drugs. One is digitalis, which slows and strengthens the heartbeat. The other is a diuretic (water pill), which reduces fluid accumulation in the body. A diuretic medication causes the client to urinate frequently to help rid the body of excess fluids. The aide should help the client remember to take medications that have been prescribed. The aide may be asked to measure intake and output. The doctor may order fluids restricted. Daily weights may need to be taken.

Diet control is an important part of the treatment for congestive heart failure. Diets usually are low in sodium and fat. A diet high in bulk helps the client avoid constipation. A person who is constipated must strain to have a bowel movement; this strain can be dangerous for any person with a heart condition. People who are overweight should restrict their calorie intake as well. The dietitian provides exact orders for diet preparation. Exercise and rest must be balanced. The correct amount of each is determined by the doctor.

Clients with congestive heart failure must stay in an upright or semiupright position (head higher than feet). They will need frequent position changes, TED hose or Ace bandages on their legs, bedside commode or bedpan, and a bed bath. The clients will need to have activities spaced throughout the day to prevent becoming overly fatigued. When sitting in a chair, the client will need to have the legs slightly elevated.

The aide must help clients limit their activities. Clients with congestive heart failure usually cannot go up and down stairs. They must lead very quiet lives because they tire easily. Such clients may get depressed because they must be dependent on others. To help reduce this feeling of dependence, the aide should give the client as much control over personal care

The symptoms are:

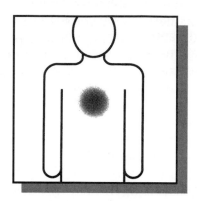

An uncomfortable feeling in your chest —
- Heaviness
- Pressure
- Tightness
- A squeezing sensation

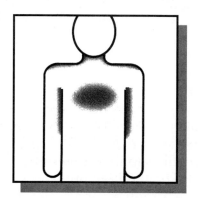

It can spread to your left arm, sometimes to both arms and to your neck and jaw.

You may also get sweaty, feel like vomiting and have trouble breathing.

Take action:

Go to the nearest hospital emergency room, or call 911 if you're too sick to go on your own. Do it right away! New treatments can save your life and help you recover. But you must act quickly. The quicker you act the better your chances. Every minute counts.

FIGURE 17-3 Symptoms of a heart attack. (Courtesy of American Heart Association, New York City Affiliate, New York, NY)

and selection of activities as possible. Refer to Figure 17-4 for a summary of the effects of congestive heart failure.

Arteriosclerosis

Arteriosclerosis is a condition in which the arteries become hard and lose their soft, rubber-like stretchiness. It is caused by a buildup of fatty deposits on the inside walls of the blood vessels.

An important aspect of client care is to increase the client's circulation. A bath not only cleans the skin but also helps to increase circulation. Even if a client does not need a complete bath daily, the aide must wash the client's feet and rub them with lotion every day. After the feet are cleaned, a pair of cotton or wool socks may be needed. Arteriosclerosis clients often complain of cold feet. **CAUTION:** The home health aide must *NEVER* apply a hot water bottle or heating pad even if requested by the client. To warm the client's feet, the aide should give the client a second pair of socks or put a blanket over the client's legs. The socks should not fit tightly. Socks or other items of clothing that are tight further restrict circulation.

Pressure sores are caused by poor circulation in particular areas of the body. Pressure sores cause worry because the healing process is so slow. As a result of worry and discomfort, clients can be short-tempered. A home health aide should communicate with the client. Recreation and diversions should be planned to keep the client's mind off the condition. An aide will need to find hobbies or activities that the client may be interested in and plan activities around these interests.

Contractures. If unable to move about, the client must be protected from developing deformities. Weight from the bedcovers can press against the feet. Bedcovers should be kept loose around the feet. Bed cradles may be used in holding bedcovers off the feet. Footboards may be placed against the soles of the feet so that the

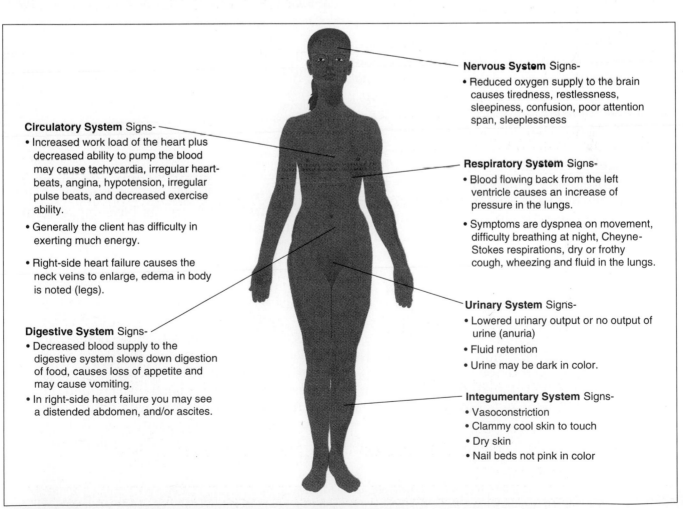

Circulatory System Signs-
- Increased work load of the heart plus decreased ability to pump the blood may cause tachycardia, irregular heart-beats, angina, hypotension, irregular pulse beats, and decreased exercise ability.
- Generally the client has difficulty in exerting much energy.
- Right-side heart failure causes the neck veins to enlarge, edema in body is noted (legs).

Digestive System Signs-
- Decreased blood supply to the digestive system slows down digestion of food, causes loss of appetite and may cause vomiting.
- In right-side heart failure you may see a distended abdomen, and/or ascites.

Nervous System Signs-
- Reduced oxygen supply to the brain causes tiredness, restlessness, sleepiness, confusion, poor attention span, sleeplessness

Respiratory System Signs-
- Blood flowing back from the left ventricle causes an increase of pressure in the lungs.
- Symptoms are dyspnea on movement, difficulty breathing at night, Cheyne-Stokes respirations, dry or frothy cough, wheezing and fluid in the lungs.

Urinary System Signs-
- Lowered urinary output or no output of urine (anuria)
- Fluid retention
- Urine may be dark in color.

Integumentary System Signs-
- Vasoconstriction
- Clammy cool skin to touch
- Dry skin
- Nail beds not pink in color

FIGURE 17-4 Congestive heart failure—systems involved

foot will not drop into an unnatural position. A contracture is a condition in which muscles become shortened and stiff. The muscles freeze in an uncomfortable position. Foot drop is a kind of contracture. The client who is unable to move in bed should be repositioned regularly every 2 hours. This increases circulation, bringing more oxygen to the cells. Prescribed exercise and repositioning help prevent pressure sores from forming.

Cerebral Vascular Accidents (CVA or Stroke)

Stroke is the common term for **cerebral vascular accident** (CVA). The blood flow to a specific area of the brain is interrupted, resulting in sudden acute symptoms such as paralysis, vision disturbances, language problems, mental confusion, or a combination of these.

Stroke is caused by a lack of oxygen and nutrients to the brain cells. This interruption of blood to the brain may be due to one of the following three reasons: an **aneurysm** (a ballooning out of the wall of an artery) that breaks open and causes a hemorrhage; an **embolus** (a moving blood clot) that causes complete blockage of an artery; or a **thrombus** (a blood clot that forms inside an artery) that can cause a blockage of blood flow to the brain cells. Brain cells deprived of circulation for even a few seconds stop functioning. If the circulation stops for a few minutes, brain cells die. This causes loss of voluntary motion and results in paralysis, often on one side of the body.

Brain cells die when they are without oxygen for 4 minutes. Once brain cells are destroyed, they cannot be brought back to life. Unlike other cells in the body, new brain cells do not form to replace damaged ones. The most common cause of a CVA is high blood pressure. A CVA does not necessarily destroy all the brain cells. Remaining cells can compensate by taking over the duties of those destroyed by a CVA. For that reason rehabilitation is of vital importance. Refer to Unit 10 for a detailed discussion on the need for rehabilitation and Unit 15 for information on the care of a client with rehabilitation needs.

Risk Factors in Stroke.* Often, long before a stroke occurs, there are conditions or symptoms that are now recognized as associated with an increased risk of stroke. These are:

- **Hypertension**—sustained elevated blood pressure. This can increase vessel lining damage, accelerating the formation of plaque (fatty deposits) in arteries. Refer to Unit 10, Procedure 12 for a description of the proper method for taking blood pressure.
- **Atherosclerosis** (often called hardening of the arteries)—a disease in which fatty materials containing cholesterol, platelets (blood cells that promote clotting), and calcium accumulate on the interior walls of the arteries. These accumulations can build up to the point where the vessel becomes obstructed.
- Heart disease—coronary artery disease, damaged heart valves
- Diabetes
- Family history of heart disease or stroke

In addition, several conditions also may be controllable risk factors. Among these are high blood fat and cholesterol levels, obesity, physical activity, cigarette smoking, and excessive alcohol intake.

An individual who has one or more of these conditions or habits has a greater risk of developing a stroke than those without them. The risk increases when several of these risk factors are found in a particular individual.

Statistics indicate that although stroke can happen at any age, strokes are more common in the elderly. Approximately 75% of strokes that occur yearly are in individuals over 65 years. African Americans have more strokes than Caucasians.

First Signs of a Stroke. A stroke can begin in several ways: with transient ischemic attacks, gradual onset, or sudden onset of symptoms.

Transient ischemic attack (TIA) consists of a brief period of weakness, loss of speech, or loss of feeling that lasts from minutes to hours and then goes away completely. These attacks are caused by a sudden but temporary decrease or stoppage of blood flow to a part of the brain. These attacks are important because they are a reliable warning of possible permanent stroke.

*The following material is adapted from and used with permission from a booklet prepared for in-service training. Courtesy of The Burke Rehabilitation Center, White Plains, NY, the Auxiliary and Fletcher H. McDowell, MD, Executive Medical Director.

Usually a person with TIA reports one or more of the following: the sudden onset of numbness, tingling, or weakness on one side of the body, or in the hand and face on one side; temporary blindness in one or both eyes; difficulty understanding words and using them correctly; dizziness; nausea; vomiting; staggering; fuzzy speech; or a combination of these symptoms. During a TIA people do not lose consciousness, and recover with no aftereffect.

Whenever the symptoms described above occur, it is important that a physician be notified, even if the episode seems to pass as quickly as it came. Knowing and heeding these symptoms can help to avoid a future stroke because treatment of the underlying conditions that caused the attack often is possible, either with medications or with surgery.

When TIAs have occurred, an individual should receive a careful neurologic examination to determine if the condition causing the TIA can be corrected. Most TIAs are caused by atherosclerosis, which may block an artery, or may break up and release bits of debris, which travel through larger arteries and may block small arteries in the brain, stopping blood flow temporarily to a part of the brain. Most commonly, the site of arterial disease is in the carotid artery, where it divides into two large vessels—one going to the brain, the other to the face, jaw, and eye. This site is important because it is accessible to surgery and often the obstruction or plaque can be removed. Also, medications that reduce blood clotting or prevent blood platelets from clumping together can help stop TIAs and reduce the chance of stroke.

Clinical evaluation of TIA usually includes an examination by a neurologist, examination of blood vessels in the arms, legs, and neck; ultrasound examination of the arteries in the neck; and often an arteriogram. The **arteriogram** is a series of x-ray pictures that show the flow of blood in the arteries, neck, and head taken after the injection of dye into the artery. The dye causes the arteries to stand out clearly in the x-ray picture, allowing the physician to identify sites of vessel disease and obstructions. This allows the physician to determine whether surgical correction of an obstruction is possible.

Multi-infarct dementia is a common form of dementia that is the result of multiple strokes that damage brain tissue. This condition may occur suddenly or develop gradually over time. Symp-

toms consist of a deterioration of mental function, confusion, memory loss, poor judgment, and changes in personality. These symptoms are progressive; however, individuals may experience periods of time when their mental condition reaches a plateau and no further deterioration occurs.

Cerebral infarction is the term used to describe the condition in which a portion of the brain dies when an artery becomes blocked and blood is prevented from reaching that part of the brain. The blockage can be the result of hardening and eventual blockage of the artery (atherosclerosis), or be caused by a blood clot in the vessel, or other substances plugging a vessel (emboli). The portions of the brain thus starved of blood, die and cannot function. The effects of the stroke, weakness, paralysis, and loss of feeling, become evident in those parts of the body controlled by the affected part of the brain. When a person has a stroke, which means that the paralysis or loss of sensation does not go away rapidly, that person should be hospitalized to be given needed care and to be sure that there is no further progression of the stroke. Treatment of a patient after a stroke is difficult because there are no known remedies that can reverse the brain damage or cause nervous system tissue to regrow. If improvement occurs in nerve function, it happens naturally. Function in a person with stroke can be adapted and improved by rehabilitation.

Risk factors that singly or in combination increase the chances of stroke caused by the interruption of blood flow to the brain, resulting in cerebral infarction, are the same as for TIA. Frequently, a person may have a stroke with no recognized underlying cause. Cerebral infarction is the most common form of stroke and is responsible for most of the partially or completely disabling strokes. The most desirable form of management of this condition is prevention.

Cerebral hemorrhage means bleeding into the brain, which destroys or disrupts brain tissue. Normally, blood flows to the brain through arteries under high pressure. In vessels with weakened walls, the pressure may cause a rupture and blood will escape into the brain. Under high pressure, blood can spread rapidly in all directions from the point of rupture and may disrupt or damage a large area of the brain, causing weakness, paralysis, loss of sensation, and, frequently, loss of consciousness. Cerebral hemorrhage has a high risk of being fatal.

High blood pressure is the main risk factor for hemorrhage into the brain because almost all cerebral hemorrhages occur in clients with high blood pressure. Treatment of high blood pressure is the only satisfactory means to deal with cerebral hemorrhage. Survivors usually have severe physical disability.

Possible Aftereffects of Stroke. Stroke can affect an individual in many different ways, depending on which part of the brain has been damaged. Among the possible consequences are:

- Physical Deficits
  —Paralysis or complete loss of strength or mobility in a part of the body, usually the arm, leg, and face on one side.
  —Weakness in a part of the body. Usually weakness is more marked in the hand than in the arm, and the arm is more affected than the leg.
  —Loss of sensation (feeling) in parts of the body, usually on one side
  —Loss of bladder and bowel control
  —Difficulty in swallowing
  —Loss of coordination, such as unsteady gait
- Perceptual/Cognitive (thinking) Deficits
  —Loss of awareness
  —Speech and language disability. Difficulty thinking of and saying words or difficulty using or understanding words
  —Denial or neglect of the right or left part of the body and environment
  —Inability to understand time
  —Difficulty performing tasks in proper sequence
  —Disrupted sleep-wake cycles
  —Uncontrolled laughter or crying
  —Confusion, forgetfulness, memory loss, impaired judgment
- Personal/Family Problems
  —Loss of job
  —Inadequate financial resources
  —Loss of independence. Dependence on others who may or may not be willing or capable of accepting the new responsibility for continuing care.
  —Loss of sexual capacity
  —Loss of self-esteem
- Psychological Problems (mood)
  —Depression, apathy
  —Anger, hostility
  —Euphoria

- Environmental Problems
  —Architectural barriers in the home
  —Lack of accessible transportation

Not all of these problems happen to each individual. When any of them do happen, there are degrees of difficulty. Most of these problems can be improved. However, after a stroke, the person will always have limitations. Those with paralysis, those whose perceptual capacities are affected, or those whose memory and orientation are diminished have the greatest difficulties.

Signs and Symptoms. The person who suffers a stroke usually loses consciousness and becomes incontinent of urine and feces. In addition, breathing becomes labored or difficult. If consciousness is not lost, the client may complain of a severe headache, slurred speech, and blurred vision. After a stroke there is usually a weakness or paralysis on one side of the body. This one-sided weakness or paralysis is known as hemiplegia (Figure 17-5). The use of muscles is temporarily or permanently lost when paralysis occurs. Thus, the client may have difficulty

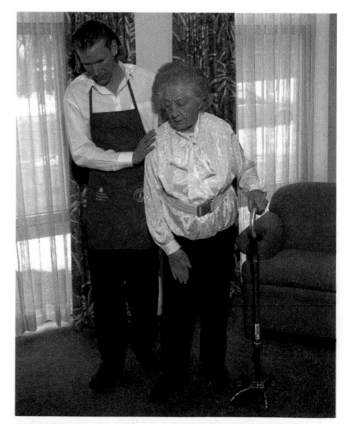

FIGURE 17-5 A home health aide is walking a client with right-side weakness. The aide is on the client's weak side. The aide is using a gait belt while walking the client.

in speaking, eating, swallowing, and even hearing. The client may take a long time to eat meals. The home health aide must be patient and permit the client to be as independent as possible. That means assisting with eating, not *force feeding*, to finish the meal.

Rehabilitation After a Stroke. A care plan will be developed by the home health team for each individual client. The plan will be implemented once the client has returned home. The goal of the plan is to have the client return to the highest level of function as possible. The client will need to be encouraged continuously to do as much as possible with as little assistance as possible from others. At times it may be easier for an aide to dress or feed the client, but it must be remembered that the goal of care is to have the client do it, not the aide.

After a stroke the client will most likely have one-sided weakness. The client will need to do exercises to regain strength and function to the side of the body that is weak. If the client is unable to do the special exercises, called range of motion exercises, the aide will need to do the exercises. The supervising nurse or physical therapist will train the aide to do the exercises (Figures 17-6A and B). If the client can do the exercises without assistance from others, the exercises are called active range of motion exercises. Passive range of motion exercises are those in which the client moves with the assistance of others. See Unit 10, Procedure 15 for the proper method of performing range of motion exercises. Exercises will be helpful in the prevention of contractures and will improve the client's self-image.

Ambulation is important in the rehabilitation of a person after a stroke. The client may need to have a brace applied to the weak leg for support before ambulating. Check to see if the brace fits properly and does not cause skin irritation. A gait belt should be applied to the client's waist before you help the client to stand. Remember to stand on the client's weak side and hold onto the gait belt when ambulating the client. Each time you ambulate the client, encourage the client to go a few steps farther. This will help the client build up strength and also make the client feel

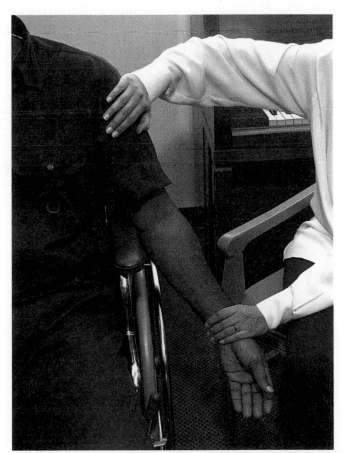 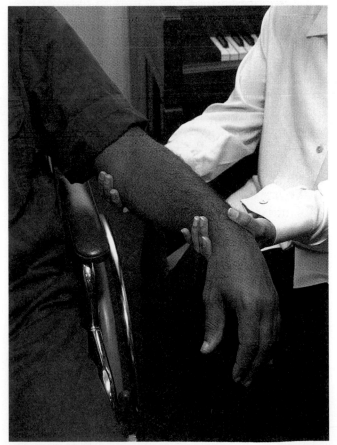

FIGURE 17-6 A. Physical therapist is performing range of motion exercises with a client who has had a stroke. B. Physical therapist is doing range of motion exercises to the client's arm.

like some progress is being made. Occasionally a client's sight may be affected after a stroke. Be sure when you walk a client there is a clear pathway without obstacles in the way. You, the home health aide may see these obstacles, but your client may not. See Unit 10, Procedure 16 on the proper method for assisting the client to walk with crutches, walker, or cane.

Dressing is another area in which the client may need assistance. If you need to assist the client to put on a shirt, remember to put the shirt on the weak arm first and then the strong arm. If the client is unable to button the shirt, Velcro closures can be substituted in place of buttons. Elasticized waist slacks will be easier to slip on and off than pants with buttons and zippers. See Unit 15, Procedure 59, for the proper method of dressing and undressing the client.

Oral care is of special importance for the client with a stroke. Before mealtime, it is important to do routine oral care, and if the client has dentures, encourage the client to wear them. Refer to Unit 14 for the proper method of assisting with routine oral hygiene (Procedure 38), and caring for dentures (Procedure 39). The client may need assistance in eating or the client may need to use one of the many assistive feeding devices now available. An **occupational therapist** may work with the client in restoring the ability to eat without the assistance of others. It will be the home health aide's job to follow through with the plan designed by the occupational therapist. The aide may need to cut the meat or open the milk carton, but once these small tasks are done, the client will be able to manage eating without assistance. Thick liquids are easier to swallow than thin liquids and less likely to cause choking. Be sure to check the inside of the weak side of the mouth for food particles after the client has finished eating. The client does not have feeling on the paralyzed side and often food becomes lodged in the cheek and the client may not know it.

Bowel and bladder retaining may also be part of the rehabilitation of a stroke client. The aide should follow a schedule suggested by the nurse. The urinal, bedpan, or commode should be presented at specific times during the day and night. For example, the client who is given the bedpan after each meal and before bedtime eventually becomes adjusted to using it at that time. The body then becomes regulated. Before the client adapts to a schedule, the aide should be sure to keep the client's bed dry and clean.

See Unit 13 for the proper method for giving and emptying the bedpan (Procedure 19), giving and emptying the urinal (Procedure 20), retraining the bladder (Procedure 25), and retraining bowels (Procedure 28).

Communication Problems. The client with a stroke often has a great deal of trouble communicating. The home health aide must be patient and understanding regarding the client's speech problems. **Aphasia** is a condition in which the ability to speak is impaired. Aphasia is common after a client has had a stroke. Aphasia can affect the ability to talk, listen, read, or write. The client's speech may be slurred, distorted, and slowed. A client who has **receptive aphasia** does not understand words someone else says. In this case, it may be better to have a communication board to point to (Figure 17-7). In a few cases the client might understand all words coming into the brain, but he is unable to respond appropriately. An example of this might be when an aide asks him if he is hungry and he responds with "no" and in reality he wanted to say "yes" but the answer came out just the opposite of what he wanted. This is extremely frustrating to both you and the client. This type of aphasia is called **expressive aphasia** because the client is unable to express himself correctly. In the majority of cases in which the client just recently suffered a stroke, a speech therapist will be assisting with communication problems. The speech therapist will inform the aide of the client's type of aphasia and how to communicate more effectively. Sometimes the only words a stroke client uses are curse words or nonsense syllables. This is called automatic speech (involuntary speech). The home health aide should avoid treating the client as a child. In speaking to a stroke client, the aide should use simple sentences that require only short and simple answers from the client. Speaking clearly and simply aids the client's understanding. Stroke clients usually need a great deal of encouragement and reassurance.

Clients who normally wear glasses should continue to wear them even if their sight has been affected by the stroke. This makes the client feel less changed in outward appearance. The same is true if the client wears dentures or a hearing aid. These courtesies show that the aide respects the client.

The home health aide should encourage clients to help themselves as much as possible. This may take more of the aide's time, but it is a form of rehabilitation. The more the clients help themselves, the more progress they will make.

Phlebitis

Phlebitis occurs when the lining of a vein becomes inflamed, causing a clot to form in the vein. This usually occurs in one leg, which may become swollen and painful to touch. The area may feel warm. The physician may order antiembolism stockings or elastic bandages (such as Ace bandages) to be applied to the affected leg or to both legs.

Venous Insufficiency

Venous insufficiency is due to damage of the veins that return blood to the heart. The symptoms are chronic aching, edema, and discoloration of the lower extremities. The client may develop leg ulcers due to lack of oxygen available to these tissues. Clients suffering from venous insufficiency are at risk of developing **thrombophlebitis,** which occurs when the vein becomes inflamed and a clot forms. The symptoms of this condition are tenderness, redness, warmth over the vein, and pain in the calf of the leg when the client flexes his or her foot. As part of the treatment for this condition the aide may have to assist clients with the application of elastic stockings, which promote venous blood return. Refer to Procedure 61. The client should be discouraged from standing or sitting for any prolonged period of time. It is important to have legs elevated when the client is sitting to help lessen pain, edema, and to encourage venous flow. A serious complication of thrombophlebitis is a **pulmonary embolus,** which is a clot that has broken away and traveled to the lungs. The symptoms of pulmonary embolus are shortness of breath, chest pain, and increased heart rate. This is a life-threatening condition that requires immediate medical attention.

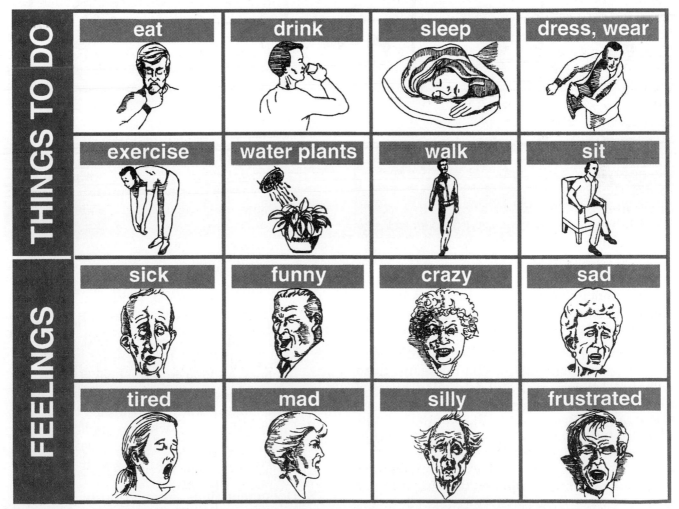

THINGS TO DO — FEELINGS

eat | drink | sleep | dress, wear
exercise | water plants | walk | sit
sick | funny | crazy | sad
tired | mad | silly | frustrated

FIGURE 17-7   A communication board is often used to increase communication with a client who has aphasia.   *(continues)*

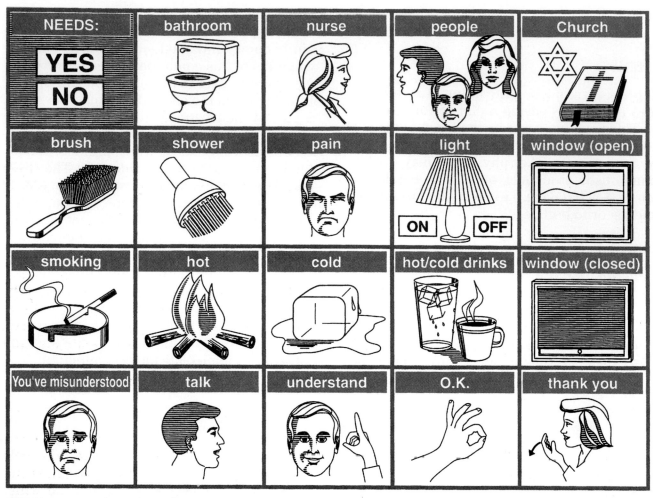

FIGURE 17-7 *(continued)*

CLIENT CARE PROCEDURE

61

Applying Elasticized Stockings

PURPOSE

- To prevent swelling of feet and ankles
- To prevent formation of blood clots in legs
- To increase blood circulation in the legs

NOTE: It is better to apply the elastic hose in bed rather than in the chair. Elastic hose should be removed and reapplied every 8 hours. Elastic hose come in a variety of sizes and lengths. They need to be supportive but not too tight. If they are too loose, they lose their effectiveness.

PROCEDURE

1. Wash your hands.
2. Tell client what you plan to do.
3. With client lying down, expose one leg at a time.
4. Turn stocking inside out to heel by placing your hand inside stocking and grasping heel. Position stocking over foot and heel of client, making sure the heel is properly placed. Continue to pull the remaining part of the hose upward over the client's leg.
5. Check to be sure stocking is applied evenly and smoothly and there are no wrinkles.
6. Repeat procedure on opposite leg.
7. Wash your hands.
8. Document time, completion of the procedure, and client's reaction.

Arterial Insufficiency

Arterial insufficiency results from a narrowing of the arteries that deliver blood to the lower extremities. When a client walks any distance, exercise increases the demand for oxygen to the tissues and muscles of the legs. Because of the narrow arteries, the blood flow is not sufficient to meet the demand. The client experiences cramping pain in the calf of the leg or thigh. This is called **intermittent claudication.** This pain should subside after the client rests for a few minutes. Treatment for mild symptoms is to encourage client to lose weight if obese, to avoid smoking, and to walk daily up to the point where pain is experienced, and then to rest. If an artery should become completely obstructed and blood not restored in 4 to 6 hours, the client is in danger of losing a limb. Signs of complete obstruction are severe pain, pallor, absence of pulse in foot and/or lower leg, numbness, paralysis, and coldness of limb. When providing care to these clients, the aide should watch for any sign of skin breakdown, especially between toes. **CAUTION:** *Do not use heating pads, hot water bottles, or hot soaks with these clients.* The client should be discouraged from wearing tight-fitting clothing, such as hose or shoes, which could further impair circulation.

Gangrene

Gangrene is the infection of damaged tissue brought on by lack of adequate blood supply. Those at risk for developing this infection include diabetics and other people with poor circulation. The lower extremities are most often affected. The home health aide must look carefully for any signs of skin breakdown, especially in diabetics, and report any sign of skin breakdown immediately to the nurse or supervisor.

DISORDERS OF THE BLOOD ⋯⋯⋯⋯⋯⋯

Blood is the life stream of the human body. Blood performs many tasks, and no part of the body can live without it. Blood supplies the cells of the body with the food and oxygen they need for work and growth. It carries waste products to specific organs that remove them from the body, or breaks them down into harmless substances. Blood also fights germs that enter the body. Blood has four main parts:

1. Plasma (the liquid part of the blood)
2. Red blood cells (carry oxygen and carbon dioxide to and from the lungs and body tissues)
3. White blood cells (fight infections)
4. Platelets (help to clot the blood)

Disorders of the blood can occur as a result of a malformation or malfunction of a part of the blood.

Anemia

Anemia occurs when there are not enough red blood cells. It may result from an excessive loss of blood, from malformation of blood cells, or from a lack of essential nutrients. If blood loss is excessive, **hypotension** (low blood pressure) may occur.

Sickle Cell Anemia

With **sickle cell anemia** the client's red blood cells are crescent shaped, like a sickle. The cells do not carry enough oxygen in them, causing anemia. This is an inherited disease for which there is no cure, but new drugs are helping clients. Infections, stressful situations, excessive exercise, and other situations that increase the client's need for oxygen should be avoided. In the United States, this disease is usually found only in African Americans.

Leukemia

Leukemia is a condition in which there are too many immature white blood cells. These excess white blood cells block the normal transport of oxygen to the body's tissues. They may also affect production of new red blood cells. Leukemia may also be called cancer of the blood.

Hemophilia

Hemophilia is an hereditary disease characterized by spontaneous hemorrhages due to a deficiency of a clotting factor in the blood. The classic form of the disease affects males only. If an individual starts to bleed, a special preparation can be given to stop the bleeding.

REVIEW

1. List six risk factors that would make a client more susceptible to having a stroke or heart attack.

2. List three signs that a client may have if suffering a heart attack.

3. List four warning signs of a stroke.

4. List three causes of stroke.

5. Explain aphasia.

6. List three possible long-term physical effects of a stroke.

7. Explain the role of the home health aide in the rehabilitation of a client who has had a stroke.

8. A client who has had a stroke or CVA has difficulty speaking, a disorder that is called:
   a. Aphasia
   b. Lethargy
   c. Paraplegia
   d. Mutism

9. As a home health aide caring for a client with congestive heart failure (CHF), which of the following would not be in the care plan?
   a. Low-salt, low-fat diet
   b. Schedule all activities for the morning.
   c. Observe for shortness of breath and retention of fluid.
   d. Assist client in maintaining an upright and semi-upright position.

10. Mr. Kane has had a stroke. Which of the following signs would you expect Mr. Kane to display?
    a. Aphasia
    b. Paralysis on one side of the body
    c. Drooping lip on one side of the face
    d. All of the above

11. T F The drug nitroglycerin may be used by clients with heart problems.

12. T F A client with a diagnosis of angina pectoris will often have mild chest pain after exercising or eating a large meal.

13. You are working with a client who has thrombophlebitis. Which one of the following symptoms would necessitate you seeking immediate medical attention for your client?
    a. Lower extremities edematous
    b. Redness and warmth over vein
    c. Shortness of breath
    d. Pain in the calf of the leg when the foot is flexed

14. Name two blood disorders caused by a malformation of the red blood cells.

15. Your client, Mr. Jones, is a 60-year-old man who recently had a heart attack and bypass surgery. His hospitalization went well and he seems to be recovering very well. On release from the

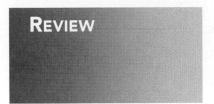

REVIEW

hospital he was given a special diet to follow, new medications to take, and an exercise plan. When you arrive at his home, you discover that he has not been exercising and appears irritable and depressed. What steps can you take to properly care for Mr. Jones? What are some of the psychological factors that might have an impact on Mr. Jones' recovery?

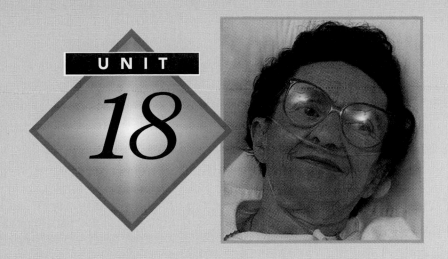

Respiratory System

asthma
chronic bronchitis

chronic obstructive
pulmonary disease
(COPD)

emphysema
pneumonia
respiratory system

LEARNING OBJECTIVES

After studying this unit, you should be able to:

- Discuss the basic function of the respiratory system.
- Name the major organs of the respiratory system.
- Define pneumonia, chronic bronchitis, emphysema, and asthma. (Include at least one symptom and one intervention for each illness.)

- Demonstrate the following:

  PROCEDURE 62   Collecting a Sputum Specimen

  PROCEDURE 63   Assisting With Coughing and Deep-Breathing Exercises

  PROCEDURE 64   Assisting the Client With Oxygen Therapy

The **respiratory system** consists of the nose, pharynx, larynx, trachea, bronchi, and lungs (Figure 18-1). Through effective air distribution and gas exchange, the respiratory system helps maintain a constant balance in the body, enabling the cells to function properly.

RESPIRATORY SYSTEM

The respiratory system is closely linked to the circulatory system. Blood is supplied with fresh oxygen by means of this system. Fresh air is inhaled into the body and carried to the lungs. The oxygen from the air is carried to all parts of the body by the circulatory system. As oxygen is delivered to the cells of the body, waste gases are picked up and carried back to the lungs, where they are exhaled from the body. The most plentiful waste gas is carbon dioxide. In short, oxygen is inhaled and carbon dioxide is exhaled. In addition to the above, the respiratory system filters, warms, and humidifies the air we breathe.

MAJOR RESPIRATORY ILLNESSES

Diseases of the respiratory system have now been classified together as **chronic obstructive pulmonary diseases (COPD).** COPD refers to the decreased ability of the lungs to perform their ventilation function, which may result from an acute infection, such as pneumonia, or a chronic condition, such as bronchitis or asthma. An example of a COPD is emphysema. Clients with breathing difficulties will need more frequent rest periods because they tire easily. In addition, they will need more time to accomplish their activities. Often, clients who experience difficulty breathing will be anxious. It is important that the aide remain calm and help the client to stay calm as well.

Clients with breathing difficulties may use inhalers, bronchodilators, nebulizers, compressors, or portable oxygen containers. These treatments are prescribed by a physician. A respiratory therapist or nurse will train the client on the proper use of equipment and medication. The home health aide may be instructed to coach the client through a breathing treatment

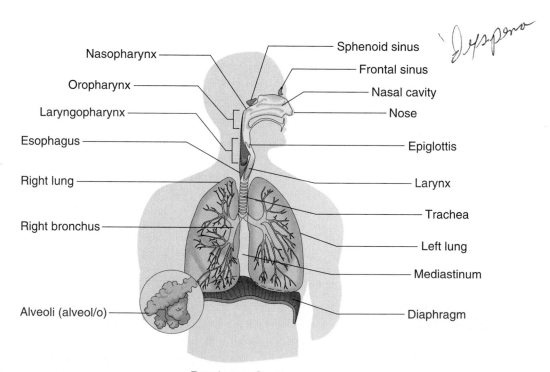

Nasopharynx
Oropharynx
Laryngopharynx
Esophagus
Right lung
Right bronchus
Alveoli (alveol/o)

Sphenoid sinus
Frontal sinus
Nasal cavity
Nose
Epiglottis
Larynx
Trachea
Left lung
Mediastinum
Diaphragm

Respiratory System

FIGURE 18-1 The respiratory system. Primary organs of the respiratory tract are the nose, pharynx, larynx, trachea, bronchi, and lungs. The upper respiratory tract refers to anything outside the chest cavity. The lower respiratory tract refers to within the chest cavity.

or to simply be supportive of the client who is self-administering a breathing treatment. Although the home health aide will not be teaching or administering a breathing treatment, it is important to observe and report to the team if a client has breathing difficulties, difficulties using equipment, or trouble taking prescribed medication.

A sputum specimen may be required to diagnose a respiratory infection and to provide a method to monitor the client's ongoing respiratory condition. Procedure 62 describes the proper technique for collecting a sputum specimen.

Pneumonia

Pneumonia is an acute infection of the lung. It is usually caused by bacteria, but there may be other causes, such as a virus. It is treated with antibiotics.

Pneumonia is a leading cause of death in the United States. Because many elderly persons already have preexisting conditions and chronic illnesses, they are more vulnerable. Also, the immune system of an older adult is compromised as well. It is critical to understand that many older adults do not always have severe early symptoms, but then can become acutely ill very quickly. This puts them in danger because of the chance for delayed or missed diagnosis. Symptoms to look for (but *not* always present in older adults) are fever, productive cough with sputum, rapid respirations, nausea, vomiting, and fatigue. Care plan includes rest, fluids (intravenous or oral), and possibly respiratory therapy with oxygen, antibiotics, and adequate nutrition.

Chronic Bronchitis

Chronic bronchitis often occurs in middle-aged or elderly persons. It can result from a number of acute conditions, asthma, bronchitis, cigarette smoking, and air pollution.

Bronchitis is an inflammation of the bronchi, and, once again, elderly persons are more vulnerable to this than younger persons. This includes, in particular, elderly individuals with a history of chronic pulmonary disease. The treatment plan is devised in conjunction with symptom relief.

Symptoms include fever (usually low grade) with productive cough, lethargy, and malaise.

CLIENT CARE PROCEDURE

62

Collecting a Sputum Specimen

PURPOSE

- To provide a sputum specimen for a diagnostic test
- To monitor the client's ongoing condition

PROCEDURE

1. Assemble supplies:
   disposable gloves
   specimen container, cover with label completed
   tissues
   moisture-proof plastic bag
   mask (optional)

2. Wash hands and apply gloves. Wear a mask if client has an infectious disease.
3. Ask client to cough deeply and bring up sputum from the lungs. Have client expectorate (spit) into the container. Collect 1 to 2 tablespoons of sputum unless otherwise directed. Be sure to have client cover mouth with tissue to prevent the spread of infections. If excess sputum contaminates the outside of the container, wipe off right away. Cover specimen container and place in moisture-proof bag.
4. Remove gloves and wash hands.
5. Document collection of sputum and when transported to laboratory.

Treatment includes rest, fluids, and cough medication to loosen secretions. If there is no mucus accompanying the cough, then a cough suppressant may be given. Medications to dilate the bronchi and facilitate more effective breathing are also ordered. Encourage clients to elevate both their head and upper torso to facilitate better breathing. Educate clients regarding the use of humidifiers, and caution them about use of any over-the-counter medications. Sometimes these symptoms are very gradual and prolonged.

Refer to Procedure 63 on the proper method to assist with cough and deep-breathing exercises.

Asthma

Asthma is a condition caused by an allergic reaction, although there are other causes. Often the specific substance causing the asthma cannot be determined. Symptoms may include coughing, difficulty breathing, wheezing, and a feeling of tightness in the chest.

CLIENT CARE PROCEDURE

63 Assisting With Cough and Deep-Breathing Exercises

PURPOSE

- To prevent congestion or infections in the client's lungs
- To expand the lungs

PROCEDURE

1. Wash your hands.
2. Tell client what you plan to do and ask for cooperation (Figure 18-2).
3. Assemble equipment:
   disposable gloves—optional
   pillow case—covered pillow
   tissues
   small basin or receptacle.
4. Have client sit up if possible.
5. If the client has recently had surgery, a pillow placed over the incision site may reduce muscle movement in the area and reduce discomfort during the breathing exercises.
6. Ask client to take as deep a breath through the nose as possible and hold it for 5 to 7 seconds and then exhale slowly through pursed lips.
7. Repeat this exercise about five times unless the client is too tired.
8. Give client tissues and instruct client to take a deep breath and cough forcefully twice with mouth open. Collect any se-

cretions that are brought up in tissues. Protect yourself from secretions and droplets.
9. Put on gloves if you will be touching or handling the tissues.
10. Dispose of tissues in plastic bag and assist client to comfortable position.
11. Remove gloves and wash hands.
12. Document procedure completed, your observations, and client's reaction.

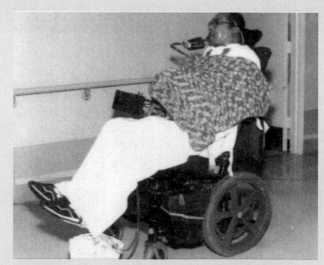

FIGURE 18-2 This client is quadriplegic and needs to be encouraged to cough and breathe deeply to prevent upper respiratory infections.

Asthma strikes more adults than once thought. Primarily asthma is associated with constriction of large and small airways causing spasms. Swelling in the airway and increased mucous productivity result in these symptoms: severe difficulty breathing, wheezing, sweating, feelings of suffocation, and anxiety. The care plan includes resolving immediate respiratory distress, elevation of client torso, and teaching the client to inhale through the nose and exhale through pursed lips. Remain calm and help client stay as calm as possible. Provide adequate humidity. Teach patient to avoid the potential allergens (the substances causing allergic reactions) if they are known.

Emphysema

Emphysema is a lung condition in which the air sacs within the lung lose their elasticity. Breathing is difficult for the person affected by this disease. Medications can relieve the symptoms of emphysema, but there is no cure.

The typical emphysema patient is a smoker 50 to 60 years of age. As the lung loses elasticity, it results in altered oxygen and carbon dioxide exchange and increased airway resistance from severe narrowing or collapse of airways. Symptoms include shortness of breath, gradually worsening, pursed-lip breathing, and increased effort to breathe, with use of accessory muscles such as the diaphragm. Later symptoms include headache, irritability, possible confusion due to poor air exchange, and leaning forward in posture. Care plan includes oxygen as ordered to facilitate breathing. (Note that too much oxygen can raise other blood gas levels too high and therefore eliminate stimulus to breathe.) Refer to Procedure 64 on the method to assist the client with oxygen therapy. The care plan also includes education regarding healthier lifestyle and abstinence from smoking.

CLIENT CARE PROCEDURE

64 Assisting the Client With Oxygen Therapy

PURPOSE

- To assist the client to receive correct amount of oxygen ordered
- To avoid misuse of oxygen equipment and careless practices that risk causing fires, explosions, or injury
- To describe two devices used to administer oxygen
- To assist with special mouth care for client receiving oxygen therapy

PROCEDURE

1. Check the meter of the oxygen tank or reservoir. If low, check to see if there is a spare tank. If there is not a spare tank, call for a replacement. **NOTE:** An oxygen concentrator is commonly used for clients with COPD who require oxygen. The concentrator lasts longer than a portable unit and is generally safer. A long tube is connected to the oxygenator, providing the client greater freedom of movement in the home than with a portable unit (Figure 18-3).
2. Wash your hands before beginning the procedure.
3. Check to see if the client's oxygen mask or cannula is placed properly (Figure 18-4). The straps on the cannula should be secure but not too tight. Check top of ears for signs of irritation. Check for signs of irritation where the prongs touch the client's nose. Be sure both prongs are in the client's nose.

   If a mask is being used, check to see whether the mask is over both nose and mouth. If inside of mask is wet, remove and dry inside.

(continues)

CLIENT CARE PROCEDURE **64** **Assisting the Client With Oxygen Therapy**
(continued)

4. Check the gauge to see if the oxygen is being given at correct amount of liter flow (Figures 18-5 and 18-6). (Oxygen therapy is delivered in liters.) The client's care plan should state the liter flow to be administered to the client. Follow any special instructions that the respiratory therapist may prescribe.

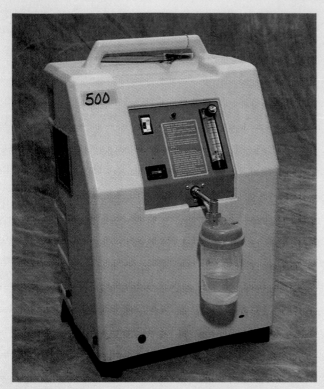

FIGURE 18-3 Oxygen concentrators are commonly used in the home for people with COPD who require oxygen.

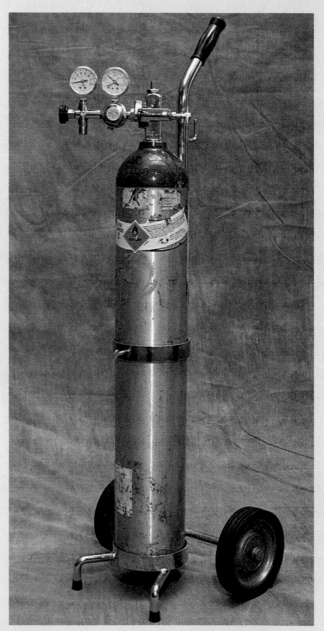

FIGURE 18-5 Portable oxygen tank

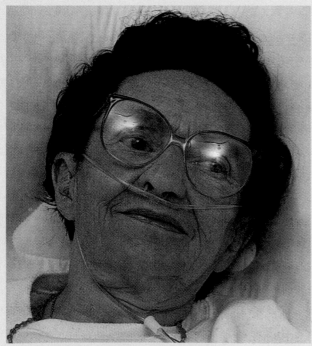

FIGURE 18-4 Client is receiving oxygen through a nasal cannula.

(continues)

CLIENT CARE PROCEDURE 64 Assisting the Client With Oxygen Therapy
(continued)

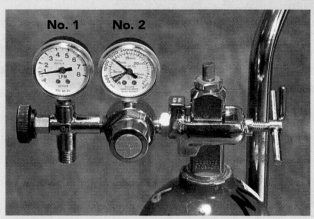

No. 1   No. 2

FIGURE 18-6 No. 1 gauge notes the liter flow. No. 2 gauge notes the amount of oxygen left in the tank.

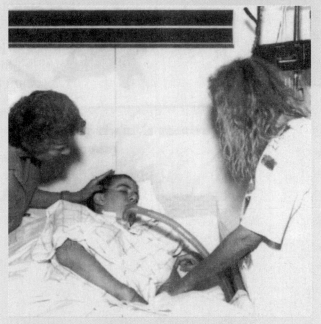

FIGURE 18-7 This young client is receiving oxygen through her tracheotomy.

5. Check the client's position. If in bed, elevate the head with three pillows to assist the client in breathing (Figure 18-7).
6. Do frequent mouth care for clients receiving oxygen therapy. The client's mouth can become dry and have an unpleasant taste. Apply lubricant to lips, if permitted, if they become dry.
7. Check that all safety precautions are being observed.
   • Do not smoke in room where client is receiving oxygen. Post "No Smoking" sign, if necessary, to warn visitors not to smoke.
   • Do not use matches, candles, or open flames where oxygen is used or stored.
   • Do not use electrical appliances during oxygen therapy. Avoid sparks. If you need to shave the client, turn off the oxygen while using the electric razor, or use a disposable razor.
   • Avoid use of woolen blankets, which may create static electricity sparks.
9. Wash your hands.
10. Document the liter flow and the device being used, your observations, and client's reaction.

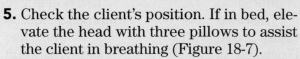

REVIEW

1. Name the major organs of the respiratory system.
2. List two purposes of the respiratory system.
3. T F A person with emphysema can never receive "too much" oxygen.
4. T F The only reason to collect a sputum specimen is to see what the sputum looks like.
5. T F Asthma is a condition caused by an allergic reaction.

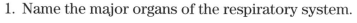

REPRODUCTIVE SYSTEM

The reproductive system consists of the external and internal sex organs of the male and female. The male organs include the **scrotum,** a saclike organ that contains the testes and other tubules; the **testes,** which produce sperm, the hormone **testosterone** and fluid; and the **penis,** which contains the **urethra** for transporting urine and sperm (Figure 19-1).

The female external organs are the **genitalia (vulva)** and breasts. The internal organs include the **vagina,** which functions as the birth canal and leads to the **cervix** and **uterus;** the cervix, which is the mouth of the womb; the uterus, located behind the urinary bladder (which functions as the womb that receives the fertilized egg and developing fetus); the **ovaries,** located on either side of the lower abdomen, which produce **estrogen** and **progesterone** hormones as well as egg cells; and the **fallopian tubes,** which carry the egg cells from the ovaries to the uterus (Figures 19-2 and 19-3).

The female has a menstrual cycle approximately every 28 days, by which the uterus is prepared to nurture the fertilized egg into a viable fetus. However, if the egg cell that is produced midcycle is not fertilized by the sperm cell, the uterine lining is sloughed off, and bleeding occurs for approximately 3 to 5 days. This is called **menstruation.**

The reproductive system is important in maintaining sexual characteristics. The hormones that produce male characteristics (such as broad shoulders, facial, chest, and pubic hair) and female characteristics (such as rounded hips, enlarged breasts, and pubic hair) are also thought to help maintain function in other systems of the body. Illness or malfunction of the reproductive system can cause emotional and physical problems. In giving care, it is important to treat the person with understanding and consideration and to give the person opportunities to express feelings about illness.

COMMON DISORDERS OF THE REPRODUCTIVE SYSTEM

Some common disorders of the reproductive system include dysmenorrhea, vaginitis, and

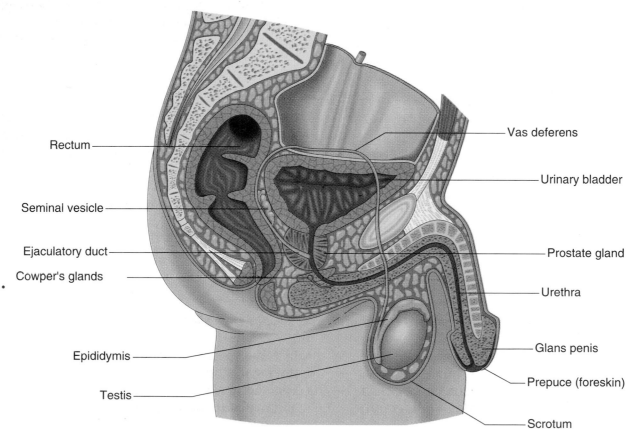

FIGURE 19-1 The male reproductive system

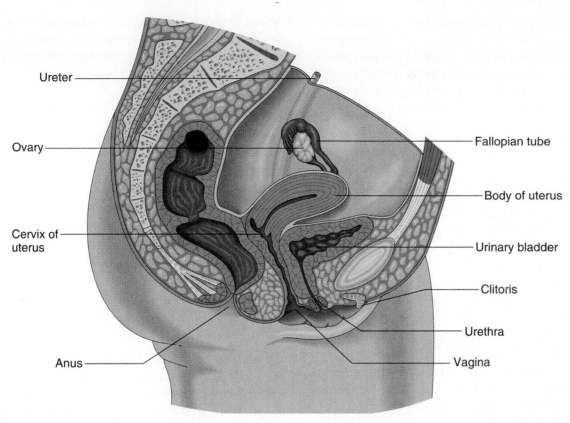

FIGURE 19-2 The female reproductive system

sexually transmitted diseases. Many of these disorders may be caused by infections or sexual activity with an infected person, and may require medication for treatment.

Dysmenorrhea

Dysmenorrhea refers to pain that sometimes accompanies the menstrual flow. Although a large percentage of women experience some minor discomfort during menstruation, it should be emphasized that menstruation is a normal process. However, any severe cramping or persistent pain should be reported to a **gynecologist,** a physician specializing in women's reproductive health.

Vaginitis

Vaginitis is an infection of the vagina (birth canal), which may be caused by bacteria, protozoa (one-celled organism), or yeast; or may

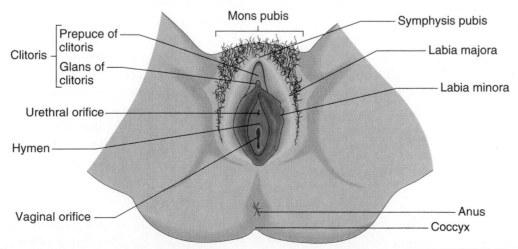

FIGURE 19-3 The female external genitalia

result from changes in vaginal secretions after **menopause** (the permanent end of menstruation). There is usually a whitish discharge with itching and burning. Treatment usually includes drugs and cleanliness, depending on the organism present.

SEXUALLY TRANSMITTED DISEASES ····

Infections spread by sexual intercourse are called **sexually transmitted diseases (STDs).** These are common worldwide, especially among young adults. In developed countries, syphilis and gonorrhea declined after World War II, increased in the 1960s and 1970s, and declined in the 1980s, and are rising again in some areas. Some STDs increase the risk of transmitting the human immunodeficiency virus (HIV). Please refer to Unit 24 for a detailed discussion of HIV and AIDS.

Pelvic Inflammatory Disease

Pelvic inflammatory disease (PID) is an infection of the upper female reproductive tract. The disorder is usually caused by chlamydial infection or gonorrhea. The diagnosis is based on the symptoms and on tests carried out on samples of cervical or vaginal discharge taken during a physical examination. PID is usually treated with a combination of antibiotics.

Complications. Pelvic inflammatory disease is serious because it can cause severe damage and scarring in the reproductive tract. Worldwide, it is the most common cause of infertility. Other complications of PID include chronic pelvic pain and abnormal menstrual bleeding. Scarring in the fallopian tubes can block passage of a fertilized egg, increasing the risk of an **ectopic pregnancy,** a condition in which the egg implants outside the uterine cavity.

Nongonococcal Urethritis

Nongonococcal urethritis, also known as nonspecific urethritis, is urethral inflammation caused by an infection other than gonorrhea. This infection is among the most prevalent of all STDs. Symptoms usually start 1 to 3 weeks after exposure. In women, the main symptom is vaginal discharge. Men, as a result of inflammation

of the urethra, commonly experience discharge from the penis and pain when urinating. Infection may cause scrotal pain and swelling. Treatment consists of antibiotics.

Gonorrhea

Gonorrhea, a bacterial infection, causes a discharge of pus from the penis or sometimes the vagina, and pain on urination. The main sites of infection are the urethra and, in women, the cervix, from where organisms can spread to the uterus, fallopian tubes, and ovaries. The rectum can also be affected. A pregnant woman risks passing the infection to her baby during childbirth. Gonorrhea is treated by antibiotics, but in some parts of the world resistance has developed to most drugs.

Syphilis

The earliest symptom of **syphilis** is usually an ulcer (chancre) on the genitals. However, an ulcer can also develop in the mouth or anus. A rash, mouth ulcers, and enlargement of the lymph nodes follow. Later effects include brain, heart, and bone disorders. A pregnant woman can pass the infection to her baby.

Genital Herpes

One of the most common STDs is **genital herpes,** and its reported incidence has increased over recent years in some countries. Caused by an organism known as herpes simplex virus, genital herpes tends to recur. The first episode is the most severe, with subsequent occurrences decreasing in severity and frequency.

During an episode, crops of small blisters form on the penis or around the vagina, then develop into shallow, painful ulcers. The first attack of herpes may be accompanied by headache, fever, and pain in the groin, buttocks, and legs.

There is no cure for genital herpes. Painkillers, such as aspirin, as well as warm baths, can help relieve symptoms. Certain drugs can provide pain relief and speed healing during an attack. Prolonged use of the antiviral drug, acyclovir, may reduce the number and frequency of occurrences.

Prevention of STDs

To prevent STDs, sexually active people should, ideally, have a single sexual partner, always use a condom when engaged in penetrative sex, and avoid practices that could damage the delicate lining of the vagina or anus. People with symp- toms of an STD or who are being treated for an STD should abstain from sex and their partners should be checked for infection.

REVIEW

1. The male reproductive system includes:
   a. Scrotum, testes, and penis
   b. Uterus and cervix
   c. None of the above
   d. All of the above

2. The female fallopian tubes:
   a. Produce estrogen and progesterone
   b. Carry egg cells from ovaries to uterus
   c. Slough off during menstruation
   d. None of the above
   e. All of the above

3. The acronym STD stands for
   a. Short-term disability
   b. Sanitize to disinfect
   c. Sexually transmitted disease

4. Match Column I with Column II.

Column I	Column II
_____ 1. uterus	a. sloughing off of uterine lining
_____ 2. scrotum	b. male hormone
_____ 3. vaginitis	c. sexually transmitted disease
_____ 4. menstruation	d. receives fertilized egg and developing fetus
_____ 5. testosterone	e. infection of the vagina
_____ 6. genital herpes	f. saclike organ that contains testes and other tubules

5. Name five sexually transmitted diseases and their symptoms.

6. T   F   Female hormones produce masculine characteristics.

7. T   F   The person with an illness or malfunction of the reproductive system may need to express his or her feelings about an illness.

8. T   F   Diseases spread by sexual intercourse are called STSs.

9. T   F   Pelvic inflammatory disease affects male and female reproductive systems.

10. John, a 23-year-old man, was recently involved in a motorcycle accident where he sustained multiple injuries and now requires the services of a homemaker home health aide. Prior to his accident, he was sexually active, with multiple partners. Now he is complaining of painful urination. The homemaker home health aide suspects a sexually transmitted disease is the cause, but John becomes defensive when the subject is mentioned. What should the homemaker home health aide do?

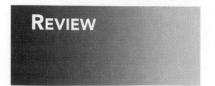

REVIEW

11. Mary's 14-year-old daughter confides to the homemaker home health aide that she has noticed a bloody discharge. She is afraid to discuss this with her mother because she is fearful of her mother's reaction. What should the homemaker home health aide do?

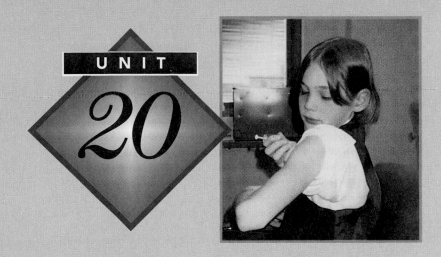

UNIT 20

Endocrine System and Diabetes

KEY TERMS

acidosis
blood lancet
cyanotic
diabetes
ducts
endocrine glands

gangrene
gestational
glucometer
glucose
hormone
hyperglycemia

hyperthyroidism
hypoglycemia
hypothyroidism
insulin
neuropathy
subcutaneously

LEARNING OBJECTIVES

After studying this unit, you should be able to:

- Name four signs and symptoms of diabetes.
- List four types of diabetes mellitus.
- Name three ways of controlling diabetes.
- Name three long-term complications of diabetes.
- List signs and symptoms for insulin shock and acidosis and the immediate care for each.

- Explain special foot care given to the diabetic client.
- Describe special techniques used in caring for a client who has vision impairment.
- Demonstrate the following:
  PROCEDURE 65 Testing Blood

ENDOCRINE SYSTEM ·······················

The **endocrine glands** are ductless glands that secrete substances within the body called hormones (Figure 20-1). The glands do not have **ducts** (little tubes) and are, therefore, unlike tear and sweat glands. **Hormones** are chemicals that are secreted directly into the bloodstream. They are carried throughout the body to regulate and control specific body functions. They are powerful substances and direct the functions of other systems. Each hormone has a special job to do (Figure 20-2). It only takes a small amount of hormone to trigger a body reaction. Most scientists agree that the brain sends messages to the endocrine glands. These messages cause the gland to secrete the hormone needed by the body. For instance, in a time of physical danger the adrenal gland secretes a hormone called adrenalin. The adrenalin causes the heart rate to increase. This forces more blood through the body, which increases the nourishment to the muscles. Sugar is released into the body, giving it quick energy. The adrenalin also speeds up the body's reflexes. All of these changes occur rapidly, making the body able to react and save itself or others from harm.

The thyroid gland regulates the metabolic rate of the body. This determines the speed that food is turned into energy.

HYPERTHYROIDISM AND HYPOTHYROIDISM ·····················

The thyroid weighs less than an ounce but all aspects of metabolism, from the rate at which your heart beats to the speed at which you burn calories, are regulated by the thyroid hormones. Some people have an overactive thyroid and their food metabolizes quickly (**hyperthy-**

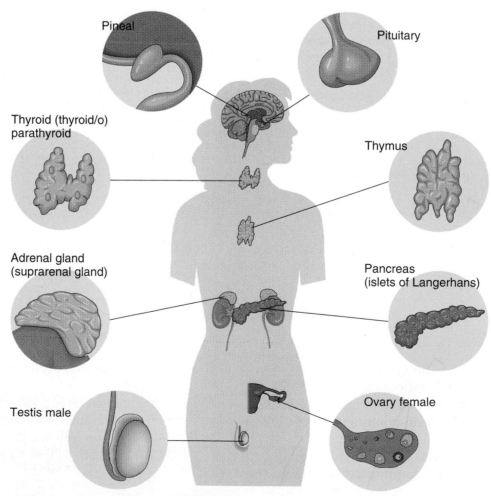

FIGURE 20-1 Location of the endocrine glands

FIGURE 20-2	Functions of the glands of the endocrine system
Pituitary gland	Once called "master gland" of the body; secretes a number of hormones that regulate many bodily processes. The pituitary is completely controlled by the hypothalamus, a part of the brain.
Thyroid gland	Helps to regulate the metabolic rate and growth process.
Parathyroid glands	Regulate metabolism of calcium and phosphorous.
Thymus gland	Regulates immunity to infectious diseases during infancy and early childhood; becomes smaller as body ages.
Adrenal glands	Adjust body to crisis and stress; increase blood pressure; speed reactions; metabolize carbohydrates and proteins.
Pancreas	Produces insulin needed to burn sugar in body. (Too little insulin causes diabetes; too much insulin causes hyperglycemia). Also produces glucagon to raise blood sugar.
Ovaries	Produce ovum (egg) for reproduction; secrete estrogen and progesterone that develop and maintain secondary sexual characteristics (breasts, pubic and underarm hair, etc.).
Testes	Produce sperm to fertilize ovum; secrete male hormone called testosterone.

roidism). They usually have a rapid heartbeat and tend to be restless and irritable.

About 7 million Americans, mostly women over the age of 40, are affected by an underactive thyroid (**hypothyroidism**). Early symptoms of an underactive thyroid, such as sluggishness and fatigue, are often vague. As the metabolism continues to be slow, signs such as chronically cold hands or feet, constipation, pale and dry skin, a puffy face, and hoarse voice may develop. There is some weight gain but usually not more than 10 to 20 pounds. Most people who are overweight have normal thyroid function.

DIABETES MELLITUS

Diabetes mellitus is a chronic disease with no cure. The disease is primarily managed through diet, exercise, and drug therapy. The pancreas either does not produce any or produces an inadequate amount of a hormone called **insulin.**

The functions of insulin are to enable the body to use **glucose** (sugar), to aid in the storage of nutrients, and to make possible the metabolism of carbohydrates and protein. When insulin is not manufactured or cannot be used correctly, a condition called **diabetes** develops. In diabetes, the person's blood sugar level is elevated (hyperglycemia) because the sugar remains in the blood instead of being absorbed into the cells and used for food. The buildup of sugar in the blood is unhealthy for a number of reasons. It disturbs the fluid balance in the body because it causes kidney problems. Diabetes suppresses the immune system and this allows infections to flourish. Sugar buildup in the blood vessels results in restricted circulation because of damage to the blood vessels. The lack of adequate blood supply to certain body areas causes many problems in the brain, extremities, eyes, kidney, and heart.

Facts and Figures*

- More than 11 million Americans have some form of diabetes—and 5 million of them do not know it.
- Diabetes is the third leading cause of death by disease in the United States.

*American Diabetes Association

- Each year, more than 150,000 people die from diabetes or its complications, such as kidney failure.
- In the 45-to-65-year-old age group, twice as many African Americans have diabetes as Caucasian Americans.
- Native Americans have a higher rate of type II (non-insulin–dependent) diabetes than any other population in the world.
- Among Japanese Americans in the West Coast cities, the rate of type II diabetes is two to three times higher than anywhere else in the United States.
- Japanese children living in Japan have a lower risk of developing type I (insulin-dependent) diabetes than do children in any other country.

Classifications

Diabetes can be classified into several types.

- Insulin-dependent diabetes mellitus (IDDM) Type I: usually occurs before age 25. The pancreas no longer produces any insulin and this person needs daily insulin injections to stay alive.
- Non-insulin–dependent diabetes mellitus (NIDDM): usually develops after the age of 40 and is commonly seen in the elderly person. Insulin is produced, but may be insufficient or ineffective in preventing hyperglycemia. This person is unable to use this insulin effectively to change glucose (sugar) into energy. People with NIDDM may need to use insulin, but usually take medication.
- Hyperglycemia: May be temporarily caused by doses of drugs such as steroids or hormones and by disease processes affecting the pancreas.
- **Gestational**-Type III: Occurs during a woman's pregnancy and usually returns to normal after delivery. However, these women often will develop diabetes later in life unless changes are made in diet and exercise.
- Glucose intolerance (impaired ability to metabolize glucose): Includes changes in insulin levels and insulin release, decreased peripheral effectiveness of insulin, or a combination of these factors. May occur more frequently in the elderly person because of age-related changes.

Signs and Symptoms

Signs and symptoms of diabetes can come on slowly and will only be detected during an annual physical evaluation. Occasionally it is caused by infection or stress and will come on suddenly. Some of the signs and symptoms to watch for are:

- Weakness
- Sudden weight loss
- Unusual thirst
- Frequent need to urinate
- Crankiness
- Itching
- Sores that do not heal
- Repeated infections

Testing

Routine testing for diabetes during an annual physical examination is important for early diagnosis and detection. Common tests used in the diagnoses and treatment of diabetes are:

- Fasting blood sample: Usually taken from the arm; tested for the level of blood glucose (type of sugar); normal is between 70 and 120 mg.
- Urinalysis: Urine sample is tested for presence of sugar or ketones.
- Insulin and glucose tolerance tests: Series of tests done on blood within designated time periods. Blood is tested while fasting and then after drinking a high-glucose solution at different time periods.
- Glycoslated hemoglobin: Blood test that will give the average blood sugar level over a period of 3 months.

Once diagnosed with diabetes, clients are taught how to test their blood or urine. However, urine testing is rarely done and only when the client cannot, or will not, cooperate with blood testing. In recent years, technology for testing blood at home has improved tremendously. Doctors prefer that people test their own blood because it is more accurate. Testing the blood gives a reading of what the blood sugar value is at the moment. Blood and urine testing kits are readily available at any drugstore. Blood testing equipment (**glucometer**) has been greatly improved in the last few years and, although the cost may be high, it is the best method to control diabetes. Procedure 65 outlines the method for testing blood.

Some machines have the ability to talk the client or the caregiver through the procedure. It is important to know when the blood sugar reading is high or low. When taking a reading, you must be aware of when the client last ate or drank anything to accurately know if the blood sugar reading is high. Your nurse supervisor will advise you when to call to report abnormal readings. A reading of 200 might be normal for one client, but it might be abnormal for another. It is the responsibility of your nurse supervisor to interpret the reading. Be sure to check the expiration date on the blood strips. Store the strips in the original vial in a cool, dry place. Do not store in a humid place, such as the bathroom. Always keep the vial capped tightly. Dispose of the blood lancet in a "sharps" container. Be sure that you are approved to do the procedure. If you are given the responsibility to do blood glucose monitoring, be sure to wash your hands before you start with the procedure and also at the completion of the task. Take time to familiarize yourself with the blood glucose monitor you are using.

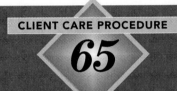

Testing Blood

PURPOSE

- To determine the blood sugar level

Testing procedures for blood sugar vary according to the type of glucometer the client has purchased. The instructions must be followed carefully to avoid an inaccurate reading. It is also important if you assist with the procedure that you follow standard precautions. *Always check with your agency to see if you are allowed to do this task.*

PROCEDURE

1. Gather necessary equipment (Figure 20-3A):
   disposable gloves
   glucometer
   blood lancet (needle)
   alcohol swab and cotton ball
   watch with second hand
   blood strips—be sure you have blood strips that correspond with your glucometer. Also check to see that the blood strips are not outdated.
2. Wash hands and put on gloves.
3. Have client wash hands with warm water; then have the client squeeze and prick the finger with the lancet (Figure

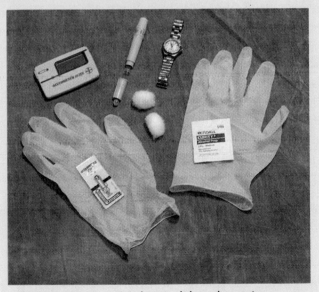

FIGURE 20-3A Diabetic blood testing equipment: glucose meter, cotton balls, lancet, alcohol, blood testing strips, gloves, and watch

20-3B). The client may use a special apparatus to prick the finger. Rotate fingers if doing this procedure daily. Use the side of finger that has less use.

(continues)

CLIENT CARE PROCEDURE **65** **Testing Blood** *(continued)*

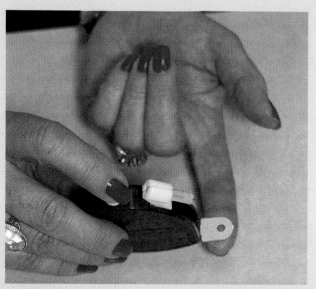

FIGURE 20-3B Client pricking finger

4. With palm facing down, firmly apply pressure to the pricked finger until a large drop of hanging blood forms. Bring the blood strip to the finger and touch the blood strip to the drop of blood. Completely cover the test zone of the strip with the blood. Gloves are worn when doing this testing for infection control purposes (Figure 20-3C).

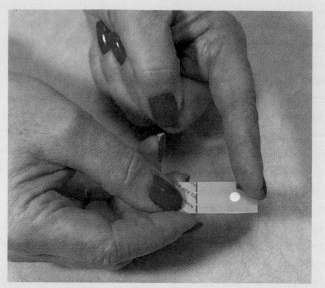

FIGURE 20-3C Drop of blood from client's finger on blood testing strip

5. Insert blood strip into machine and observe read-out.
6. Record reading and discard blood strip and lancet in proper container.
7. Remove gloves and wash hands.

Emergency Treatment

A home health aide needs to be alert for signs and symptoms of diabetic coma or insulin reaction and to follow the emergency plan of care for your client. The blood sugar level must be kept in a certain range or problems will occur in the diabetic client. If the blood sugar goes too low, a condition called **hypoglycemia** occurs. This condition results when there is an imbalance between food intake and the appropriate dosage of drug therapy-oral hypoglycemics, insulin, or both. Exercise, alcohol, or decreased kidney or liver function can make this condition worse. Some of the signs of hypoglycemia are:

* Change in mental functioning
* Tachycardia (fast heart rate)

* Palpitations
* Increased sweating
* Hunger
* Shaking

If it is confirmed by a blood glucose reading below 60, this is an emergency. In a conscious person, you should give some form of sugar, fruit juice, sugar cubes, or glucose tablets. If a person is unresponsive, call 911 or emergency response.

If a client's blood sugar is high, he or she has **hyperglycemia.** The signs of hyperglycemia are:

* Increased thirst, hunger, and urination
* Weakness
* Abdominal pain
* Generalized aches, including headaches
* Heavy breathing
* Nausea and vomiting

The blood sugar level is usually over 250. The client lacks an adequate supply of insulin. You can confirm this by doing a blood sugar check. You will need to contact your nursing supervisor. Hyperglycemia may develop into a complication of diabetes called **acidosis.** Here you may find the blood sugar over 350 with accompanying signs of dehydration, abdominal pain, vomiting, rapid or deep breathing, and changing mental status. This is a serious condition. Your supervisor should be contacted immediately. If the person is unresponsive, you should call 911 or the emergency response. Insulin is needed as well as a fluid replacement and blood tests to evaluate the client's metabolism. If either insulin reaction or acidosis is not corrected immediately, coma or death can occur.

Loss of vision is a common complication of diabetes. A few older clients with diabetes may have vision problems and be unable to read directions to do blood sugar testing or to read the numbers on the insulin syringe. Because of these vision problems, you may need to read the directions to them and also double-check their readings. The majority of the clients you will be working with will be able to do their own insulin injections and their own blood testing.

Diet

Diet is the cornerstone to the management of diabetes. The diet should contain necessary elements of good nutrition, maintain blood sugar levels, and be acceptable to the client's preferences. The diet needs to contain a defined number of calories and consist of 50% to 60% carbohydrates, 12% to 20% protein, and 30% to 36% fat. The food intake should be distributed throughout the day and accommodate the client's lifestyle, activity, and diabetic medication. Because 80% of diabetics are classified as type II diabetics, they will also need to have their calories limited to maintain their ideal weight. The American Diabetes Association has developed exchange lists of foods that can assist the aide and the client in meal planning.

An important duty of the aide is to prepare meals using the diet prescribed by the medical professional and exchange list. The aide must be sure the foods selected for the meals includes items on the food pyramid and are allowed on the exchange list and diet. The aide needs to encourage and reinforce the impor-

tance of abiding by this diet. A diabetic client also needs to remember to eat meals and snacks at the same time every day. Occasionally the client will try to deny the disease and not follow the prescribed diet. There is little you can do in the client's own home to force the individual to eat the correct foods. Many times the client will eat the correct foods when you are there, but when you leave he or she does not follow the prescribed diet. If you become aware of this it is important to document and notify your supervisor.

Obesity and poor nutrition are two common problems in diabetes. Using the prescribed diet can limit these problems. Most diabetics who stick to a diet, take medication, and exercise moderately have fewer health problems. The diabetic client who does not follow the doctor's orders risks serious problems.

Can you imagine how difficult it would be for children to have diabetes and not eat candy bars, cookies, and potato chips like their peers? It is very easy for them (and also adults) to go off the prescribed diet and eat some form of concentrated sugar, such as pie or cake. As a home health aide, you need to be supportive and give your client constant encouragement to follow the prescribed diet.

Exercise

Regular exercises are often recommended in the daily routine of clients with diabetes. The benefits of exercise are many. Exercise can improve the client's circulation, assist in maintaining ideal weight, increase a person's well-being, and improve control of glucose in the body (in type II diabetes). A home health aide should encourage and assist the client in doing the prescribed exercises. There will be a wide range of exercises that you might become involved in, depending on the client's mobility and environment. If the client is unable to walk or do the exercises, you will need to do the prescribed passive range of motion exercises for the client. Refer to Unit 10, Procedure 15 for the proper method of performing passive range of motion exercises. If your client is able to do the exercises with little assistance, you will need to encourage the client to do exercises on a regular basis. Your nurse supervisor will assist you in setting up an appropriate exercise plan for your client.

Drug Therapy

Treatment of diabetes depends on the type of disease. For example, a type I diabetic is always treated with insulin injections. However, a person with type II diabetes may need to take oral hypoglycemic drugs (which stimulate the pancreas to make more insulin), insulin injections, or both.

Type I Diabetes.   Type I diabetes is always treated with a drug called insulin, which needs to be injected **subcutaneously** (under the skin). It cannot be taken orally because the stomach juices will dissolve the drug. The person with diabetes is taught where, when, and how to inject the medication (Figure 20-4). If a diabetic person is unable to self-inject, another member of the family might be taught to give the injections. Some diabetics are too young to give themselves injections; other clients with diabetes may have poor eyesight or be uncoordinated. Most diabetic clients, if instructed properly, are able to inject their own insulin.

CAUTION: A home health aide is *not* permitted to inject insulin. The aide's responsibility is limited to bringing the medication and necessary supplies to the client (Figure 20-5).

You should always check the expiration date on the insulin bottle. The insulin should not be used if it is past the expiration date because it might not be effective any longer. It is not necessary to refrigerate insulin, but it should be kept in a cool place and where the temperature stays the same. Most clients prefer to keep their insulin in the refrigerator. The three most important factors to remember about insulin are:

1. Measurement must be *accurate*.
2. The drug must be taken at the same time every day. The client should be eating on a regular schedule.
3. Sterile technique must be maintained when injecting the drug.

The physician may prescribe different kinds of insulin. Some insulins are fast acting and some are slow acting. The physician will prescribe the type of insulin needed, the frequency, time, and amount of insulin.

Sites recommended for injections include the abdomen, upper arms, and thighs. Most clients are encouraged to rotate injection sites on a daily or weekly basis to avoid changes in the skin tissues, which can alter the rate of absorption of the drug. It is a good idea to keep a record of where the injection was given to assist the client in rotating sites.

The insulin pump is a recent development, but use is limited because of the cost of the

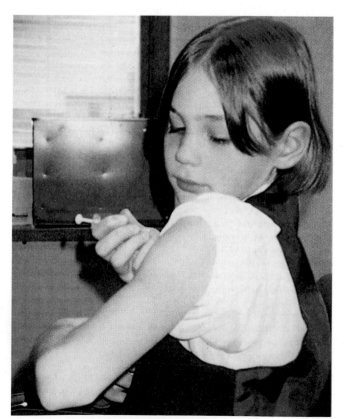

FIGURE 20-4 This young diabetic is self-injecting insulin into the upper arm. (Courtesy of The Diabetes Center of Albany Memorial Hospital, Albany, NY)

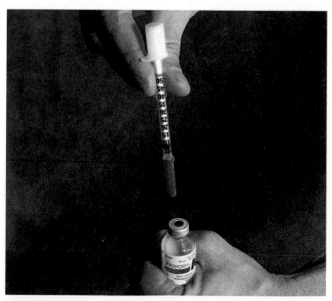

FIGURE 20-5 Bottle of insulin and insulin syringe

equipment and the vigorous participation that is required by the client for safe maintenance and monitoring. A small needle is inserted in the abdomen. The needle is connected to a pump worn on the waist, which holds the insulin supply. This device administers insulin continuously. A control button or a switch allows the client to adjust the release of insulin. This device may be implanted in diabetic clients just as pacemakers are now implanted into clients with heart disease.

Experiments are now being conducted with pancreatic transplants. The purpose of the transplant is to replace non–insulin-producing cells with insulin-producing cells.

Type II Diabetes. Type II diabetes can be treated in three ways. One way is by diet alone. Once individuals have reached their ideal weight and eat the proper foods, they may be able to maintain their blood sugar level without drugs. The second way is by taking oral hypoglycemic drugs daily. These drugs stimulate the pancreas to make more insulin available. Examples of hypoglycemic drugs are:

Generic Name	Brand Name
tolbutamide	Orinase
acetohexamide	Dymelor
tolazamide	Tolinase
chlorpropamide	Diabinese
glyburide	DiaBeta

As a home health aide you need to remember to encourage your client to take the prescribed drug as ordered. Generally, the drug is taken once a day, but it is not uncommon for a physician to order the drug two (bid) or three (tid) times a day. You should be sure the client has an adequate supply of drugs on hand. These drugs are costly and, occasionally, a client will want to save money and stop taking the medication. If this does happen, be sure to notify your nurse supervisor. There are ways your agency can help find assistance with the cost of medications.

The third way of treating type II diabetes is with insulin injections. There is another class of drugs whose purpose is to assist with the utilization of glucose. These drugs can be used alone or in conjunction with hypoglycemics or insulin. One of the most frequently used drugs is Metformin, otherwise known as Glucophage. There are other drugs in this class being developed.

Long-term Complications

Untreated or improperly treated diabetes can lead to many physical problems. Abnormal conditions that occur after a person develops diabetes are called diabetic complications. In some cases, even a well-cared-for diabetic may develop serious complications. The most common complications are vascular (blood vessel) disease and a high risk of infections. The most common long-term complications are described in Figure 20-6. Although many long-term disorders cannot be avoided, the home health aide can help the client manage them.

Special Nursing Care

Because diabetes can have serious consequences, it is important that the home health aide be particularly observant for signs and symptoms of health problems in the client. Special attention must be paid to the lower extremities, especially the feet, for signs of redness, swelling, and cracked or open skin that can easily become infected. Any abnormalities must be reported immediately to the nurse.

Neuropathy in the Diabetic. Neuropathy is defined as a destructive disorder of the nerves. Diabetic neuropathy is the loss of sensation in nerves. These individuals may be unable to feel pain or differentiate between hot and cold temperatures. This can be extremely dangerous. For example, a diabetic injures a foot or leg and, because no pain is felt, continues to use the limb. An infection can occur and the diabetic does not even realize there is a problem. Cuts or wounds not felt and thus not cared for can become infected. A home health aide carefully and routinely must check the client's feet and legs for any sign of redness, any "warm" area, any swelling, or any open cuts. Many diabetics have poor eyesight, or have difficulty bending their legs, and are unable to see to check their feet. They rely on the aide to do the checking.

Foot Care. The home health aide should give special attention to the diabetic's feet every day. A client's feet and legs need to be examined daily for signs of dry, scaly, itching, or cracked skin; blisters; corns; infections; blueness and swelling of the ankles; and discolored nails.

Any abnormality must be reported to the nurse supervisor. Feet are bathed and soaked

FIGURE 20-6	Complications of diabetes			
Long-Term Disorders	**Cause**	**Symptoms**	**Treatment**	**Aide's Care**
1. Blindness	Cataracts, glaucoma, hemorrhage	Partial or total loss of sight, client drops items, stumbles or falls; develops tunnel vision	Surgery can remove cataracts; medication or surgery for glaucoma	Assist in activities of daily living
2. Gangrene	Poor circulation; skin breakdown; invasion of tissue by bacteria	Heat in area, skin reddened, formation of ulcers that do not clear up; foul odor and spread of infection and tissue destruction	Medication under physician's order; may require amputation of limb	Assist with dressing changes and rehabilitation
3. Kidney disease	Too much sugar free in urine; filtering system works inefficiently	Frequency, pain, burning while voiding; retention of urine may occur	Diet modification and medication	Observe and record intake/output; note color and composition of urine.
4. Vascular disease and nerve degeneration	High sugar level; poor fat metabolism; poor tissue repair; poor circulation	Open lesions form on skin tissue as vascular degeneration occurs; nervous system functions at decreased level—sight, sound, taste, touch, smell may be affected	Bed rest, moist heat/dressings, diet and medication	Give proper foot care; assist in activities of daily living

in warm water with mild soap and then dried with a soft towel. A good lanolin-based lotion is then applied starting at the client's toes and working toward the ankles. This helps stimulate the blood circulation to the feet. If the areas between the toes are moist due to perspiration, a very small piece of lamb's wool or cotton can be placed between the toes. Bunions and corns must be treated by a podiatrist (foot doctor). See Unit 14, Procedure 41 for the proper method of performing a warm foot soak.

In the aged, the nails become thick and difficult to cut. Nail care (both fingernails and toenails) must be carefully done by a registered nurse or someone who has been taught to do it correctly. Unit 14, Procedure 42 discusses the proper method for giving nail care. **CAUTION:** The aide may NOT cut the diabetic client's nails. There is danger of infection from skin cuts around the nails. In addition, improper cutting may cause ingrown toenails, which easily can lead to infection. If the client's feet are well cared for and examined daily, infection is unlikely to develop. The following foot care guide will help reduce injury to the feet:

• Bathe the feet daily in warm, not hot, water.
• Pat the feet dry with a soft towel, especially between the toes.
• Massage the feet to increase circulation.
• Wear clean white cotton socks and change daily.

- Do not apply iodine or carbolic acid to cuts on feet.
- Avoid walking barefoot.
- Always wear comfortable, well-fitting, leather shoes.
- Do not use commercial corn pads.

Prevention of Infections. Clients with diabetes are very susceptible to any type of infection. If they do get the flu or a cold, their blood sugar levels usually decrease and increase erratically. Diabetic clients need to have their blood sugar monitored closely if they have even a mild cold or fever.

Diabetic persons also have problems with small cuts or abrasions healing. Special attention by the aide to keep the cut or abrasion as clean as possible will assist in the healing process. Slow healing is due in part to poor circulation. Breakdown of the blood vessels prevents nutrients from being carried to the injured tissue; this delays the healing process. The slow healing process leaves the skin open to infection. The risk of infection is also increased because of the extra sugar in the blood. The extra sugar creates an ideal environment for bacteria to grow. Bacteria can multiply quickly before the body is able to defend itself. Poor circulation delays the transport of substances needed to fight off the bacteria. It is of the utmost importance to report any sign of infection early to your nurse supervisor.

Good skin care is vital in preventing the skin from developing pressure sores and other skin lesions, and is an especially important safety precaution for the diabetic client. Remember to use only a mild soap sparingly when bathing the client and use a good lanolin-based lotion on the client's body. Keep bed linens dry, clean, and wrinkle free, and turn and reposition your client every 2 hours (q2h) to avoid pressure spots.

When blood vessels are injured or diseased, the surrounding cells die from lack of nutrition and oxygen. A large area of dead tissue is called **gangrene.** Gangrene is a serious condition because it is easily infected with certain bacteria. Gangrene is a form of an infection. The bacteria causing gangrene thrive in dead tissue. The bacteria spread quickly, causing severe pain and greater tissue damage.

The aide should check the client's feet and broken skin areas for signs of gangrene (Figure 20-7). The first sign is a hot and reddened skin area. This area becomes cold and bluish (**cyanotic**). After the tissues are dead, they turn black

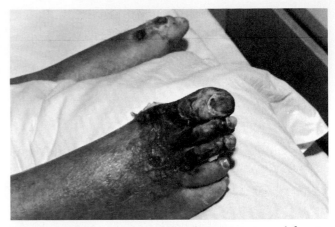

FIGURE 20-7 Gangrene of the toes and foot often requires eventual amputation.

and flake off. Drainage from the area may be bubbly and emit a strong, foul odor.

Identification Tag

All diabetics should wear a Medic Alert identification tag. The ID is a labeled tag worn as a bracelet or necklace (Figure 20-8). The ID tag

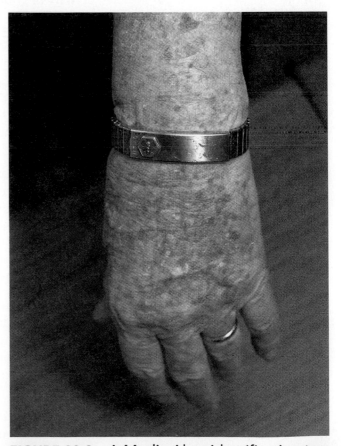

FIGURE 20-8 A Medic Alert identification tag provides essential information in case of an emergency.

should be worn by the diabetic individual at all times. The label indicates the person's:

- Name
- Address
- Telephone number
- Medical condition
- Physician's name

In emergencies, the Medic Alert ID informs emergency personnel, police, health care providers, and others of the diabetic's medical condition. A diabetic who develops acidosis or insulin shock needs immediate help. The ID tag notifies health personnel that the person's emergency is possibly a diabetic condition. If the person is unconscious, the tag may provide information necessary to save the person's life. Medic Alert tags are also worn by persons with epilepsy and with allergies to certain drugs.

REVIEW

1. List five signs or symptoms of diabetes.

2. What three treatments are used to control diabetes?

3. Explain the steps involved in testing a client's blood for a blood sugar reading. When is the reading abnormal?

4. What are the symptoms of insulin shock? What is the immediate care given?

5. What are the signs and symptoms of acidosis? What should the aide do if these symptoms appear in the client?

6. Why is good foot care important when caring for a client with diabetes?

7. Why is it important to have a client with diabetes exercise on a routine basis?

8. List three complications of diabetes.

9. Name two signs/symptoms of high blood sugar and two of low blood sugar that a home health aide may observe in a diabetic client.

10. All the following are true statements regarding foot care for the diabetic client except:
    a. Toenails should be cut frequently by the home health aide.
    b. Feet should be soaked in warm water daily.
    c. Have client wear shoes.
    d. Feet should be rubbed with lotion to keep skin in good condition.

11. Which of the following is not a common complication of diabetes?
    a. Blindness
    b. Vascular diseases
    c. High risk of infections
    d. Loss of memory

12. Diabetes can be treated by:
    a. Special diet
    b. Oral medication
    c. Insulin injections
    d. All are correct

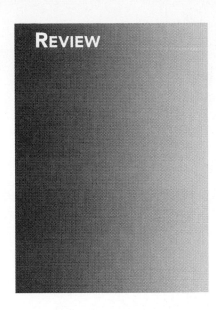

REVIEW

13. In a client with diabetes the ___ is not producing adequate amount of a hormone called insulin.
    a. Thyroid
    b. Pancreas
    c. Adrenal gland
    d. Liver

14. You are with your client, Mrs. Jones, who is a known diabetic. You notice that she is increasingly confused and is somewhat shaky. She is also perspiring. Is this a life-threatening situation? What would you do to assist Mrs. Jones?

15. Mr. Smith is complaining to you about blurred vision. In addition, he is always thirsty and needing to use the bathroom. What would you suspect is causing these problems for Mr. Smith? What steps would you take to make sure Mr. Smith gets the proper medical help?

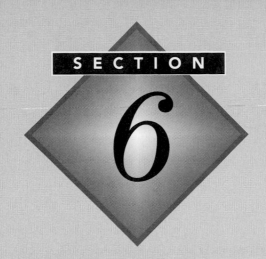

SECTION 6

Clients Requiring Special Care

Units

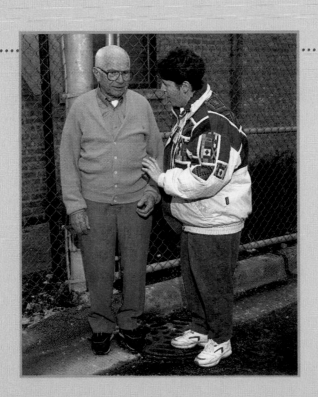

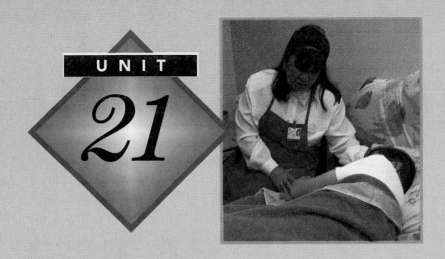

UNIT 21

Caring for the Client Who Is Terminally Ill

KEY TERMS

advance directives
autopsy
durable power of attorney
embalming

grieving
hospice
living will

Patient Self-Determination
  Act
terminal

LEARNING OBJECTIVES

After studying this unit, you should be able to:

- Identify some cultural influences surrounding practices related to death.
- Identify the five stages of dying described by Dr. Kübler-Ross.
- Identify the home health aide's responsibilities when the client dies.
- Identify ways in which a person may react to the death of a family member or friend.

- Become familiar with the needs of a dying client.
- Explain the Patient Self-Determination Act.
- Explain the purpose of hospice programs.
- Explain the importance of grieving.
- Understand different reactions to dying.

Most people in our society feel uncomfortable talking or thinking about death. This is more true today than in earlier times in history. Gathering in the room of a dying relative was a custom practiced no more than 40 years ago. Death was accepted as the natural end to life. Children openly shared the final moments of life with a dying grandparent, parent, or sibling.

This is the first time in society that three or four generations of one family are living at the same time. Death experiences in some families have been rare. For many individuals, death is extremely difficult to deal with. In the 1980s, 80% of deaths occurred in the hospital setting and few people assisted their loved ones in their last days. In recent years there has been a reversal of the trend of transferring a loved one to the hospital to die. Families are now allowing their loved ones to die in their own home in a familiar environment. This is due primarily to the expansion of the **hospice** program.

A hospice program provides care for dying persons and their families. Some hospices are small, independent programs offering services in the client's home; others are part of a hospital or health care facility. Often, hospice care is begun in the client's home. In some cases, when the client becomes very ill, he or she may continue to receive care in a hospice facility, ideally with the same caregivers. The hospice movement began in Europe, but has recently expanded in this country.

Hospice offers a combination of physical and emotional care that involves not only the client, but also friends, family, volunteers, and home health aides. The criterion to enter a hospice program is that the client's life expectancy is less than 6 months due to a terminal illness. The client is in the **terminal** stage (final stage) of a fatal illness. The goal of hospice is to control uncomfortable symptoms such as nausea and make the client as comfortable and pain free as possible (Figure 21-1). The primary concern of hospice is quality of life and not prolonging the client's life.

ADVANCE DIRECTIVES

Medical science has made treatments more available and more effective. Because of these

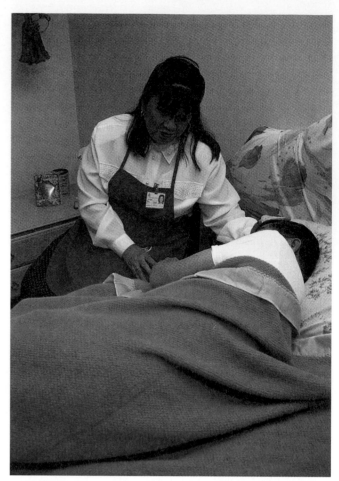

FIGURE 21-1 A hospice worker comforts a dying client.

and other changes, people can expect to live for many years. Diseases once incurable have been conquered. New medicines and surgical techniques have been developed that save thousands of lives daily. Most of these medical advances improve the quality of life. However, some of the medical advances prolong life but do not always improve the quality of life. The value of life support systems is being questioned today. At times a client is kept alive by machines but has no awareness of being alive. These machines take over the vital functions for the client (Figure 21-2). Because of problems with the making of decisions regarding use of life support machines and other life-prolonging measures, in 1991 the **Patient Self-Determination Act** was passed. This law requires home health agencies receiving Medicare and Medicaid to implement procedures to increase public awareness regarding the rights of clients to make choices. The law is concerned primarily

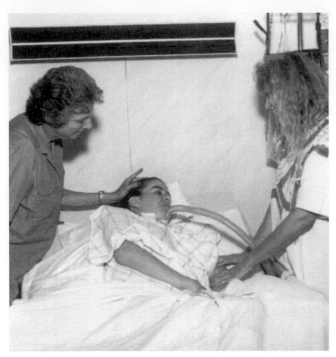

FIGURE 21-2   Sometimes machines take over the vital functions for a person.

with **advance directives,** papers that specify the type of treatment clients want or do not want under serious medical conditions in which they may be unable to communicate their wishes to the doctor or family.

Advance directives can be done by a **living will** or by **durable power of attorney.** Before you start caring for a client, the decision may already have been made by the client what he or she wants done when seriously ill. One of these forms has probably been completed already by the client. Your case manager will inform you of your client's wishes. You may have two clients with the same serious illness; one client may have mechanical life support and the other one only pain medication to keep him or her comfortable. The doctors are just following the client's wishes. This eases the burden on the family and also the doctor in making the decision to use or not use mechanical life support.

Changing attitudes toward death have appeared partly as a result of increased life expectancy. People seem to fear death as never before. They want to hold on to life and try not to think about death. Children are sometimes protected from the facts of death. When a beloved grandparent dies, children may be told that the grandparent has gone away. Because families

are often separated by great distances, some children believe that their grandparents have just moved. How a family deals with death is a personal matter. A home health aide must respect the wishes of the family in dealing with the death of a family member. The aide must be aware of the needs of the dying person and the family.

STAGES OF ADJUSTMENT TO DYING AND DEATH

Dr. Elisabeth Kübler-Ross has made careful studies of dying persons and their families. She has described a general pattern common to persons facing death. The pattern may apply to both the dying person and the person's family. Dr. Kübler-Ross has noted five stages of psychological adjustment to death.

1. Denial—This can't be happening to me; perhaps someone else, but not me.
2. Anger—An extension of denial; feeling that this death is unfair; bitterness and loss of faith; fighting against death or loss of a loved one.
3. Bargaining—"I promise to live a better life if I can just get better now."
4. Depression—Brooding, withdrawal, lack of communication; thoughts of suicide–"I'd rather kill myself than die from this disease" or, "I can't go on living if Mama dies."
5. Acceptance—Calmly facing what is to be or feeling a sense of peace; looking forward to release from pain and sorrow; hoping for the release of a loved one to a better world.

Home health aides who are in an environment of expected death may see these patterns develop or may find themselves experiencing these stages. The aide should not offer advice to the family or client. The aide should be understanding, kind, and empathetic. By knowing what to expect in the way of reactions, the home health aide is better prepared to adjust to the situation.

Sometimes a client may die suddenly and unexpectedly. Other times death is preceded by a long illness. Some people are relieved that life is ending. Some clients become unconscious just before death. Of the five senses (hearing, taste, touch, sight, smell), the last to be lost is hearing. For this reason when working with an unconscious client, the home health aide should be careful what is said in the client's presence. It would be cruel if the last words a client heard were, "Well, she's almost gone; she'll be dead by morning." The home health aide's first duty is to keep the client clean and as comfortable as possible. The client should be treated with kindness and dignity at all times. In addition, the aide should provide emotional support to the client and the family. Good communication skills are needed when dealing with the dying client and the family.

Signs of Approaching Death

Certain signs indicate that death is approaching. A person does not necessarily go through these stages in order; they may skip a stage and return to it later, or not return to it at all. These signs are:

- Noisy, labored, irregular respirations
- Irregular and weak pulse
- Cool, moist, and clammy skin
- Incontinence (bowel and bladder)
- Body muscle relaxation, open jaw
- Diminished sense of pain

When death occurs, family members may be highly emotional. The home health aide must remain calm because many details must be taken care of. Death is a legal event that calls for certain formalities. Before a funeral can take place, a physician must complete a death certificate that states the cause of death, and formally register the death. In some cases, a death may have to be investigated by a medical examiner or a coroner, and an **autopsy** (a detailed examination of the body to determine the exact cause of death) may be ordered. An autopsy provides more information about the person's illness and may either be requested by the family or required by law in the event of an unexpected or unexplained death. Funeral directors can be helpful in making these arrangements and will come to the home or hospital to remove the body and take it to the funeral home. Figure 21-3 lists the duties of a home health aide when the client dies. A home health aide may be asked to remain on duty to help the family prepare for the funeral.

FIGURE 21-3   What to do when a client dies

Postmortem Care

1. Call the case manager at once. A death certificate must be filed by a physician. Write down the time of death.
2. Do not touch the client until the case manager tells you to.
3. Call a family member after the doctor has been notified of the death.
4. Follow the case manager's instructions and clean the client's body. At death, all body functions stop.

RELIGIOUS AND CULTURAL INFLUENCES

Cultural and family differences will influence the death and dying process, including the public behavior of grieving. For example, Native Americans and Inuit people followed customs that today may be thought of as uncivilized. The aged, ill members of Inuit tribes were taken to an iceberg and left alone with a small amount of food. This was the accepted way to die. In certain Native American tribes, people who were ill and unable to do their share of work were taken to an isolated spot to await death. These customs were accepted as a natural and respectable way for life to end. Native Americans felt that it was good to allow life to end naturally. When human power to cure with herbs and medicines was not effective, it was time for death to come.

Among some Jewish families, burial occurs within 24 hours after death. Jewish religious practice forbids **embalming** (treating the body with preservatives to prevent decay) the body and requires that the casket remain closed. After the funeral the family may have a period of formal mourning. During this time, friends and relatives come to the home to comfort each other.

In other Jewish families and in Catholic or Protestant families, the body is usually taken to a funeral home. Friends and family meet at the funeral home during the 2 or 3 days before the body is buried.

Religious practices differ from one group to another and even from family to family. Most people do recognize the need for sharing grief.

This is part of the final acceptance of death. Some people weep, others are angry. Some are very quiet. As people work through their emotions, they come to accept the loss. Many believe that the death of an older person is less tragic than the death of a younger person. A death that is sudden is more difficult to accept than one following a long, painful illness. Mixed emotions may be felt by families when a client dies after a long illness. On the one hand, families are glad that their loved one is no longer suffering, yet on the other hand, their loved one will be missed.

The **grieving** process is the physical and emotional response to a loss, and the process of accepting it. The grief process can take a long time, and it is hard work. It can take from several months to a year to readjust to the loss of a loved one. Often, the first several months are the most difficult. Grief is a private journey that is different for everyone, influenced by cultural and family differences. Although life is never the same when a loved one dies, not all the changes experienced after a death are negative. Often a person grows in new ways, developing new coping styles, and becoming introspective, questioning values and life-styles. Grieving can help a person discover inner strength and resiliency, emerging as a more caring and compassionate person. Although all people cope with grief in different ways, grief needs to be expressed, or processed, so it can be healed. If grief is not expressed, symptoms of erratic behavior or failing health may appear. Today there are special support groups for individuals to assist them in the grieving process. Your agency's social worker can help you find support groups in your area.

REVIEW

1. List the five stages of psychological adjustment to death.

2. What should the home health aide do if the client dies while the aide is on duty?

3. List three cultural influences surrounding death and dying.

4. List three ways in which a person may react to the death of a family member or friend.

5. List two goals of the hospice organization.

6. Explain what the grieving process is.

7. Describe two ways a home health aide can comfort a dying client.

8. List four signs of approaching death.

9. T   F   Two examples of advance directives are durable power of attorney and living will.

10. During which of the five stages of dying would a client most likely say, "If only I could live to see my oldest daughter get married"?
     a. Denial
     b. Anger
     c. Bargaining
     d. Acceptance

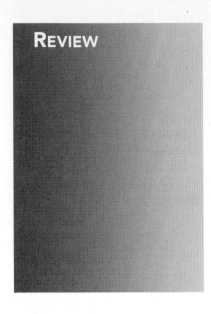

REVIEW

11. When a client is dying and a family member is always present, one important thing that the home health aide can do is to:
    a. Tell the family member all the details about the client's illness.
    b. Ask the family member questions on how the illness started in the client.
    c. Try to cheer the family member up by talking about current events in your life.
    d. Provide emotional support for the family and not offer any advice.

12. You are caring for Mr. B when he dies. His wife is very quiet and does not seem to show any emotion. What can you do for her?

13. Two weeks after Mr. B's death, Mrs. B calls you, saying that she does not know how she can cope with her husband's death. What kind of assistance can you provide for her?

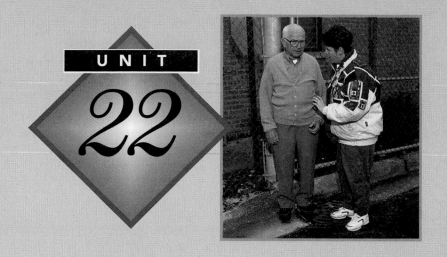

Caring for the Client With Alzheimer's Disease

KEY TERMS

Alzheimer's disease
dementia
disruptive behaviors

reality orientation
reminiscence

validation therapy
wandering

LEARNING OBJECTIVES

After studying this unit, you should be able to:

- Describe five symptoms of Alzheimer's disease.
- Understand the 10 warning signs of Alzheimer's disease.
- Name at least five interventions to take to promote the safety of a client who wanders.
- Describe several causes of wandering and disruptive behaviors.

- Describe validation therapy, reminiscence, and reality orientation and their value with the Alzheimer's client.
- List 10 tips for communicating with the client who has Alzheimer's disease.

ALZHEIMER'S DISEASE

An illness that has received much publicity in the past few years is **Alzheimer's disease,** a progressive, degenerative disease that attacks the brain and results in impaired thinking, memory, and behavior. It affects an estimated 4.4 million American adults. It is the fourth leading cause of death among the adult population. Men and women are affected almost equally. There is no known cause for this debilitating illness, characterized by loss of memory and diminished mental capacity. The only identified risk factors for Alzheimer's disease are age and family history. Most people experience Alzheimer's after age 65. However, people in their forties and fifties have also been diagnosed with the disease. Symptoms include gradual memory loss, decline in the ability to perform routine tasks, disorientation, personality changes, difficulty in learning, loss of language skills, and impairment of judgment and planning. Figure 22-1 identifies the 10 warning signs of Alzheimer's disease. The rate of change varies from person to person. The time from onset of symptoms until death can range from 3 to 20 years. In the severe, advanced stage of the disease, people are totally incapable of caring for themselves.

When it was first described by Dr. Alois Alzheimer in 1907, it was considered a rare disease. Today, it is the most common form of **dementia** (progressive mental deterioration). No single clinical test can identify Alzheimer's disease. A comprehensive evaluation to establish diagnosis will include a complete health history, physical examination, neurologic and mental status assessments, and other diagnostic tests. In addition, documenting symptoms and behavioral incidents over time, in a diary fashion, will assist a physician in making a probable diagnosis. Although these evaluations may provide a clinical diagnosis, confirmation of Alzheimer's disease requires examination of brain tissue, which is done by an autopsy, after death.

CARING FOR A CLIENT WITH ALZHEIMER'S DISEASE

Taking care of a person with Alzheimer's disease is difficult and requires a great deal of patience, empathy, and understanding of the disease process.

The majority of clients with dementia you will be caring for in the home will be moderately impaired. The following list will give you hints on how to care for them. Please remember that every client is unique and the following are only general suggestions on how to manage their care.

1. Do not argue with or confront a client.
2. Promote frequent periods of rest.
3. Do not restrain client unless absolutely necessary.
4. Limit client's intake of liquids that contain caffeine.
5. Play music for the client rather than have client watch television.
6. Provide a quiet, calming environment.
7. Serve meals at the same time every day. If restlessness makes it difficult for the client to stay seated for meals, offer finger foods or sandwiches, which allow the client to eat while moving around.
8. Do not try to reason with the client.
9. If client becomes upset over something, try to distract with something else.
10. Let client wander in a safe area.
11. Maintain eye contact with client.
12. Demonstrate how to do a task before having the client do it.
13. Give very short simple instructions to client.
14. Limit outings to small groups of people. Avoid large crowds.
15. Involve client in activities that are simple— looking through a scrapbook or a magazine, walking, dancing, gardening, or performing familiar household tasks.
16. Keep the environment as unchanging as possible.
17. Take client to bathroom at frequent intervals.

There are support groups in many communities. Family members can meet to share common problems and learn more about how to cope with their parent or relative as well as face up to their own feelings and fears. The Alzheimer's Association can link families with resources in their community to help them cope with this disease. The national toll-free number to the Alzheimer's Association is 1-800-272-3900.

FIGURE 22-1   The 10 warning signs of Alzheimer's disease

TEN WARNING SIGNS OF ALZHEIMER'S DISEASE

To help you know what warning signs to look for, the Alzheimer's Association has developed a checklist of common symptoms (some of them also may apply to other dementing illnesses). Review the list and check the symptoms that concern you. If you notice several symptoms, the individual with the symptoms should see a physician for a complete examination.

1. **Memory Loss That Affects Job Skills**
   It's normal to occasionally forget assignments, colleagues' names, or a business associate's telephone number and remember them later. Those with a dementia, such as Alzheimer's disease, may forget things more often, and not remember them later.

2. **Difficulty Performing Familiar Tasks**
   Busy people can be so distracted from time to time that they may leave the carrots on the stove and only remember to serve them at the end of the meal. People with Alzheimer's disease could prepare a meal and not only forget to serve it, but also forget they made it.

3. **Problems With Language**
   Everyone has trouble finding the right word sometimes, but a person with Alzheimer's disease may forget simple words or substitute inappropriate words, making his or her sentence incomprehensible.

4. **Disorientation Of Time And Place**
   It's normal to forget the day of the week or your destination for a moment. But people with Alzheimer's disease can become lost on their own street, not knowing where they are, how they got there or how to get back home.

5. **Poor Or Decreased Judgment**
   People can become so immersed in an activity that they temporarily forget the child they're watching. People with Alzheimer's disease could forget entirely the child under their care. They may also dress inappropriately, wearing several shirts or blouses.

6. **Problems With Abstract Thinking**
   Balancing a checkbook may be disconcerting when the task is more complicated than usual. Someone with Alzheimer's disease could forget completely what the numbers are and what needs to be done with them.

7. **Misplacing Things**
   Anyone can temporarily misplace a wallet or keys. A person with Alzheimer's disease may put things in inappropriate places: an iron in the freezer, or a wristwatch in the sugar bowl.

8. **Changes In Mood Or Behavior**
   Everyone becomes sad or moody from time to time. Someone with Alzheimer's disease can exhibit rapid mood swings—from calm to tears to anger—for no apparent reason.

9. **Changes In Personality**
   People's personalities ordinarily change somewhat with age. But a person with Alzheimer's disease can change drastically, becoming extremely confused, suspicious, or fearful.

10. **Loss Of Initiative**
    It's normal to tire of housework, business activities, or social obligations, but most people regain their initiative. The person with Alzheimer's disease may become very passive and require cues and prompting to become involved.

(Courtesy of The Alzheimer's Association)

In some areas there are special day-care centers where Alzheimer's disease clients can be taken for a few hours a day. These centers provide supervision, and clients will often enjoy talking, playing cards, playing the piano, or singing with others. Because the progression of the disease varies, clients may have "good" days or weeks when they function reasonably well at such centers. On the other hand, if the group activities have a negative effect on the client and make the person more agitated or fearful, the activity should be stopped immediately.

The home health aide helps the family members by providing respite care. That is, while the home health aide provides care, the family may take advantage of these few hours to take care of errands or just experience freedom from caregiving responsibilities.

Keeping the home environment safe is an important role for the home health aide, especially when working with a client who suffers from memory problems or who may wander away. The aide should look for safety hazards in the home and remove them. If your client smokes, urge the family to keep all smoking materials away from the client, who may forget and leave a lit cigarette unattended. If possible, restrict access into the kitchen where there are likely to be many opportunities for danger. Remove knobs from the stove, and disconnect appliances that are not in use. Be sure that all poisons, cleaning products, and medications are kept in a locked cabinet. Potential falls can be avoided by eliminating throw rugs and clutter on stairs and floors. Lighting should be improved if an area is particularly dark or full of glare. It is important for clients to maintain independence as much as possible. Belt restraints should not be ordered for a person who has had a few falls but continues to walk independently.

Figure 22-2 provides many helpful tips for the home health aide working with the Alzheimer's client.

FIGURE 22-2 Guidelines for working with the Alzheimer's disease client (up to terminal stage)

ALZHEIMER'S DISEASE

Client	HHHA Actions/Responsibilities
Has difficulty communicating . . .	• Approach the client with a friendly facial expression. • Be calm. • Stand in front of the client. • Try to maintain eye contact; touch the client to attract attention or regain it. • Speak in a low, calm, reassuring tone of voice (if the client has a hearing problem, follow the instructions in the care plan). • Speak slowly and give the client time to answer. • If necessary, repeat the statement or question—do not change the wording. • Keep the language simple and express only one idea at a time. • Lead the client in answering if he cannot find the right words—point to objects to provide cues. • Do not become impatient.
Has difficulty walking . . .	• Provide a safe environment: —Remove scatter rugs. —Do not wax floors. —Pick up and put away objects the client may not see and thus trip over such as small footstools, doorstops, plants, pet toys, and dishes.

(continues)

FIGURE 22-2 *(continued)*

Client	HHHA Actions/Responsibilities
	—The client is to use only chairs with arms for support. • Show the client what you want him or her to do and provide support. • Do not hurry the client. • If the client is unsteady and is using an aid (cane, walker) do not let the client out of your sight. • Be sure the client's shoes fit properly. • Always use proper body mechanics when helping the client. • Keep the client walking as long as possible (as the disease progresses).
Experiences changes in eating patterns . . .	• Meals must be served at the same time each day. • Meals should look appetizing and be served at the proper temperature. • Give the client one course and one utensil at a time; do not give the client a choice of foods. • If the client must be fed, do so slowly and cut the food into small pieces. • Nutritious snacks should be kept on hand. • Always encourage fluids. • As the client loses the ability to chew, soft foods are introduced; a blender can be used to liquefy foods. • As the client loses the ability to use utensils, finger foods can be used. • Maintain the diet plan included in the overall care plan. • Weigh the client regularly (at least once weekly) and record the weight.
Tends to wander . . .	• Be sure the client wears an ID bracelet or necklace. • Sew labels to each piece of clothing—labels should have the name of the client, address, and telephone number. • Keep doors locked; make sure the bell or chimes are in working order. • Place large print signs on doors—"DO NOT GO OUT," "TURN AROUND." • If the client insists on going out, do not argue—go with him (lock the door and take keys). • After a few minutes, suggest returning to the house to rest. • Try to distract the client from leaving—try another activity you know the client enjoys (Alzheimer's disease clients often respond to music). • Keep a recent photograph of the client at hand in the event the client does wander off and is not in the immediate neighborhood. • If the client does leave unnoticed and you cannot find him—call family members, police, and your agency.
Experiences incontinence . . .	• Remember that the client cannot control this behavior. • Do not scold or punish the client. • Treat the client with respect. • Set up a regular schedule for toileting and follow it. • Encourage fluids as usual to prevent dehydration. • Mark the bathroom clearly with a large print sign and a picture. • Keep the client clean and dry; use simple washable clothing. • Recognize the client's verbal and nonverbal language. • Check the skin regularly for signs of irritation.

(continues)

FIGURE 22-2 *(continued)*

Client	HHHA Actions/Responsibilities
Exhibits restlessness and agitation in late afternoon (sundown syndrome) . . .	• Decrease the level of activity in late afternoon to reduce potential stress. • Play soft, soothing music. • Do not try to reason the client out of this behavior—the client has no control over his or her actions. • Do not institute sudden changes into the routine that will confuse and upset the client. • Appointments and trips should be scheduled for morning and early afternoon. • Do not restrain or argue with the client. • Try to distract the client with quiet, simple activities. • Make sure the client has adequate exercise during the day.
Experiences sleeping disturbances . . .	• The client may exhibit less need for sleep. • Try to keep the client active during the day so he or she will feel the need for sleep. • The client should drink caffeine-free beverages. • Establish a bedtime routine and follow it. • Make sure the client is toileted before going to bed. • Make sure there are no loud noises; soft music may help. • The client may feel more secure with a night-light. • Keep a night-light on in the bathroom and keep the door open.
Needs help with bathing and oral hygiene . . .	• Permit the client to do as much as he or she can—suggest steps if necessary. • Ensure the client's safety when bathing—use hand holds, nonslip mats, tub seats, etc. • Organize all the necessary equipment before you bring the client to the bathroom. • Stay calm and pleasant; try to make this a pleasurable experience for the client. • Do not leave the client alone when bathing. • Schedule bathing when the client is least agitated. • Do not force the client into bathing; wait until the client is calm and try again. • Give the client a sponge bath if all attempts to tub bathe or shower fail. • Cleanliness must be maintained—consult with your supervisor if the client continues to exhibit resistance to bathing. • If the client cannot provide oral care, even with coaxing, brush his or her teeth yourself or clean the dentures.
Experiences delusions, hallucinations and inappropriate catastrophic) reactions to normal events . . .	• What the client sees or hears is real to him. • Do not argue or reason with the client. • Maintain a calm, ordered environment. • Reassure the client that you are there to protect him. • If the client becomes violent, stay out of his or her way. • If the client becomes agitated, try to distract him or her with an activity you know he or she likes; a small snack of a favorite food may distract him or her sufficiently to restore calm. • If the client attacks you verbally, do not take it personally. • The client may accuse you of stealing; again, do not take it personally.

(continues)

FIGURE 22-2   *(continued)*

Client	HHHA Actions/Responsibilities
Exhibits improper sexual behavior . . .	• Remember, the client is confused and disoriented. • Do not overreact—remain calm. • Do not scold or argue with the client. • Do not try to reason with the client. • If the client undresses, provide a robe or redress him or her. • If the client is in public when inappropriate behavior takes place, distract the client and remove him or her from the scene. • Plan ahead ways you can distract the client. • Provide appropriate touching to show that you care for and value the client.

(Adapted from "How to Care for the Alzheimer's Disease Patient: A Comprehensive Training Manual for Homemaker-Home Health Aides" Copyright 1986 by the Foundation for Hospice and Homecare)

BEHAVIORAL CONSIDERATIONS

An Alzheimer's patient who is confused, frightened, or in pain might demonstrate behavior that would be troublesome. If possible, the aide should identify and remove the cause of problem behavior. Sometimes when behavior management does not work, a physician may order medication or physical restraints to control the problem behavior. Almost all medications have some side effects. Occasionally the side effects may be worse than the behavior itself. Therefore, if a client is put on medication, the time, dose, and side effects of the drugs should be closely monitored. Physicians should be notified of any adverse reactions.

Wandering

Wandering is the most common agitated behavior among people with Alzheimer's disease. Frustration, fear, confusion, fatigue, and discomfort of the client can increase wandering. Often, the client is looking for something, for example, the bathroom, food or drink, a remedy for pain and suffering, a place to lie down, or a familiar face. Other times the client may wander because he or she is playing out an old routine, such as leaving work for home or going to get a loved one. At times a client wanders to escape a task or activity or to avoid noise or tension. A safe wandering area should be provided for clients to move about freely without risk of injury (Figure 22-3). Simplify the environment to minimize confusion or distraction. Avoid the use of child-gates because the client may climb over them or kick them down. If possible, walk with the client when he or she begins to wander, gently redirecting the client back home or to a task or activity. In fact, it may be helpful to schedule regular times for walks in or outside the home.

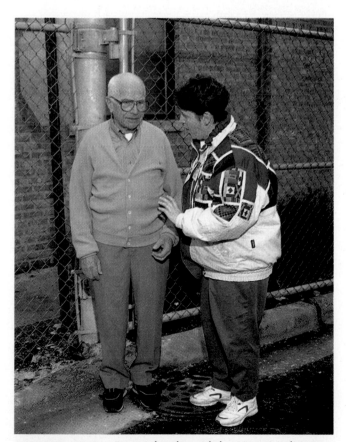

FIGURE 22-3   Provide the Alzheimer's client with a safe area to wander.

Disruptive Behaviors

Sometimes a person with Alzheimer's disease will display **disruptive behaviors,** including screaming, cursing, threatening, hitting, or biting. The causes for this behavior can relate to any number of physical, psychological, or environmental factors including fear, anger, hunger, the need for attention, or feelings of powerlessness or despair. It will be important to note what appears to trigger these behaviors and to take steps to involve the client in situations that are less likely to lead to disruptive behaviors. To interrupt the behavior, try to gain the person's attention in a calm and nonjudgmental manner. Ask the person the reason for the behavior, and listen carefully to what the client says both verbally and nonverbally. Respond to the client's requests promptly so that the behavior does not escalate. Encourage alternative expressions of anger and frustration. Often the family or other caregivers will be able to give you successful approaches they have used to diminish these types of behaviors.

INTERVENTIONS

At the present time there is no cure for Alzheimer's disease. However, good planning, medical care, and a well-structured environment can ease the burden to the client and family. For example, it is a good idea to consider health directives for the Alzheimer's client in the early stages of the disease, while the client still has the mental capacity to make choices. Physical exercise and good nutrition will help maintain the client's health. A physician can determine if medications can be helpful in managing some behaviors. A calm and well-structured environment may help the client continue functioning. As long as the client continues to understand words, it may be helpful to use reminders such as signs, labels, clocks, calendars, and family pictures to orient the client to the present.

Validation Therapy

Validation therapy is a communication technique that is used for moderately to severely disoriented clients with diagnosed dementia.

The goal of this therapy is to increase self-esteem and validate the client's feelings. The basic premise is that if the client wishes to remain in the past, that should be allowed and no attempt should be made to reorient the client. An example of this type of communication technique is: An 80-year-old client with Alzheimer's disease, is telling you (after her bath and shampoo) not to set her hair because her mother will be coming to do it. You know her mother died 20 years ago. Instead of telling her that her mother is dead, which might make her feel bad, the aide asks the client something about her mother such as her mother's name or her mother's hobbies. This will help relay a message to the client that you are concerned with her wishes and will make her feel good about herself. Once clients have Alzheimer's or another type of dementia, the ability to reason with them has diminished. Often, if you try to reason with them, they become more agitated and combative. Figure 22-4 identifies some useful techniques for communicating with a person with dementia.

Reminiscence

From the time of diagnosis until the end of life, the clients with Alzheimer's disease and their families are victims, suffering from pressures and strains of this disease. These clients have poor short-term memory, but long-term and deep-seated memories may remain. These memories, whether pleasurable or sad, can be recalled by reviewing past life history. **Reminiscence** helps the person with Alzheimer's experience being cared for with compassion.

Family involvement can be an important part of this therapy. This time for reclaiming the past creates connectedness. The present moment of a relationship increases family and client satisfaction. Sharing of information might be done by reviewing the old movies, videotapes, pictures, songs, popular radio programs, or even using scrapbooks in which to write and draw. See Unit 8 for more reminiscence techniques.

Reality Orientation

For those clients with mild to moderate memory loss, and particularly for those who continue to understand words, it may be helpful to provide simple memory aids to assist the client in day-to-day living. For example, a prominent calendar,

---

FIGURE 22-4 Tips for communicating with a person with dementia

1. Make sure you have your client's attention *before* you begin to speak: make sure that she can see and hear you, and that she knows that you are talking to her.
2. Face your client when you speak to her, and speak slowly and clearly.
3. Do not talk too much! Give one instruction at a time.
4. Speak in positives instead of in negatives. Your client will respond better to, "Come with me," than she will to "Come away from there!"
5. Listen carefully to what your client is saying. She may be telling you something important.
6. Respond to your client's feelings, not just to her words.
7. For clients with severe memory loss, focus on validation, not on reality orientation.
8. Be aware of body language—yours and your client's.
9. If your client is frustrated by not being able to make you understand her, then reassure her that you still care about what she feels: "I'm sorry I can't understand what you are saying. Why don't you wait a while and try to tell me later?" Then, move on to another activity.
10. *Never* ask, "Do you remember . . .?" It may embarrass your client if she can't remember. Instead, tell your client what you want her to remember: "We went to your doctor's office on Tuesday, and he said that you need to drink more water."

---

lists of daily tasks, written reminders, signs, labels, clocks, and even family pictures can help to orient the client to the present. This process of orienting the person to the present moment is known as **reality orientation.** This technique would not be appropriate, however, for someone with a more severe memory loss and may cause frustration, agitation, and loss of self-esteem. The home health aide must use imagination, patience, kindness, and understanding to give the Alzheimer's client the service and care that best meets the individual's needs.

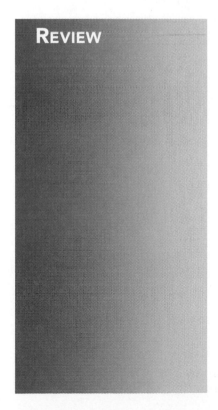

REVIEW

1. T F Occasional forgetfulness is a sign of having Alzheimer's disease.
2. T F Alzheimer's disease affects memory, personality, behavior, communication, and the ability to perform routine tasks.
3. T F A belt restraint should be ordered for a person who had a few falls but continues to walk independently.
4. Name the 10 warning signs of Alzheimer's disease.
5. Choose the best statement:
   a. Alzheimer's disease is a hereditary disease and results in irregular involuntary movements of extremities.
   b. Alzheimer's disease is caused by a lack of dopamine, which is the neurotransmitter substance in the central nervous system.
   c. Alzheimer's disease is a progressive, irreversible disease that gradually affects cognitive intelligence, memory, and functional abilities.
   d. Alzheimer's disease is caused by an obstruction in the normal flow of spinal fluid, which in turn causes fluid accumulation in the brain.

REVIEW

6. The primary reasons for wandering are:
   a. Looking for food or drink
   b. Looking for a familiar place
   c. Trying to escape a task or an activity
   d. All of the above

7. Alzheimer's disease affects an estimated _____ American adults.

8. _____ is a communication technique that is helpful with clients who are moderately to severely disoriented with diagnosed dementia.

9. A useful tool to increase the self-esteem of dementia clients by sharing past events is called _____ .

10. A strategy used to orient a client to the present, which is useful only if the client continues to understand words, is called _____ .

11. You are assigned to a new client, Mrs. Stone, who has a moderately severe case of Alzheimer's disease. What safety recommendations could you make to the family that ensure a safe environment for your client?

12. You are taking care of a client with Alzheimer's disease. During the middle of the night, he wakes up and wants to leave the house. What steps could you take to help your client and redirect him back to his bed?

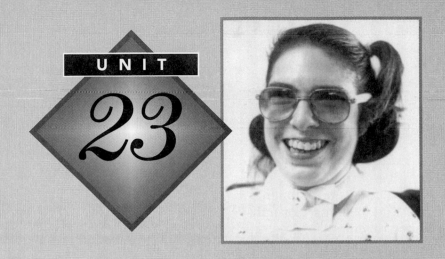

UNIT 23

Caring for the Client With Cancer

KEY TERMS

articulates
benign
biopsy
cancer
carcinogen
chemotherapy
colostomy
expectorate
hysterectomy

ileostomy
irrigation
laryngectomy
larynx
lobectomy
lumpectomy
malignant
mammogram
mastectomy

metastasis
pneumonectomy
prosthesis
remission
stoma
trachea
tracheostomy

LEARNING OBJECTIVES

After studying this unit, you should be able to:

- Identify three diagnostic tests for cancer.
- Identify six surgical procedures used in cancer treatment.
- List seven warning signs of cancer.
- Define metastasis, benign tumor, remission, and malignant.

- Name three types of treatment for cancer.
- Describe the care given to a client with cancer.
- List two precautions for an aide to take when caring for a client who is on chemotherapy.
- List side effects commonly demonstrated by clients receiving cancer treatments.

CANCER

Cancer is the uncontrolled growth of abnormal cells. In healthy tissue, body cells grow, die, and are replaced by new cells. This is a normal process that goes on day after day. Sometimes cells do not follow the rules of the body; they begin to divide quickly, stealing nourishment from surrounding cells, and pushing normal cells out of the way. They prevent normal cells from doing their regular jobs. Finally, these cells cause changes in the body, which produce signs and indicate something is wrong. Any one of the warning signs listed in Figure 23-1 should be called to the supervisor's attention as soon as possible.

The exact cause of cancer is unknown. However, studies are beginning to determine some factors that lead to the formation of cancer cells. A substance or agent that produces cancer is called a **carcinogen.** The general group of carcinogens are chemicals, environmental factors, hormones, and viruses. A chemical could be ingested with food such as red dye #2. The chemical could be inhaled as tar or asbestos. Environmental factors include such physical agents as x-rays, sunlight, or trauma. Hormones may be cancer causing because of their excess, deficiency, or imbalance. Viruses seem to upset the functions within a cell.

The way that carcinogens change normal cells into cancer cells is unclear. Therefore, a cure is not yet possible. Most physicians agree, however, that the sooner cancer is detected, the less chance it has of spreading to other parts of the body. Some tumors may interfere with body functions and require surgical removal, but they do not spread to other parts of the body. These are known as **benign** tumors. **Malignant** or cancerous tumors not only invade or destroy normal tissues, but the cells break away from the original tumor and move to other parts of the body by a process known as **metastasis** (Figure 23-2A and B). There they may form other tumors. (A cancer originating in the brain, for example, can spread or metastasize to the lungs, kidneys, or other parts of the body.) When cancer is treated early and does not reappear for 5 years, the cancer is considered to be cured or in remission. **Remission** means no longer growing or spreading.

It has been estimated that in the United States alone more than 1,400 people a day die from some form of cancer. Since 1949, there has been a sharp rise in the number of men who develop cancer. Cancer of the lung has risen sharply in women also. Cancer of the breast, colon, and rectum occur most often among women. There are more than 100 types of can-

FIGURE 23-1   Warning signs of cancer
Warning Signals
1. Unusual bleeding or body discharge
2. A lump or thickening in an area of the body
3. A sore that does not heal
4. A change in bowel or bladder habits
5. Hoarseness or a chronic cough
6. Indigestion or difficulty in swallowing
7. A change in size, shape, or appearance of a wart or mole

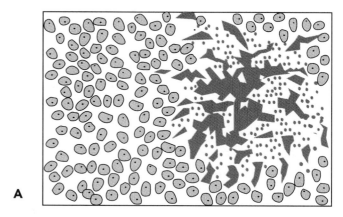

A

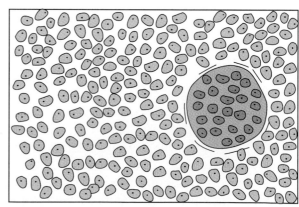

B

FIGURE 23-2 Growth of cancer cells. A. Malignant cancer growth (no capsule with random growth). B. Benign tumor growth (with capsule around it).

cer. Cancer is second only to heart disease as the leading cause of death each year. However, statistics also show that deaths due to cancer are increasing, whereas those due to heart conditions are decreasing. Research continues into the causes and possible cures for cancer.

CANCER TREATMENTS

Several kinds of treatments may slow or stop the growth of cancer cells. Surgery is used to remove tumors and organs of the body that have become cancerous. Sometimes surgical procedures alone are used. At other times, radiation therapy may be used after surgery to kill any cancer cells around the surgical area. Radiation therapy is sometimes the only treatment used. The rays are aimed deep in the body to reach cells that cannot be removed surgically. Often, however, surrounding normal cells are destroyed in the rays. The site of the therapy is marked in ink on the body. The home health aide must be careful not to remove these marks when bathing the client. The marked area should not be touched by the home health aide. Side effects of radiation therapy may include nausea, skin damage, itching of the area, and loss of hair.

Chemotherapy is the use of one or a combination of drugs to attack cancer cells. Chemotherapy may be used after surgery or in combination with radiation therapy. In some cases chemotherapy works only for a short time, after which it no longer kills cancer cells. New combinations of chemicals are then prescribed. This treatment, too, can cause unpleasant side effects. All of the cancer treatments cause damage to healthy cells around the cancer site. If you are caring for a client who is undergoing chemotherapy, you should take certain precautions to protect yourself. These precautions need to be taken the first 48 hours after the client has received chemotherapy. You need to wear gloves when handling urine or stool material. When you empty the bedpan or urinal you need to be careful that you do not splash the contents on the toilet seat, floor, or yourself. You will need to flush the toilet twice after emptying the contents of the bedpan or urinal or after a client uses the bathroom.

After 48 hours these precautions are no longer necessary.

Common side effects of chemotherapy include nausea, vomiting, diarrhea, anemia, rash, susceptibility to infections, loss of hair, bleeding, and mouth sores. Hair loss caused by chemotherapy is usually temporary.

So-called miracle cures for cancer are sold in many forms. Most people who market these products are only interested in making a profit from the misfortune of others. Some people with cancer choose to take experimental drugs. However, a person is wiser and safer to follow the advice of a trustworthy physician. The best treatment plans are based on sound research.

CARING FOR A CLIENT WITH CANCER

Proper nutrition and special diets are important parts of cancer care. Clients should be given foods they like unless otherwise ordered by the doctor. Four to six small meals a day are usually preferred. If meals look attractive and are served nicely they may stimulate the client's appetite. Usually these diets are high in protein and calories. It is often necessary to supplement the diet with nutritious liquid supplements such as Ensure or similar products. The client's appetite is usually better in the morning. Be sure to give your client good oral care to stimulate the desire to eat, then follow with foods the client likes.

Clients in the later stages of cancer become very thin and weak. They will need assistance in all their activities of daily living. They will need excellent skin care to prevent skin breakdown. Their bodies need to be bathed with a mild soap and gently rubbed with lotion frequently during the day. They need to be positioned every 2 hours. It is recommended that at least twice a day the client be allowed to sit in a comfortable chair to give the back a rest and also to increase the circulation. An air mattress, eggcrate mattress, or sheepskin can be used on the bed to try to make the client as comfortable as possible.

It is not uncommon for cancer clients to have a distinguishing odor even after a bath. Occasionally the room where the client sleeps may need a room deodorizer. As a home health aide you can place a deodorizer in the room to mask this odor.

The goal of cancer therapy in the final stages is to keep the client as comfortable as possible with the least amount of pain. Your nurse supervisor will discuss with you when the client may have the pain medication. If the pain is not controlled by the medication that is ordered, you will need to inform your nurse supervisor. As the cancer spreads in the client's body, the pain may become more severe and less tolerated by the client. Sometimes patients may choose to enter into hospice care. Hospice is designed to relieve the physical and emotional suffering of terminally ill persons. This is usually done in the home or a homelike environment. The main goal is to provide comfort, peace, and dignity to the dying person and emotional support to the family and loved ones. Unit 21 discusses hospice and caring for the terminally ill client in greater detail.

CANCER OF THE FEMALE REPRODUCTIVE SYSTEM

Among women in the middle years, problems may occur in the reproductive system. All women should have an annual physical examination, including a Pap smear. A Pap smear detects early cellular change in the cervix. A microscopic examination is made of cells scraped from the uterus. If repeated Pap smears show cellular changes, the physician takes a biopsy. A **biopsy** is a sample of tissue cut from the area where cellular change is present. Through a microscopic examination of the tissue, the biopsy determines the seriousness of the cell changes. Sometimes a cone-shaped section is cut out for examination. If cancerous cells are found, a partial or complete hysterectomy may be performed. A **hysterectomy** is a major surgical procedure in which the uterus, and sometimes the ovaries and fallopian tubes, are removed.

Some women develop fibroid tumors in the uterus. These tumors are benign or noncancerous. They can become large or cause heavy bleeding during menstruation, or cause pain. When these problems exist, a hysterectomy may also be needed. After any major surgery it

may take from 9 to 12 months for full health to return. Very often women are depressed after a hysterectomy. If the ovaries have been removed, hormones may be prescribed to replace those normally produced. The hormone pills help the body to adjust physically and help restore a sense of well-being. Although a hysterectomy prevents further childbearing, it does not physically prevent enjoyment of sex.

Cancer of the Breast

Another area in which women develop cancer is the breast. An excellent method of detecting breast cancer is self-examination. Each woman should self-examine her breasts monthly about 7 to 10 days after each period. A woman stands in front of a mirror with her arms raised above her head (Figure 23-3A). She checks for changes in the shape of each breast, swelling,

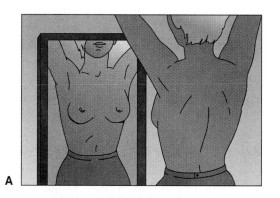

A

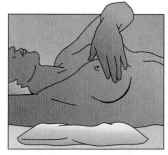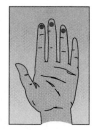

B Finger pads

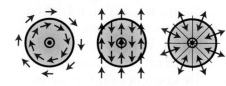

C

FIGURE 23-3A–C Self-examination helps to detect breast cancer at an early stage. (Courtesy of American Cancer Society)

dimpling of the skin, or changes in the nipple. She checks for lumps while lying on her back with a pillow under her right shoulder (Figure 23-3B). Using the finger pads on the three middle fingers on her left hand, she moves around the breast in a set way (Figure 23-3C). If a lump is noticed, she should go to her gynecologist for further examination. Not all lumps are malignant (cancerous). Many women have simple, benign breast tumors. Sometimes it is necessary to remove the benign tumors through surgery.

One diagnostic technique used in suspected breast cancer is an x-ray called a **mammogram.** Special x-ray studies can detect unhealthy or cancerous cells. In some cases, a biopsy is ordered if there is a suspicion of cancer of the breast. An incision (cut) is made in the breast and a microscopic examination of tissue is made at once. If cancer is diagnosed, some doctors remove only the growth itself. This can only be done when the diagnosis is made early. This procedure is sometimes known as a **lumpectomy.** Sometimes it is necessary to remove the entire breast tissue, underlying muscles, and the lymph glands under the arm. This procedure is called a radical **mastectomy.** If there is any sign that the cancer cells have metastasized (spread), both breasts may need to be removed. A woman's self-image is often decreased after a mastectomy. She may see the altered shape of her body as a deformity. However, an increasing number of women who have had this surgery can talk about it quite openly. Because they have talked about their own surgery, other women have become more aware of the need to examine themselves. As a result, many breast cancers are discovered early enough for successful treatment.

Following a mastectomy, there is often a time of depression. It is very important for a mastectomy patient to have the support of her loved ones. She must understand that her life can continue as before. Part of this is accepting that she is just as much a woman as she was before surgery. Because the surgery may involve the underarm glands and muscles of the chest and underarms, rehabilitation is very important. Special exercises are prescribed by the doctor. After a mastectomy patient returns home, these exercises must be continued regularly. After the incision is healed, most patients are encouraged

to have a **prosthesis** (artificial breast) made. In some cases, the prosthesis may be surgically fitted under a flap of skin. Other prosthetic devices shaped as cups are fitted into a special bra.

Many women who have breast surgery are helped by the American Cancer Society's *Reach to Recovery Program*. This is a free service to help meet the physical, emotional, and cosmetic needs of women who have had breast cancer. The Cancer Society carefully trains select volunteers who have a previous history of breast cancer and have coped well with their own breast cancer. This volunteer and the client can talk over fears arising from this disease, the impact on a client's body and self-image, and concerns for her future. The volunteer can talk about the need for exercises and how to adjust to the prosthesis that replaces her breast. This has been a successful program and has given many women the courage to accept the loss of a breast.

CANCER OF THE RESPIRATORY SYSTEM

The respiratory system is on duty 24 hours a day from birth to death. Fresh air is inhaled into the body and carried to the lungs. The oxygen from the air is carried to all parts of the body by the circulatory system. As oxygen is delivered to the cells of the body, waste gases are picked up and carried back to the lungs. Carbon dioxide is exhaled and expelled from the body.

Many infections and disorders can affect the respiratory system. Everyone has had a common cold. Flu, pneumonia, bronchitis, and upper respiratory infections are some of the illnesses affecting this system. Cancer, too, can start to grow in the lungs. Signs of lung cancer are:

- A persistent, hacking cough
- Pains in the chest area
- Tiredness
- A low-grade fever
- Sudden weight loss
- Coughing up blood
- Wheezing
- Recurrent bronchitis or pneumonia
- Difficulty swallowing

If a biopsy shows cancer cells, surgery can sometimes be done to remove all or part of a lung. Removal of part of the lung is called a **lobectomy.** Removal of the entire lung is called a **pneumonectomy.** Lung cancer grows slowly at first. However, by the time it is diagnosed, 7 of 10 patients are not helped by surgery. A person with lung cancer must be kept as comfortable as possible. Most clients with lung cancer are cared for in the home setting. The client will require oxygen therapy throughout the day. The client will most likely need to sit in the chair to breathe. If the client does go to bed, the bed will need many pillows because the client cannot breathe well lying down. The client will also most likely **expectorate** (spit) thick sputum. Remember to use standard precautions when handling the client's sputum.

Cancer of the Larynx

The **larynx** (voice box) is located at the top of the **trachea** (windpipe or airway between the nasal passages and the lungs). Cancer of the larynx occurs in men more often than in women. In addition, 75% of the people who develop cancer of the larynx have been heavy smokers. A common treatment for cancer of the larynx is surgical removal of the larynx, called a **laryngectomy.** To remove the larynx, a tracheostomy must be performed. A **tracheostomy** is a surgical opening made into the trachea below the larynx. The tracheostomy is an artificial airway that can be used to supply oxygen to the lungs. A tracheostomy tube is placed into the artificial airway to keep it open (Figure 23-4). In some instances the tracheostomy tube is no longer being used. Instead, a **stoma** is created surgically. An opening is made in the rear wall of the trachea and the front wall of the esophagus. A small tube is placed into these openings, allowing air to pass into the esophagus and keeping the opening clear and the trachea free of food and liquid. Sometimes, a valve can be placed on the stoma. When this valve is closed, the air that passes through the device into the esophagus permits esophageal speech.

After the tracheostomy has been done, the second part of the surgery is completed and the cancerous larynx is removed. The tracheostomy

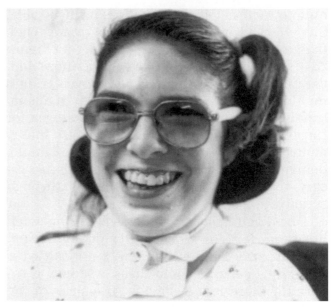

FIGURE 23-4 A tracheostomy tube provides an airway for this client.

tube remains in place permanently in a laryngectomy patient. After the patient has recovered from surgery, rehabilitation starts.

Speech therapy is needed to teach the patient how to talk. One of the methods is to gulp air in through the tracheostomy tube, swallow it, and then burp out words. It takes a great deal of practice to relearn speaking. Another method the laryngectomy patient may use to aid speech is an artificial larynx. A battery-powered vibrator is one type of artificial larynx. When wishing to speak, the patient places the vibrator against the side of the neck. The vibrator vibrates the air inside the patient's mouth as the patient **articulates** (or makes sounds).

A home health aide must be tactful when caring for such clients. It may be hard to understand what the client is saying. The aide should report to the nurse supervisor immediately if the client has any difficulty breathing. Crusting or bloody discharge from the tracheostomy also must be reported immediately.

GASTROINTESTINAL CANCER

More new cases of gastrointestinal (stomach and colon) cancer occur in the United States every year. At least 93% of these individuals are over 50 years of age. Women are slightly more likely than men to develop the disease. Only lung cancer exceeds colon cancer in the number of new cases and number of deaths each year. Early detection of such cancer is an important factor in survival. One treatment for this type of cancer is to remove the diseased part of the large intestine (Figure 23-5). An opening, called a **colostomy,** is made through the wall of the abdomen. The cancerous portion of the intestine is removed. The end of the intestine remaining is pulled to the outside of the abdomen. The body wastes are expelled through this opening into a colostomy collection pouch attached to the abdomen. The area where the intestine opens to the outside is called the stoma.

The client with an ostomy is usually taught to care for it before going home. If more care is

needed at home, the nurse will provide it, or teach the family and clients to take over the care. The patient is also taught how to irrigate the colostomy. **Irrigation** is the use of water to clean out the remaining colon.

In some cases, a colostomy is temporary. It may be possible to reconstruct and reconnect the intestine after several months. When this is not possible, the client's rectum is surgically closed and the colostomy becomes permanent. The feces from a colostomy are fairly solid. The kind of diet prescribed for these clients helps control the type of bowel movement. Each client needs to experiment with diet and bowel habits until the best balance is found. Some people with a colostomy may be able to regulate bowel movements very well. They may only need to keep a gauze pad over the stoma.

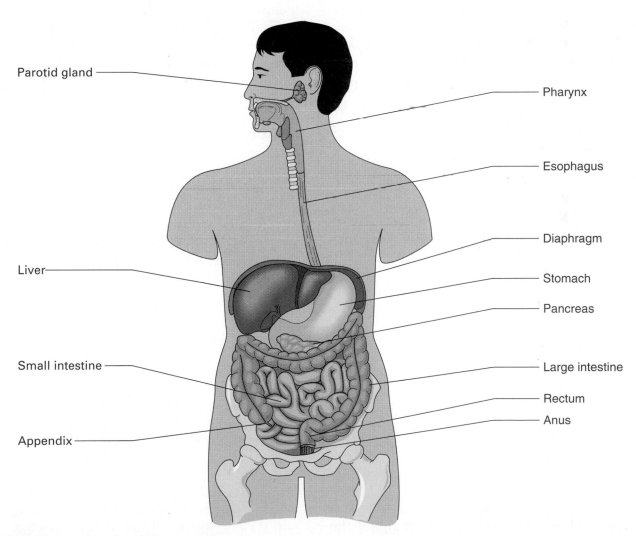

FIGURE 23-5 The digestive system

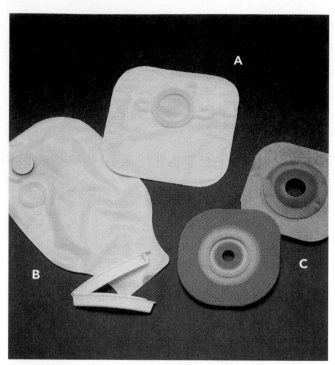

FIGURE 23-6 A. Closed stoma bags used for stool collection. (Permission to use this copyrighted material has been granted by the owner, Hollister Incorporated.) B. Karay seal drainable stoma bags for the loop colostomy C. A colostomy irrigating set

Cancer can destroy the functioning of the entire large intestine. When this occurs, the small intestine is cut and brought to the outside through the abdomen. This procedure is called an **ileostomy**. Most ileostomies are permanent. The waste discharge from an ileostomy remains liquid and drains constantly. The drainage irritates the skin.

Odors from the bag may be controlled by oral medications taken by the client or a deodorizer put into the container bag. Many different stoma appliances are on the market today, available for the client to select and use. Figure 23-6 shows an example of a closed stoma bag. Your nurse supervisor will instruct you on the type of appliance your client chooses to use.

Client Care

The home health aide should assist the client in cleaning around the stoma and changing the dressings and stoma bags. The aide can also help with colostomy irrigations and sitz baths. The aide may be asked to help the client clean the skin or to dispose of the contents of the bag. Some points to remember are:

- Bags with end openings can be rinsed out as needed and do not need to be changed as often, which reduces skin irritation.
- The client may want two bags so that one can air out while the other is worn.
- Some clients with colostomies who have good bowel regulation prefer to wear only a gauze dressing over the stoma.
- Clean and dry the skin around the stoma and cover it with a 4 × 4 dressing held in place by tape.
- Some clients may prefer an elastic supporter or a homemade muslin binder with ties to keep the dressing in place.
- Use care not to spread germs when changing the dressing; put the soiled 4 × 4 dressing into the trash.
- The ileostomy and ostomy bags require a tight fit because of the liquid contents and constant drainage; the appliance or bag must be changed when there is leakage; it should be emptied when one-third to one-half full and changed every 5 to 7 days.

See Procedure 31 in Unit 13 for the correct method to assist with changing an ostomy bag.

Clients are sometimes embarrassed or ashamed of the odor and the appearance of the stoma. A home health aide must be careful not to offend the client. Aides should never show disgust at the odor or shy away from helping the client.

SKIN CANCER

Skin cancer is becoming a common type of cancer, especially among the elderly. Skin cancer is most often caused by excessive exposure to ultraviolet radiation in the younger years. The lesion can be either benign or malignant. There are definite signs to watch for on the client's skin (Figure 23-7). If you notice any of these signs while bathing or working with your client, report the abnormal sign to the nurse supervisor. If detected and treated early enough, the prognosis is usually good.

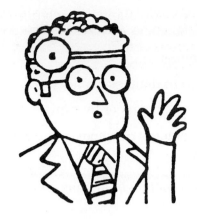

See your doctor or clinic if you notice changes in your skin moles such as:

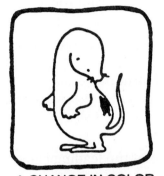

A CHANGE IN COLOR
(especially new black areas)

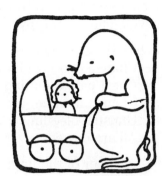

A NEW MOLE

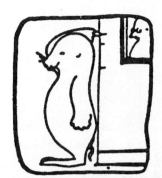

A MOLE THAT RISES IN HEIGHT

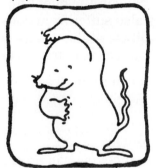

A CHANGE IN SENSATION
(especially new itching)

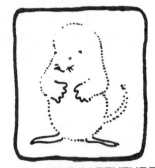

A CHANGE IN TEXTURE

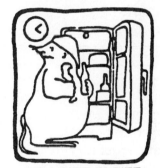

A CHANGE IN SIZE

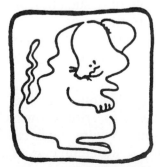

CHANGES IN SHAPE

See your doctor or clinic if you notice any other changes in or on your skin that you can't explain, and that last for more than 30 days.

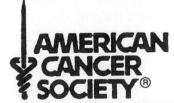

AMERICAN CANCER SOCIETY®

(Adapted from the New Mexico Skin Cancer Project)

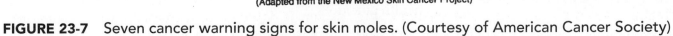

FIGURE 23-7 Seven cancer warning signs for skin moles. (Courtesy of American Cancer Society)

REVIEW

1. List four common side effects of clients receiving cancer treatments.

2. List seven warning signs of cancer.

3. List three diagnostic tests used to diagnose cancer.

4. List six surgical procedures used in cancer therapy.

5. List two nonsurgical types of cancer treatment.

6. Define hospice.

7. Describe specialized care a cancer client may need from a home health aide.

8. List two precautions to take when caring for a client who is receiving chemotherapy.

9. Which of the following is not a warning sign of cancer?
   a. Change in bowel habits
   b. Chest pain radiating down arm
   c. Change in mole
   d. Unusual bleeding
   e. All are correct

10. T F Cancer of the lung is one of the leading causes of death from cancer in men.

11. T F In the later stage of the cancer, the client may become very thin. The client may also suffer from constant pain. The goal of care in this phase of the disease is to keep the client as comfortable and as pain free as possible.

12. T F A deodorizer is often used in a room of a cancer client to diminish the odor due to the client's cancerous condition.

13. Match Column I with Column II.

Column I	Column II
_____ 1. remission	a. substance that can produce cancer
_____ 2. benign	b. no longer spreading
_____ 3. carcinogen	c. sample of tissue cut from an area of the body
_____ 4. colostomy	d. an opening into the colon
_____ 5. malignant	e. noncancerous
_____ 6. biopsy	f. cancer

14. Ms. Patterson, 43 years old, has a colostomy that was the result of colon cancer. The colostomy was a terrible blow to her pride and self-esteem. She returned home, where she lives alone, and plans were made to have a home health aide come daily to assist her with her colostomy care. However, Ms. Patterson refused all attempts of assistance by the home health aide. She refused to look at the colostomy, touch it, or even talk about it. She seemed to withdraw more each day. What should the home health aide do?

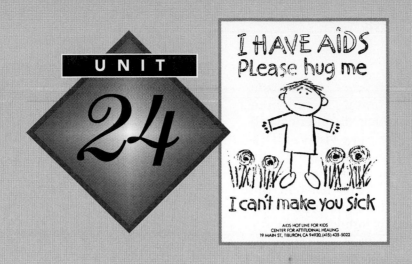

I HAVE AIDS
Please hug me

I can't make you sick

AIDS HOT LINE FOR KIDS
CENTER FOR ATTITUDINAL HEALING
19 MAIN ST, TIBURON, CA 94920, (415) 435-5022

Caring for the Client With AIDS

KEY TERMS

acquired immunodeficiency
   syndrome (AIDS)

human immunodeficiency
   virus (HIV)

sexually transmitted
   disease (STD)

LEARNING OBJECTIVES

After studying this unit, you should be able to:

- Understand how HIV is transmitted.
- Understand symptoms of HIV.
- Understand symptom-specific nursing care
  for clients with HIV.

- Understand necessary precautions to prevent
  the spread of HIV.

AIDS

Acquired immunodeficiency syndrome (AIDS) is a severe immunologic disorder caused by the **human immunodeficiency virus (HIV).** In this disease, the body's immune system becomes severely depressed and unable to fight any type of infection. The HIV virus lives in the infected person's blood, semen, and other body fluids. It can be transmitted by intimate contact—oral, vaginal, rectal—or by direct contact with body fluids or blood. In most cases, AIDS is transferred by sexual contact and drug users sharing needles. AIDS can also be transmitted to newborn babies during delivery or through the mother's milk. A new mother infected with the virus can pass the disease by breast-feeding her infant. Prior to 1985, AIDS was also transmitted through contaminated blood transfusions. Contaminated blood is no longer a concern because the American Red Cross now tests all blood donations for HIV.

At this time AIDS is considered to be the most dangerous of the **sexually transmitted diseases (STD).** Before 1981, AIDS was unknown in this country. Today AIDS is epidemic. From June 1981 through January 1995, more than 450,000 Americans were diagnosed with this disease. Of this group, over 60% have already died. Many others still carry the HIV virus and will eventually develop AIDS. According to the World Health Organization there are 3 million cases of AIDS worldwide. About 1.5 million people in the United States, and 15 to 17 million worldwide are estimated to be carriers of the virus. It has been found in persons of both sexes and in homosexuals and heterosexuals from all walks of life.

After the original infection with the HIV virus, the incubation period before AIDS develops is 7 to 15 years. Once an individual has been diagnosed with AIDS, the client may display swollen lymph glands, diarrhea, skin lesions (Figure 24-1), fever, chills, night sweats, nausea and vomiting, mouth sores (Figure 24-2), difficulty breathing, cough, hair loss, fatigue, difficulty walking, memory loss, and confusion. Death usually follows within 2 to 3 years after the appearance of these symptoms.

Your nursing care will be designed around these problems. Remember no two clients will be alike. Some may be confused, whereas others will be alert and oriented. Each care plan will need to be individualized to meet the client's physical and emotional needs (Figure 24-3).

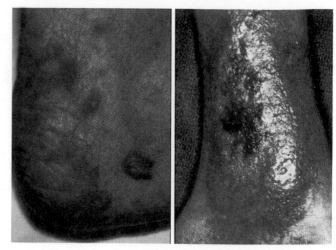

FIGURE 24-1 Typical skin lesions of Kaposi's sarcoma (Photos courtesy of The Centers for Disease Control and Prevention, Atlanta, GA)

Diagnosis of an infant with AIDS is difficult during the first year of life. Nonetheless, every effort is being made to make an immediate diagnosis of the newborn because it is hoped that experimental drugs, AZT and DDZ, may arrest the disease if given immediately after birth.

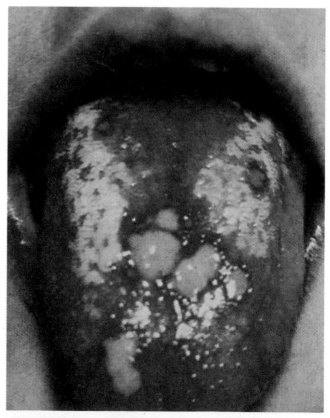

FIGURE 24-2 White patches on the tongue are evidence of the infectious process called thrush.

FIGURE 24-3   Working with the AIDS client

1. Listen to the client. Do not lie or give false encouragement. Empathize rather than sympathize.
2. Get the client to participate in care planning.
3. Encourage as much independence as possible and assist only as necessary.
4. Encourage participation in social, recreational, and occupational activities.
5. Encourage the client to talk and listen, but be sure not to pass judgment.
6. Do not start working with an AIDS client if you think you may not be able to handle it. If you take an AIDS client, work with your supervisor and plan a regular rotation so that the client has consistent care.
7. Do not try to become the client's "best friend," but do try to establish a good relationship and develop mutual trust.
8. Allow your client to feel anger and frustration and recognize that he may take it out on you. Let the client vent the anger or frustration—but do not take it personally.
9. Do not condemn or blame yourself if you feel fear, anxiety, or discomfort. Working with terminally ill clients is difficult. Such feelings are natural. Discuss your feelings with your supervisor. Learn as much as you can about the illness. Facts can fight fears!

Children with AIDS need special attention and care (Figure 24-4).

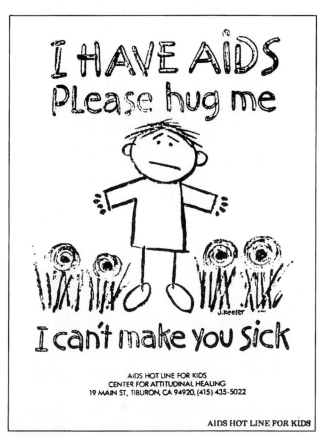

FIGURE 24-4 Love might be the hardest thing to get. (Courtesy of the Center for Attitudinal Healing, 33 Buchanan Drive, Sausalito, CA 94965. 415/331-6161)

Because the incubation time for the virus can be as long as 7 to 15 years, it is possible that individuals who received blood transfusions as far back as 1981 may be at risk for AIDS. Anyone who feels that he or she has been exposed because of sexual contact, blood transfusions, or drug use can be tested for AIDS. The results of such tests must be kept confidential.

As more information has come to light about AIDS, the public is more aware of what is and what is not true. According to Dr. C. Everett Koop, former Surgeon General of the United States, we must come to terms with the fact that we are fighting a disease, not the people who have AIDS. He also said that those who are already afflicted need to be cared for like any other sick individual.

HOW TO PROTECT AGAINST AIDS

At this time there is no vaccine to prevent AIDS and there is no cure for AIDS. Experimental drugs are being used, and a great deal of research is being done to isolate the virus and discover effective treatments.

The only way to lessen the impact of the AIDS virus is to avoid situations that are dangerous and take precautions, for example, practicing safe sex by using condoms, practicing abstinence, not "shooting" drugs intravenously, not using "dirty" needles (best of all, not getting involved in drug use of any kind), and using precautions when caring for an AIDS client. Refer to Unit 9 for a detailed discussion on the principles of infection control and standard precaution guidelines (Figure 24-5).

The Surgeon General states that quarantine has no role in the management of AIDS because AIDS is not spread by casual contact, unless the AIDS victim deliberately exposes others by sexual contact and sharing drug equipment.

CARING FOR THE AIDS CLIENT

AIDS is a debilitating disease with no cure. Dealing with the effects of AIDS can be difficult for the client and family alike. AIDS often afflicts young adults at their most productive time of life, making it especially difficult for the client and their loved ones to face death. The emotional and physical support of caregivers, family, and friends is crucial in helping those with AIDS lead as normal a life as possible, for as long as possible.

One of the major concerns of the Department of Health is to provide proper care for the AIDS client while protecting the health care workers. At this time the Centers for Disease Control and Prevention (CDC) indicates that one cannot get AIDS from casual social contact (shaking hands, hugging, coughing, sneezing, or kissing), contact with tears of an AIDS individual, or from their perspiration. AIDS is not spread by swimming in pools, bathing in hot tubs, or from eating food prepared or served by an AIDS victim, or from health team members working with AIDS clients. You will not get AIDS from handling bed linens, towels, cups, straws, dishes, or other eating utensils. You do not get AIDS from toilet seats, telephones, or household furnishings. However, until definitive answers are found, it is strongly recommended that health care workers always follow standard precautions.

What an Aide Can and Should Do

When working with an AIDS client it is important to know that many misconceptions about the disease exist. The home health aide should learn the facts about AIDS and remain nonjudgmental of the client, regardless of how the disease was contracted. A home health aide must never reveal to friends, neighbors, or anyone else the nature of a client's illness. That is considered an invasion of privacy and the client can file a complaint with the State Department of Human Rights if such information is revealed by the agency or the aide.

The home health aide should create a comfortable and pleasant environment for the client. Personal hygiene is crucial to maintain the client's comfort and to promote health. Regular bathing will be necessary if the client suffers from night sweats. Practicing good oral hygiene will go a long way in maintaining good nutrition. Figure 24-6 shows a sample care plan for the client with AIDS.

Your employer must provide you with basic training on AIDS. The training program must cover topics such as how it is spread, signs and symptoms, and necessary precautions to be aware of while caring for the client.

FIGURE 24-5 Preventing the transmission of HIV

To prevent transmission of infection:

1. Wear a gown if there is a possibility of soiling your clothing with blood or body secretions of client.
2. Wear gloves when touching blood or body secretions.
3. Wash hands before and after client contact and immediately if they are potentially contaminated with blood or body fluids.
4. Discard articles contaminated with blood or body secretions and secure in red biohazard bag or container.
5. IF YOU HAVE AN OPEN CUT OR WOUND, DO NOT CONTAMINATE THE WOUND WITH CLIENT'S BODY FLUIDS. Cover the area with an adhesive bandage and wash immediately if open area becomes contaminated with client's body fluids.
6. Follow any additional instructions by your supervisor or case manager.

FIGURE 24-6   Sample care plan for client with AIDS

Sign/Symptom	Care to Provide	Purpose
Weakness/ tiredness	High-calorie diet with in-between meal high-protein snacks	To provide protein nutrition and to slow muscle deterioration
Fever	Sponge baths, give additional fluids by mouth; cover with blankets during chill periods	To lower the temperature and to prevent complications. To get client comfortable
Night sweats	Sponge baths, frequent linen changes, give additional fluids to avoid dehydration	To provide comfort and to return skin to normal condition
Cough	Observe and record patterns and changes and report findings. Offer cough medicine if prescribed. Gloves required when working.	To make the client comfortable and to obtain relief from strain
Dyspnea	Note patterns and changes—record and report. Calm client and avoid exertion by client and help with breathing exercises	To provide breath control and relaxation
Skin lesions	Keep client from scratching—be sure nails are properly cut by nurse—wear gloves when working with client with lesions and wash hands carefully after contact with client	To prevent infections
Dry hair and hair loss	Avoid too frequent shampooing—use mild shampoo containing no alcohol. Use hair conditioner	To prevent further hair loss and to avoid scalp irritation
Mouth lesions	Provide saline or anesthetic mouthwashes; brush teeth gently. Check to be sure client can swallow without difficulty—observe, record and report to supervisor. Avoid spicy, acid foods and carbonated beverages. Gloves are required when giving mouth care.	To provide infection control, client comfort, and maintain adequate nutrition
Diarrhea	Encourage fluid intake; change linens as needed; apply brief if required; observe, record and report; gloves required	To maintain nutrition and fluid balance. To prevent pressure sore formation
Impaired immune system (when client picks up any infection around)	Give daily shower or bath; both client and aide wash hands frequently; request nurse to apply sterile dressings as needed with gloves; do not allow visitors who have infections, such as colds; do not come to give client care if you are suffering from any infection.	To prevent infection and to assist in client protection
Unstable emotional responses	Be aware of client's feelings as well as your own. Be honest with client and accept him as a person, not as an AIDS victim. Offer emotional support, kindness. Communicate by touching client's hand, pat on back, etc.	To create an atmosphere of mutual trust

SPECIAL PRECAUTIONS ·····················

For the safety of the home health aide, and the AIDS client, it is important to follow standard precautions at all times.

1. Wash hands properly before and after client's care, before and after food preparation, and before and after using the bathroom. If the client's home has no provision for handwashing, your employer must provide either antiseptic hand cleanser with paper towels or antiseptic towelettes.
2. Wear disposable gloves when handling blood or body fluids. A gown needs to be worn only if the client has severe diarrhea or if there is a chance of blood or body fluids being splashed. Masks or goggles will not need to be worn unless one expects to be splashed with blood or body fluids, such as when the client has a wet cough and cannot cover his mouth.
3. Discard any sharp item such as needles and razor blades in puncture-resistant, closable, leak-proof containers. These containers must be labeled and color coded.
4. It is recommended that the primary cleaning product be household bleach. At the beginning of each visit, the home health aide should prepare a solution of 1:10 bleach and water. Gloves should be worn when using this bleach solution because it may be very harsh on the skin. Do not mix bleach with anything other than water. Be careful not to splash in the eyes. This solution can be used to clean the bathroom, counters, and floors.
5. Laundry can be done in the home, making sure you wear gloves if the laundry is soiled with urine or blood. If the laundry is to be sent out, you will either have to double bag it or place it in a strong plastic bag and mark the linens "contaminated."
6. A home health aide who has an infection or illness should follow reverse isolation procedures—putting on gloves, gown, and mask before giving client care, and removing those items after completing client care. However, in the interest of the client, it is best for the aide to stay away from work until the aide is well again. This is especially true in the case of an AIDS client because such individuals have a damaged immune system unable to fight off germs or infections carried by the aide.
7. If the home health aide has open cuts or skin sores oozing fluid, he or she should not give direct client care. This is for the safety and health of both the aide and client.
8. The aide may not tell anyone of the client's diagnosis unless a special release form has been signed by the client.

AIDS clients should also be educated about prevention of the transmission of the disease. It is their responsibility to practice commonsense hygienic measures to protect others with whom they live in close contact.

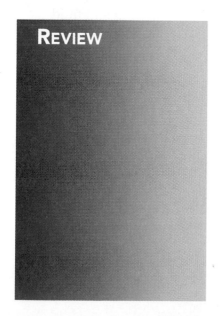

REVIEW

1. List two ways AIDS can be transmitted from one person to another. 326
2. List three signs and symptoms of AIDS. 374
3. Describe the care an aide would give to a client with AIDS. 378
4. List six guidelines or rules to follow when caring for a client with AIDS 378 - 2 4 5
5. List six rules to follow for the prevention of the spread of infections. 378
6. AIDS is not spread by:
   a. Sexual contact with a client with AIDS
   b. Sharing needles of infected client
   c. Holding a baby that is infected by the AIDS virus
   d. Having infected blood from an AIDS client enter an open sore on the aide's body

REVIEW

7. Signs and symptoms of AIDS is/are:
    a. Swollen lymph glands
    b. Diarrhea
    c. Skin lesions
    d. All are correct

8. T   F   The incubation time for the AIDS virus can be as long as 15 years.

9. You are caring for Mr. H, who has AIDS. While you are caring for him, you cut your finger and start to bleed. What are your next steps? *370 — #7*

10. One day, while caring for Mrs. P, who has AIDS, she starts shouting at you, saying things like, "You don't know what you are doing! It's your fault my condition hasn't improved!" She then bursts into tears. How should you respond? What might be the reason for this client's outburst?

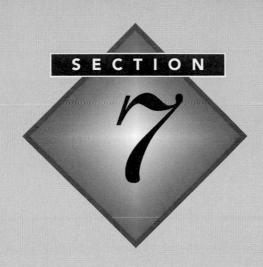
Maternal/Infant Care

Units

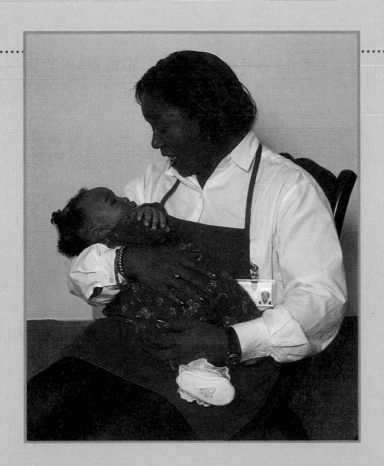

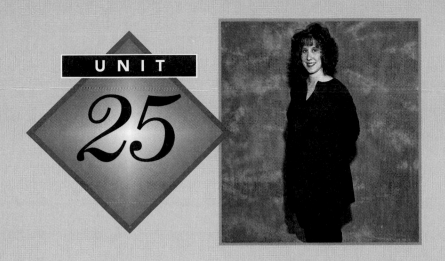

25

Maternal Care

KEY TERMS

breast engorgement
Down's syndrome
edema
engagement
fetal alcohol syndrome

flatulence
heartburn
hemorrhoids
high-risk pregnancies
lochia

postpartum
postpartum blues
varicose veins

LEARNING OBJECTIVES

After studying this unit, you should be able to:

- List common pregnancy symptoms and their treatments.
- Identify high-risk pregnancies.
- Recognize danger signals in pregnancy.
- Describe mechanisms for caring for the expectant mother.

- List common postpartum discomforts and their treatments.
- Recognize abnormal postpartum problems.

The goal of every expectant mother and the professionals who care for her is the delivery of a normal, healthy baby. A key element in normal fetal development is an expectant mother in good physical and emotional health.

COMMON PREGNANCY SYMPTOMS····

Pregnancy today is regarded as a normal and natural stage of a woman's life cycle (Figure 25-1). At the same time, the woman must realize that extra demands are being placed on her body by the growing fetus. Regular medical care should be sought as soon as a woman realizes she is pregnant and should continue throughout the pregnancy. Even with regular medical care, often discomforts are involved with pregnancy. Most women experience at least one of the symptoms listed below at some point during their pregnancy.

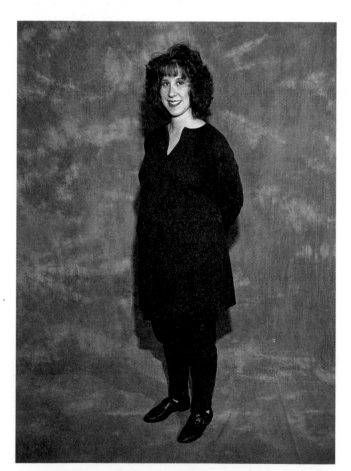

FIGURE 25-1 Pregnancy is regarded as a normal and natural stage of a woman's life cycle.

Frequent Urination

Frequent urination is caused by pressure of the enlarged uterus on the bladder. This usually subsides by the second or third month of pregnancy, when the uterus rises in the abdominal cavity. However, in the last week of pregnancy, when the uterus drops into the pelvic cavity—a condition known as **engagement**—both urgency and frequency of urination can be a problem.

Morning Sickness

Morning sickness is one of the most common symptoms of pregnancy. It is characterized by nausea and, sometimes, by vomiting. Although it usually occurs in the morning, it can happen at any time of day, most often lasting for a 4- to 12-week period during the first trimester. Hormonal changes can contribute to morning sickness.

Some techniques for alleviating nausea include remaining in bed and resting for half an hour after awakening. During this period the expectant mother should try to eat dry toast or a cracker.

Heartburn/Flatulence

Diminished gastric motion during pregnancy may cause stomach contents to back up into the esophagus. This is commonly called **heartburn.** Nervousness and emotional upsets can contribute to this symptom. Fried and fatty foods should also be avoided. Sitting up for 30 minutes after eating will also help to alleviate this condition. Antacids should be used only with a doctor's prescription.

Feelings of gassiness, referred to as **flatulence,** may also be present because of gas-forming bacterial action in the intestines. One way to alleviate gassiness is to eat slowly, chew food thoroughly, and avoid gas-forming foods, such as beans, corn, and fried foods. Yogurt will help to inhibit gas formation.

Constipation/Hemorrhoids

Constipation can result from the pressure of the uterus on the intestines. Pressure exerted by the pregnant uterus can interfere with circulation in the veins. In the anal area, coupled with constipation, this can result in **hemorrhoids.** Suppositories or other medications, including those available over the counter, should be used only when prescribed by the physician.

Varicose Veins

Varicose veins (swollen veins) can develop during pregnancy. This can be caused by pressure on the great veins of the pelvis, a hereditary predisposition, constrictive clothing, and prolonged standing, and can affect the lower extremities. Legs should be elevated, and rest should be encouraged.

Breathlessness

The pressure of the enlarged uterus on the diaphragm can cause respiratory discomfort. The expectant mother should be reassured that, with the birth of the infant, or even before, the symptom will resolve itself. About 2 to 3 weeks before the onset of contractions, the fetus descends into the pelvis. This process is called lightening and usually alleviates respiratory discomfort of the mother.

Backache

Backache is a common complaint of pregnant women and results from adjustments in posture caused by carrying the baby's weight, the changes in the mother's center of gravity, and the relaxation of the joints at the base of the spine. Wearing flat, firmly balanced shoes and a properly fitting maternity support garment may help, as well as practicing good posture, proper body mechanics, and getting adequate rest.

Leg Cramps

Leg cramps can be another discomfort of pregnancy. Leg cramps may be caused by inadequate calcium, excessive amounts of phosphorus, fatigue, tense muscles, and chilling. This symptom can be addressed through frequent rest periods, with the feet slightly elevated. The physician should be consulted to be certain that the proper amount of calcium is being taken and absorbed through diet.

Edema

Edema, or swelling, of the lower extremities can also occur, particularly in hot weather. Rest, elevation of the legs, and use of an abdominal support or support hose, as directed by the physician, are the most frequent ways of alleviating the swelling (Figure 25-2).

Vaginal Discharge

Although an increase in vaginal discharge, requiring a perineal pad, is normal during pregnancy, a discharge that is irritating, excessive, has a bad odor, and is yellow or green can be an indication of a problem. Among the causes could be venereal disease or yeast infections. Medical attention should be sought.

COMPLICATIONS OF PREGNANCY

Although the vast majority of pregnancies progress quite naturally, occasionally complications may develop. Complications of pregnancy may be the result of the age of the mother, the use of harmful substances during pregnancy, or certain medical factors. Complications of pregnancy can affect the health of the mother and the baby. For this reason it is important that women receive medical care throughout the pregnancy.

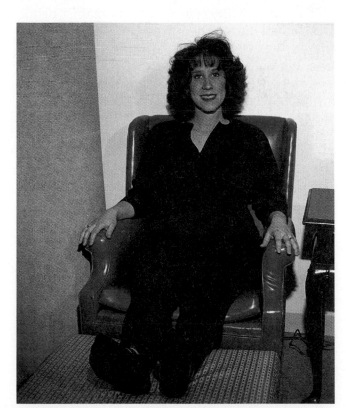

FIGURE 25-2 Elevation of the legs is a common method to reduce edema.

High-Risk Pregnancies

When physical, emotional, or environmental situations compromise the mother's well-being, a **high-risk pregnancy** can result. These pregnancies can cause low birthweight, premature or brain-damaged babies, and maternal complications. These complications increase the chances of infant and maternal mortality (death).

The age of the mother can have a significant influence on the outcome of the pregnancy and its identification as a high-risk event. Statistically, women over age 35 are more likely to give birth to babies with **Down's syndrome,** a form of retardation. Prenatal (before birth) tests are offered to pregnant women in high-risk categories. These prenatal tests include ultrasound, amniocentesis, and blood tests that can determine the health of the fetus.

Mothers who are too young are also at risk. Frequently, the pregnant adolescent does not seek prenatal care or first sees a doctor late in her pregnancy due to fear, denial, or lack of knowledge. Very young mothers often suffer from malnutrition, anemia, vitamin deficiency, excessive weight gain, drug abuse, and infections. Deficiencies in the expectant mother's diet can cause low birthweight in her baby.

Pregnant women are advised against drinking alcohol during their pregnancy. Heavy drinking during pregnancy can result in several serious complications known as **fetal alcohol syndrome.** This condition produces infants who are born underweight, usually mentally deficient, and with multiple deformities (Figure 25-3). Cigarette smoking can also lead to a variety of pregnancy complications. Tobacco use is one of the leading causes of prenatal problems, such as vaginal bleeding, miscarriage, and early delivery. If the expectant mother is a substance abuser, her chances of problems during pregnancy are increased. Drug-addicted women can, and often do, give birth to drug-addicted babies.

Women can be placed in the high-risk group because of medical factors, such as having a history of spontaneous abortions, stillbirths, premature births, or difficult pregnancies in the past. Women who have cardiac, respiratory, or renal disease, or who are diabetic or hypertensive, fall into the high-risk category, as do those who have experienced vaginal bleeding during pregnancy, who are Rh negative, or have been pregnant five times or more. A history of psy-

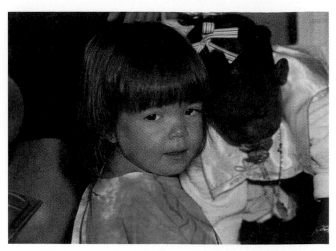

FIGURE 25-3 Facial abnormalities typical of fetal alcohol syndrome (FAS) include characteristics of eyes, ear, and smooth upper lip.

chiatric disorders and exposure to hazardous environmental factors also increase the risk of complications in pregnancy.

Danger Signals

Many expectant mothers fear miscarriage during their first trimester of pregnancy. Some possible signs of miscarriage include bleeding associated with abdominal cramping, severe abdominal pain that does not go away, heavy vaginal bleeding or light spotting that continues for several days, and passing blood clots or grayish pink material. Other danger signals include persistent vomiting, chills and fever, sudden escape of fluid from the vagina, swelling of face or fingers, severe and continuous headaches, and blurred vision. If any of these situations arise, medical attention should be sought immediately. Whenever in doubt, the physician should be notified.

CARING FOR THE EXPECTANT MOTHER

In many parts of the country, demand for home health care services for the expectant mother and for new families is growing. Home health care services for a pregnant mother can occur if a pregnancy is high risk, the mother is under unusual stress, or the mother is on complete bed rest.

When taking care of a pregnant woman in the home setting, some important things for the home health aide to remember are:

- Encourage a balanced diet; this is important for the mother and especially for the growth of the fetus.
- Encourage regular medical checkups.
- Follow the care plan carefully, which will include activity orders. Bed rest is sometimes ordered for high blood pressure or vaginal bleeding, with a threat of miscarriage.
- Make sure the physician is aware of *any* medication the mother-to-be might be taking because birth defects can result from taking certain medicines.
- Discourage smoking and drinking of alcohol; growth of the baby can be affected, and birth defects may arise from these practices.
- Observe the mother-to-be carefully for signs of bleeding. If there is a threat of miscarriage or any severe pain, report these immediately.
- Encourage good personal and dental hygiene and exercise, as allowed.
- Try to help the mother-to-be feel as optimistic as possible; provide a calm environment to help promote a general feeling of well-being.
- Help her maintain a good fluid intake for her general health.
- Teach her how to use good body mechanics.

Exercise is important, but it must be undertaken only with the physician's permission, in moderation, and designed for each woman's needs. Age, physical condition, previous exercise history, and the stage of pregnancy all influence the type and amount of exercise allowed.

While meeting the expectant mother's medical needs is important, her personal needs relative to good hygiene and life-style cannot be neglected. As her body changes, she needs to feel good about herself and the way she looks. Attractive nonrestrictive clothing will help her feel physically and emotionally comfortable. An abdominal support may be necessary in the last stages of pregnancy to prevent fatigue and backaches.

CARING FOR THE POSTPARTUM MOTHER

Labor and delivery are exhausting physical and emotional experiences. In the past, new mothers remained in the hospital for 5 to 7 days after delivery. Today, new mothers are released to their homes within 24 to 48 hours after vaginal deliveries and in 3 to 4 days after cesarean sections. As a result, many new mothers are choosing to hire home health aides to assist them during the first several weeks postpartum. The **postpartum** period is defined as the period after childbirth, usually lasting 6 weeks.

Postpartum Discomforts

Frequently, first-time mothers are unprepared for the discomforts of the postpartum experience. The home health aide should be supportive and reassure the new mother that her feelings—physical and emotional—are considered normal postpartum experiences. The home health aide must also be aware of abnormal postpartum danger signals and should seek medical attention whenever in doubt.

Exhaustion. The postpartum mother is usually exhausted as a result of labor and delivery and her role as a new mother. She should be encouraged to get as much rest as possible so that she can regain her strength.

Lochia. **Lochia** is the bloody vaginal discharge that is secreted by postpartum women. Although bright red at first for several days, it should turn light pink, brown, then yellow by the end of 2 weeks. Sanitary napkins should be used to absorb the flow. Excessive bleeding should be reported as well as lochia with a foul odor. Pads should be changed frequently and the area should be kept clean.

Incisional Pain. Incisions (episiotomy or cesarean section) can be extremely painful. Encourage and assist the patient with cool sitz baths to ease the pain, and offer ice packs during the first 24 hours to reduce swelling and numb the pain. A physician will determine what, if any, pain medication should be used.

Breast Engorgement. A few days after delivery, breast milk comes in, causing **breast engorgement.** If bottle-feeding, this can be a painful experience for postpartum women. A sports bra or a tight wrap and ice packs will minimize the pain. Reassure the patient that engorgement should last only 12 to 24 hours. A physician may prescribe pain medication. If breast-feeding, warm showers and compresses will help the milk flow.

Difficulty Walking and Sitting. Assist with walking and sitting. Remind the patient to walk as upright as possible and, if desired, to sit on a foam cushion.

Abdominal Cramping. Abdominal cramps are believed to be caused by the uterus as it contracts to its normal size. Cramping could be felt more during nursing. Medical attention should be sought if pains persist for more than several days.

Sweating. The body rids itself of pregnancy-accumulated fluids during the postpartum period, frequently during the night. The patient's temperature should be taken to check for a fever. Fever should be reported to the physician.

Difficult Urination. Difficulty with urination is a common postpartum condition. This temporary condition should last only approximately 24 hours. If urinating is still difficult or unusual, the physician should be notified to check for a urinary tract infection.

Depression/Mood Swings. Postpartum blues, or postbaby blues, are experienced by many women during the first few weeks after delivery. Some women feel anxious, tired, and weepy or experience mood swings. The home health aide should provide support and reassurance. If the postpartum mother feels that she is likely to hurt herself or her baby, professional assistance should be sought.

The following are factors to be considered when caring for the new mother:

- Encourage the new mother to get as much rest as possible to regain energy.
- Emotional changes may range from depression to elation in both parents; the mother may be irritable and weepy at times; be understanding and patient.
- Involve the family in care of the new baby to help in family adjustment.

- Help with home management activities as needed.
- Encourage the mother to eat a balanced diet, get adequate rest and exercise, interact with the family unit, and take time to get to know her baby.
- Watch for signs of infection (pain, elevated temperature, or foul odor of the vaginal discharge) and report any of these signs or symptoms immediately.
- Watch for vaginal bleeding; the discharge should change from bright red to pink to white within several days; report excessive bleeding immediately.

Nutrition and Breast-Feeding

If a mother is planning to breast-feed her baby, she will need to pay close attention to her diet. The mother's diet will influence both the amount and quality of the milk she produces. Some tips to maintain the best nutrition for a breast-feeding mother are:

- Consume about 500 to 800 additional calories per day.
- Eat three regular meals and a bedtime snack. Avoid going too long between meals.
- Additional protein in the diet is needed; eat generous servings of meat, milk, eggs, or cheese.
- Additional calcium will help meet vitamin D needs.
- Calcium, iron, and vitamin supplements may be continued (as prescribed by the mother's physician).
- Avoid trying to lose weight too quickly after the baby's birth.
- Caffeine and alcohol are passed from the mother's blood into the milk and should be avoided.
- Some drugs are passed from the mother's blood into the milk, and should only be taken if prescribed by a physician.
- Drink plenty of fluids.

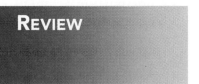

REVIEW

1. T F Pregnancy is a normal, natural stage of a woman's life cycle.

2. T F Regular medical care is not necessary during pregnancy.

3. T F Edema is a common pregnancy symptom.

REVIEW

4. T F Women are advised against drinking alcohol or smoking cigarettes during pregnancy.

5. T F Lochia is considered a normal postpartum discomfort.

6. T F Persistent vomiting, chills and fever, and swelling of the face are some danger signals during pregnancy.

7. Backache, nausea, and leg cramps are all common symptoms of:
   a. Pregnancy
   b. The postpartum period
   c. A high-risk pregnancy
   d. Miscarriage

8. Some possible signs of miscarriage are:
   a. Difficulty with urination
   b. Severe headache and blurred vision
   c. Bleeding with abdominal cramping and spotting for several days
   d. Leg cramps

9. Common postpartum discomforts include:
   a. Depression/mood swings
   b. Incisional pain
   c. Breast engorgement
   d. All of the above
   e. None of the above

10. Match Column I with Column II.

Column I	Column II
_____ 1. flatulence	a. swelling of lower extremities
_____ 2. lochia	b. danger signal during pregnancy
_____ 3. edema	c. feelings of gassiness
_____ 4. blurred vision	d. bloody vaginal discharge
_____ 5. morning sickness	e. vomiting and nausea

11. You are caring for an expectant mother who is categorized as high risk. She is on complete bed rest. What should you do to assist her in maintaining a safe pregnancy until her due date?

12. Mrs. Smith was released from the hospital 24 hours after her first baby was born. She hired you to assist her during her first 3 weeks at home. She is exhausted and is depressed. What should you do?

13. The postpartum mother for whom you are caring is complaining of having some difficulty with urination 7 days after delivery. She cannot describe exactly what is wrong. What should you do?

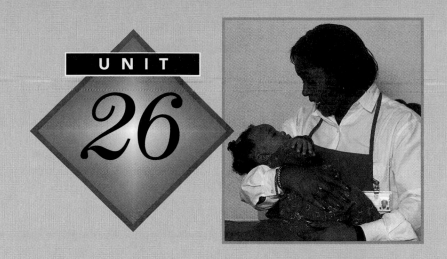

UNIT
26

Infant Care

KEY TERMS

bottle-feeding
breast-feeding

circumcision
foreskin

glans
lactose

LEARNING OBJECTIVES

After studying this unit, you should be able to:

- Understand the proper technique to bottle-feed an infant.
- Identify the procedures for breast-feeding an infant.
- Describe three techniques for burping an infant.
- Describe the steps to bathe an infant.
- Define circumcision and identify the appropriate care for the circumcised/uncircumcised penis.

- Identify safety precautions to be taken with each infant care procedure.
- Demonstrate the following:
  - **PROCEDURE 66**   Assisting with Breast-Feeding and Breast Care
  - **PROCEDURE 67**   Bottle-Feeding an Infant
  - **PROCEDURE 68**   Burping an Infant
  - **PROCEDURE 69**   Bathing an Infant

INFANT CARE

The birth of a baby is a time of adjustment for both the baby and the new parents. The newborn must now learn how to live in a new environment, outside the womb, where its needs are not automatically met; and the parents must learn how to care for their new baby. During the first year of life, the child is totally dependent on the care of others. Physical and emotional well-being are intimately related to each other. The individuals who meet the infant's primary needs significantly influence its physical and emotional development. Caring for a newborn baby can create anxiety for the new parents. The home health aide should try to reduce these anxieties by becoming familiar with basic infant care procedures, such as feeding, burping, bathing, caring for the circumcised or uncircumcised penis, and caring for the umbilical cord.

FEEDING THE INFANT

The newborn infant will approximately triple its birthweight during the first year of life. The nutritional needs during this rapid growth period are greater than at any other time in its life. Feeding the infant should be an enjoyable, relaxing time. Hold the infant close, cuddle, and make eye contact while feeding. There are two ways to feed the infant: **breast-feeding** and **bottle-feeding.** Either method can be used independently or in combination.

Breast-Feeding

Human milk is the best possible food for any infant. Its major ingredients are **lactose** (sugar), protein (whey and casein), fat, and numerous vitamins, minerals, and enzymes, all appropriately combined to suit an infant's nutritional needs. The home health aide should assist the new mother with the breast-feeding technique, as outlined in Procedure 66.

It is not necessary for the nursing mother to wash the nipple before each feeding, which can lead to drying and cracking. After nursing it is important to keep the nipple as dry as possible. Exposing the nipple to air is recommended and reduces the risk of developing cracked nipples and breast infections. Cracked nipples are common among breast-feeding women. Sometimes the nipple may bleed, making nursing painful. Bacteria can enter the breast through the

---

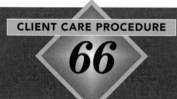

CLIENT CARE PROCEDURE

66

Assisting with Breast-Feeding and Breast Care

PURPOSE

- To provide for cleanliness and prevention of infection to the breasts
- To protect the nipples and observe for cracking or signs of soreness
- To protect the infant from bacterial infection
- To provide for the mother's comfort before, during, and after nursing the child
- To nourish infant
- To promote mother-child interaction

PROCEDURE

1. Provide supplies.
   mild soap
   warm water in basin
   clean washcloth and towel
   clean nursing bra (or well-fitting support bra)
   nursing pads
   cotton balls
   rinse water in basin (at feeding time)
   clock or watch to time nursing period
2. Wash your hands thoroughly before beginning the procedure.
3. Help the mother to wash her hands before handling the breasts.
4. Have the mother open the front of her dress or shirt top, if needed.

(continues)

5. Have the mother sit in comfortable position in a rocking chair with armrest and footstool to support the feet. If mother is still on bed rest, help her lie on one side.

6. Bring child to mother. Make sure infant's nose is not pressed against the mother's breast. The nostrils must be free so the infant can breathe as it nurses. Follow procedure as taught in hospital. There are three positions for breast-feeding: side-lying, football hold, and cradle hold (Figures 26-1A–C). Rotate positions to reduce breast tenderness in one particular area.

7. The nursing period is gradually built up from just a few minutes to a maximum of 20 minutes. Some mothers prefer to let baby nurse at both breasts (one at a time) during one feeding period. Others will feed the infant only at one breast for each 20-minute feeding period. They alternate breasts at different feedings.

8. To remove the baby's mouth from the breast, have mother insert finger in baby's mouth to break suction.

9. Burp the baby. This may be done over the shoulder or sitting up. Change diaper if necessary.

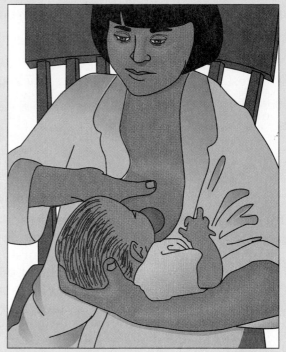

FIGURE 26-1B Football hold position for breast-feeding

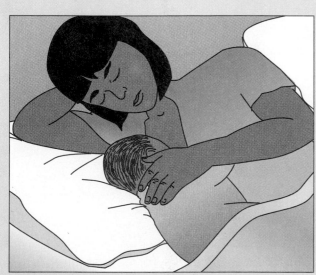

FIGURE 26-1A Side-lying position for breast-feeding

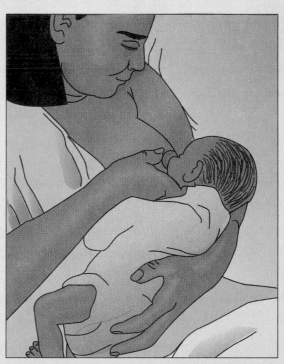

FIGURE 26-1C Cradle hold position for breast-feeding *(continues)*

CLIENT CARE PROCEDURE **66**   **Assisting with Breast-Feeding and Breast Care**
(continued)

10. Wash your hands before continuing with the procedure.
11. Help the mother with her bra, putting fresh nursing pads over the nipples if necessary. If nipples are sore or cracked, have the mother contact the nurse. An ointment or medication may be pre-scribed. Report these problems to the case manager. An over-the-counter oint-ment called Lanisol may also be used for sore or cracked nipples.
12. Return supplies to storage.
13. Wash your hands following the procedure.

cracked nipple and lead to an infection. Symp-toms of a breast infection include red, tender, or painful swelling or lumps in the breast. In addi-tion, swollen glands in the armpit or fever can also signal a breast infection. If a nursing mother has a cracked nipple, contact the physi-cian, who can recommend a soothing lanolin cream that can be applied several times daily (not before nursing). This type of cream can help the nipple heal within a few days.

Bottle-Feeding

Infant formula used in bottle-feeding combines all the nutrients found in breast milk; however, it does not provide the antibodies found in the mother's breast milk. Bottle-feeding allows all members of the family to participate in the feed-ing process. The home health aide can feed the infant or assist the new parents, following the guidelines outlined in Procedure 67.

CLIENT CARE PROCEDURE

67

Bottle-Feeding an Infant

PURPOSE

- To provide nutrition
- To give the infant the security of being held, cuddled, and bonded
- To provide opportunity to observe infant's responses, color, skin condition, etc.

PROCEDURE

1. Wash your hands before beginning the procedure.
2. Prepare formula as directed and pour into baby bottle (Figure 26-2). Put lid on bottle (Figure 26-3).

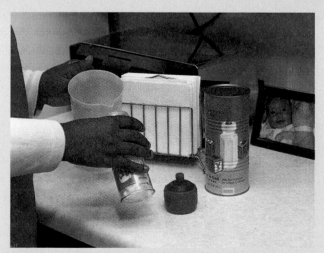

FIGURE 26-2   Prepare formula as directed.

(continues)

CLIENT CARE PROCEDURE ◆ *67* ◆ **Bottle-Feeding an Infant** *(continued)*

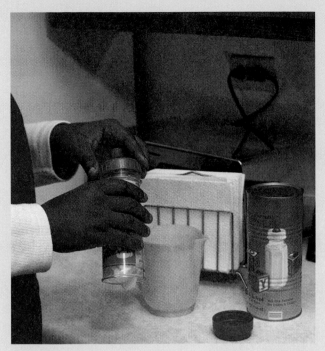

FIGURE 26-3 Put lid on bottle.

a. Test the temperature of the formula before feeding.

3. Change infant's diaper, if necessary, so infant will be comfortable, clean, and dry while eating. Wrap infant loosely in a clean receiving blanket. Leave infant in crib with side rails up.

4. Wash your hands.

5. Bring warm bottle of formula to a comfortable rocker or armchair.

6. Support the child's head and back when picking the infant up from the crib. Sit comfortably in chair, holding child securely in a comfortable position for taking nipple; start to feed the infant. Keep the nipple full of formula. Do not prop bottle (Figure 26-4).

7. When infant has had 2 to 3 ounces, either sit the infant upright on your lap and gently pat back (Figure 26-5) or hold the infant over the shoulder and pat the baby's back until the infant burps.

8. Continue feeding and burping (Figure 26-6) until infant is finished or shows no interest in eating. Do not force infant to take more than he or she wants.

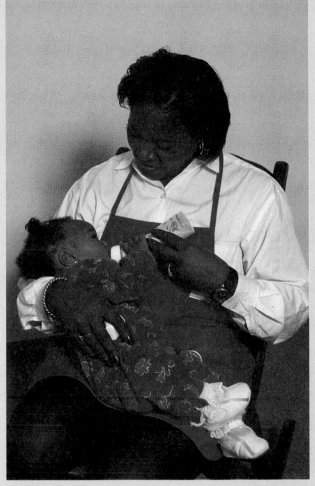

FIGURE 26-4 Sit in a comfortable chair to feed the infant, preferably a rocking chair.

9. When the baby is finished, burp him or her once more, then place in the crib, the infant lying on the side or back. *Do not place the infant on his or her stomach!* Exceptions are in the cases of:
   —Premature infants
   —Excessive spitting up or vomiting
   —Pediatrician's recommendation
   —Facial deformities that make infant susceptible to airway blockage

10. Wash your hands after the procedure. **CAUTION:** Do not put infant to bed with bottle and do not prop bottle.

(continues)

CLIENT CARE PROCEDURE **67** **Bottle-Feeding an Infant** *(continued)*

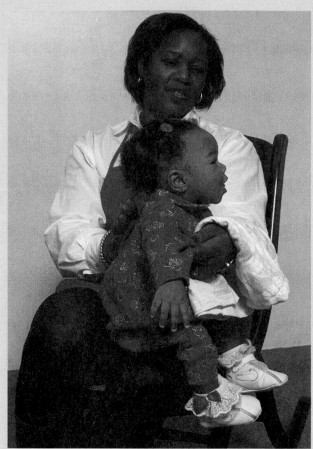

FIGURE 26-5 Burp the infant after every 2 to 3 ounces.

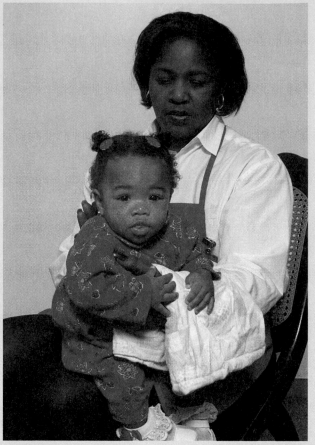

FIGURE 26-6 When you finish feeding the infant, rub the infant's back a few seconds. An infant can also be burped in this position.

Spend as much time as you can with the infant and interact with the infant (Figures 26-7, 26-8, and 26-9).

Burping the Infant

Both bottle-fed and breast-fed babies swallow air while feeding. Infants may fuss or become cranky if they need to burp. It is a good idea to burp the bottle-fed baby after the baby drinks 2 to 3 ounces and the breast-fed baby between breasts. If the infant does not burp after several minutes, continue feeding and try again when the baby is finished. Refer to Procedure 68 for techniques for burping an infant.

CARING FOR THE NEWBORN INFANT

In addition to feeding and burping the infant, the care of an infant will include bathing, care of the penis, and care of the umbilical cord.

Bathing an Infant

The newborn infant does not require much bathing as long as the diaper area is cleaned thoroughly during diaper changes. Sponge baths should be given until the stump of the umbilical cord has fallen off and the circumcision is healed (for males). Refer to Procedure 69 on how to bathe an infant.

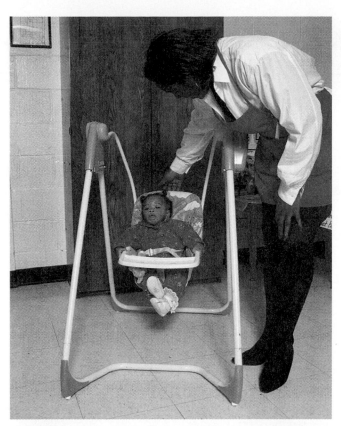

FIGURE 26-7 An infant may be placed in a swing at periodic intervals during the day.

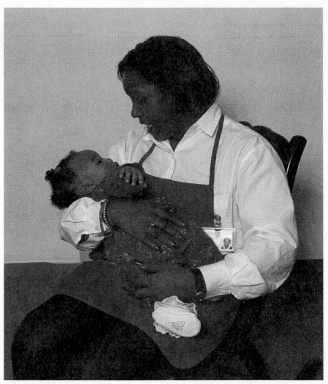

FIGURE 26-9 Infants like to be held and talked to.

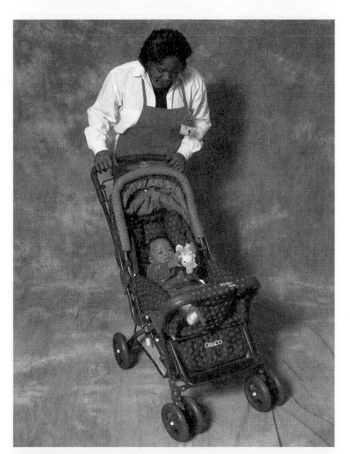

FIGURE 26-8 Infants do enjoy a short ride in a baby stroller.

Care of the Penis

At birth, the boy's **foreskin** is attached to the **glans** (head) of the penis and cannot be pushed back. Urine flows through the small opening at the tip. **Circumcision** is a procedure in which the connections between the foreskin and the glans are separated, and the foreskin is removed, leaving the glans visible. Parents may choose to have their sons circumcised in the hospital, 1 to 2 days after birth. Some Jewish parents may have circumcision done during a religious ceremony 7 days after birth.

Caring for the Circumcised Penis. A light gauze with petroleum jelly will be placed over the glans of the penis after the circumcision procedure. At each diaper change, the dressing should be changed, as recommended by the physician (usually 2 to 3 days, or until healed). The area should be kept clean, and sponge baths should continue until healed. The tip of the penis may appear red, and a yellow secretion may be noticed. This indicates the normal healing process. The redness and secretions should disappear within a week. If there is swelling, the redness persists, or crusted yellow sores appear, there may be an infection. The physician should

Burping an Infant

TECHNIQUE A—THE SITTING POSITION

1. Sit the infant in your lap.
2. Support the infant's head and chest with one hand.
3. Pat or rub the infant's back gently with the other hand (Figure 26-10).

TECHNIQUE B—THE SHOULDER POSITION

1. Put the burp cloth or pad on your shoulder.
2. Hold the baby upright, with his or her head on your shoulder (your shoulder will provide support for the baby's head and neck).
3. Gently pat or rub the baby's back (Figure 26-11).

TECHNIQUE C—THE LAP POSITION

1. Place the burp pad in your lap.
2. Place the baby in your lap, face down, with his or her head turned to one side.
3. Support the baby's head so that it is higher than the chest.

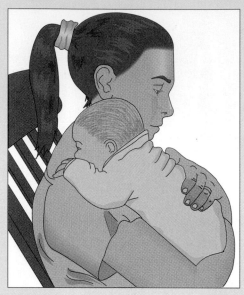

FIGURE 26-11 Hold the baby upright with baby's head on your shoulder, supporting the head and back, while you gently pat the back with your other hand.

4. Gently pat or rub the baby's back (Figure 26-12).

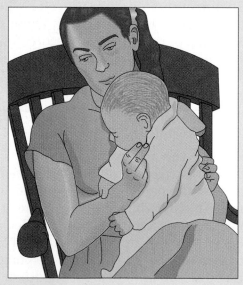

FIGURE 26-10 Sit the baby on your lap, supporting the chest and head with one hand while patting his back with your other hand.

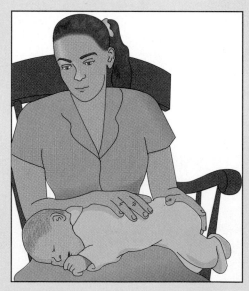

FIGURE 26-12 Lay the baby on your lap, on the baby's stomach. Support the head so it is higher than the chest, and gently pat or rotate your hand on the baby's back.

69

Bathing an Infant

PURPOSE

* To clean and refresh the infant
* To observe skin tone, activity, and signs of abnormality or unusual changes in behavior

PROCEDURE

1. Bring needed supplies to kitchen table or baby's bath table.

   warm water in basin (test temperature)
   towel and washcloth
   bath sheets
   diapers (cloth or disposable paper)
   bath oil
   baby lotion
   baby shampoo
   change of clothing (undershirt, gown, etc.)
   mild soap

2. Wash your hands thoroughly before beginning the procedure.

3. Lower side rail of crib. Keep the rail raised to its highest position whenever infant is in crib. Bring infant to bathing area.

4. Place infant on bath sheet and undress (Figure 26-13). Drop soiled diaper into diaper pail. If diaper pins are used, close diaper pins and keep out of baby's reach. **CAUTION:** *Never* leave the baby unattended while it is on the bath table or in the bath basin.

5. Place infant in bath basin one-third to half filled with warm water (Figure 26-14). Be sure to test the temperature of the water before placing the infant in the basin. Carefully supporting the baby with one hand, use your free hand to wash the infant's face with warm water only. Do not use soap on the face. Pat face dry. Make sure ears are carefully dried. Wash and rinse neck.

6. Gently apply a small amount of soap over baby's head and lather well to remove

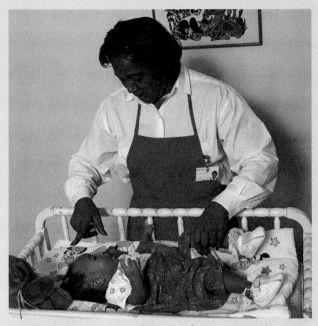

FIGURE 26-13 Undress infant. Note home health aide is talking to infant.

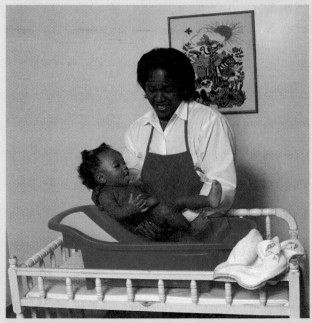

FIGURE 26-14 Slowly place the infant into basin half filled with warm water. Be sure to test temperature of water before placing infant in basin. *(continues)*

CLIENT CARE PROCEDURE **69** **Bathing an Infant** *(continued)*

crust, if present (Figure 26-15). Rinse soap away by holding head over basin as you repeatedly wipe head with wet washcloth. Keep soap out of infant's eyes. If soap is left on scalp, it will cause scales to crust and collect. Dry scalp carefully.

7. Apply soap to the infant's hands, arms, and chest. Rinse completely with washcloth.

8. Apply soap to abdomen and legs and lather well. Rinse with washcloth.

9. Turn the infant on his or her stomach and lather the back; rinse with washcloth.

10. Wash and rinse genital (perineal) area last (Figure 26-16). Wash the penis and folds of the scrotum. Dry infant (Figure 26-17).

11. Dress infant (Figure 26-18). Play and talk with infant if time allows.

12. Return supplies to storage. Clean up area where bath was given.

13. Wash your hands after the procedure.

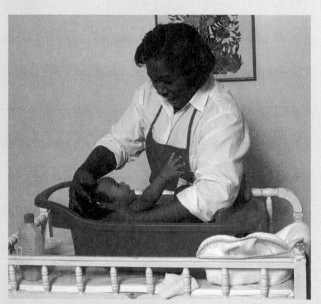

FIGURE 26-15   Massage scalp gently.

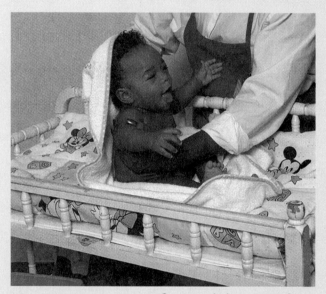

FIGURE 26-17   Dry infant with large, soft towel.

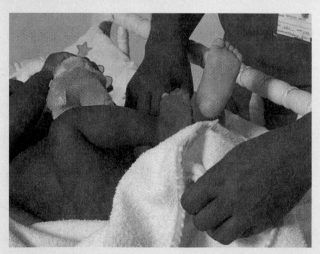

FIGURE 26-16   Wash, rinse, and dry genital area.

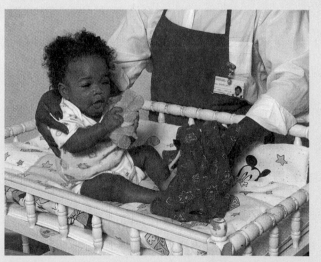

FIGURE 26-18   Dress infant. Talk and play with infant if time allows.

be notified. The penis requires no special care after the circumcision has healed.

Caring for the Uncircumcised Penis. During the first few months, the uncircumcised penis should be cleaned with soap and water. The foreskin is connected by tissue to the glans so it should not be pulled back. Once the foreskin separates naturally (could be several months to years—the physician will determine this), the foreskin should occasionally be pulled back to cleanse the penis underneath.

Care of the Umbilical Cord

During pregnancy the fetus receives its nourishment from the mother through the umbilical cord. When the baby is born, the umbilical cord is cut about 2 inches from the baby's abdomen. The remaining stump of the cord begins to dry up and then falls off within 12 to 15 days after birth, leaving the navel. Care of the umbilical cord is easy. In fact, many physicians advise not to cover the area at all and to keep the area dry. When diapering the baby, fold the top of the diaper over so that it does not cover the navel. This will promote the healing of the site. If necessary, the baby can be sponge bathed until the cord drops off. Some physicians may recommend swabbing delicately around the end of the stump with a piece of cotton dipped in alcohol. Gently pull on the stump and swab the base of the navel.

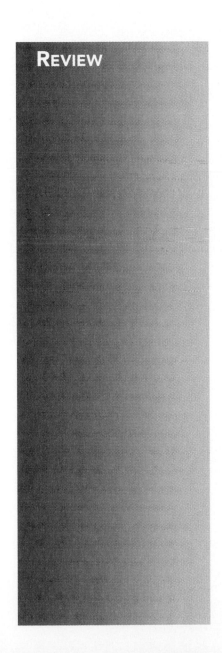

REVIEW

1. Identify at least one safety precaution associated with each of the four procedures described in this chapter.

2. T F Infants cannot be both bottled-fed and breast-fed.

3. T F Infants should be burped frequently.

4. T F Sponge baths should be given until the umbilical cord stump falls off.

5. T F All infants must be circumcised.

6. Bottle feeding:
   a. Allows other family members to feed the infant
   b. Contains antibodies not found in breast milk
   c. Is the only way to feed an infant
   d. None of the above

7. The following holds can be used by the breast-feeding mother:
   a. Football hold, upside-down hold, cradle hold
   b. Side-lying hold, football hold, cradle hold
   c. Cradle hold, side-lying hold, baseball hold
   d. The side-lying hold is the only way to hold a baby while breast-feeding.

8. Match Column I with Column II.

Column I	Column II
_____ 1. lactose	a. a hold used for breast-feeding
_____ 2. Lanisol	b. sugar
_____ 3. circumcision	c. ointment
_____ 4. cradle hold	d. a medical procedure performed on males

9. It's your first day working for a new mother/newborn. The newborn is 2 days old. The new mother is exhausted but is committed to breast-feeding her baby. She is having difficulty breast-feeding, and the baby begins crying uncontrollably. She then, in frustration, begins crying herself. What should you do?

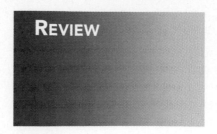

REVIEW

10. Your client, Mrs. Jones, delivered a healthy baby boy 1 week ago. On your first visit to her home she is concerned because the tip of her son's penis is still red, and she has noticed yellow secretions. She fears that he has developed an infection from the circumcision. Are these signs of an infection or is this part of the normal healing process? What signs should Mrs. Jones' watch for that would indicate an infection?

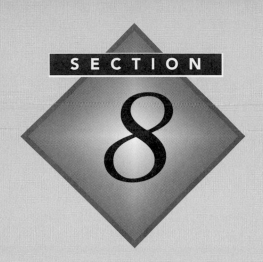

SECTION

8

Employment

Unit

27 Job-Seeking Skills

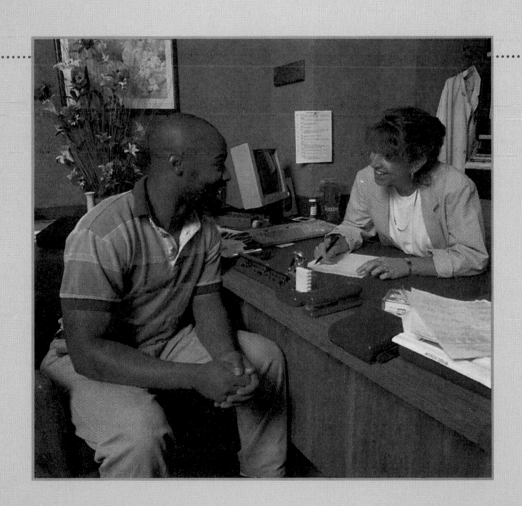

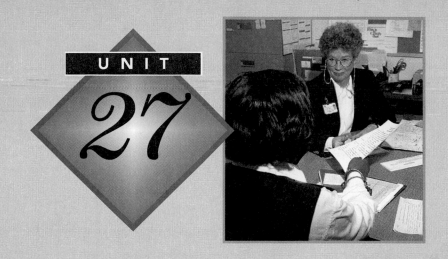

UNIT
27

Job-Seeking Skills

KEY TERMS
....

diagnosis-related group
   system (DRGs)
information sheet

infraction
misconduct

personal reference
registry service

LEARNING OBJECTIVES
....

After studying this unit, you should be able to:

- Identify three trends affecting home health care employment.
- List potential employment sites that hire homemaker/home health aides.
- Prepare a personal information sheet.
- Describe how to present yourself in a professional manner during an employment interview.

- Complete an employment application accurately.
- Give five examples of misconduct on the job.

407

One of the more difficult tasks faced by anyone is entering a new situation. As a student, you were probably afraid you would not be able to pass the tests, recite in class, or demonstrate a skill to the teacher in front of the other students. However, if you have passed your course for home health aide, you have already met these challenges. Now as a graduate, you are facing a new challenge—putting your newfound skills to work.

Until now, you have been guided by your instructor(s) and for the most part have worked in a team situation with your fellow students. Now you are on your own. You must "sell" yourself and your skills to an employer.

You must make your own decisions as to what kind of clients you prefer to work with. Do you want part-time or full-time work? Do you want a sleep-in job? Would you rather work with elderly clients who mainly need companionship and minimal care, or do you want to use all your skills and deal with complex medical problems? Do you prefer working with children or are you willing to take whatever jobs are open?

These questions must be answered by you so that you can conduct an effective job search that will result in employment.

TRENDS AFFECTING EMPLOYMENT ····

During the past 15 years, the need for home health care services in the United States has increased. In October 1983, the **diagnosis-related group system (DRGs)** for reimbursing hospitals was enacted to control costs. This system has encouraged early discharge of patients who are sicker and in need of special care. Medicare-covered home health visits have increased from 31 million in 1984 to 209 million in 1996. An estimated 9 to 11 million individuals need assistance with daily living activities. Sixteen percent of those individuals are institutionalized, whereas 84% live in the community.

Another trend is that hospitals are changing their focus from acute care to a community concept of care. A few hospitals are now offering or sponsoring adult day care, home health care, and continuing care retirement communities. Other housing arrangements that allow the person to remain at home and maintain independence are also becoming popular. A few examples of these options are: house sharing, where two or more unrelated people live together in a combination of shared and common space; board and care homes that provide a room, three meals a day, and personal care services; congregate housing facilities that offer independent living with central dining and social and recreational programs.

Government programs also provide funds for home-delivered meals, friendly visits, telephone reassurance, and chore services. (Chore services done by the chore aide usually include services such as shopping, marketing, transportation, and heavy cleaning.) These services may be offered free of charge or on a sliding scale fee basis. In some cases, both cost savings and increased independence can be achieved by using various home health care services plus housing options instead of nursing homes. These different housing options provide a variety of employment opportunities for the home health aide.

The demand for home health care and assistance with activities of daily living by the young as well as the old will continue to increase. Americans age 85 and older are the fastest growing segment of our population, and 49% of these individuals will need some assistance with their personal care needs. The rise in the number of individuals with AIDS will also increase the need for additional home health aides. Health care services rank in the top five in the nation as far as job opportunities are concerned.

CONTACTING PROSPECTIVE EMPLOYERS·······

Your first step toward finding a job is to research your community's job market. Local and national agencies in most areas are listed in the telephone directory. Your instructor may also be able to provide you with a list of possibilities. You can look in the employment section of your local newspaper; you can contact your local department of social services; and you can see if area hospitals have a **registry service** or home health agency where you may apply. Some medical groups also have lists of clients who need home health aides.

Make a list of those places you plan to contact; then keep a record of the date you called and any appointments you may set up. Remember, you may register at several agencies and you may work for more than one agency on a part-time basis. When you telephone for an appointment, know what you want to say. "I am a graduate of the ABC home health program, and I am looking for work. May I have an appointment to discuss job opportunities in your agency?"

THE JOB INTERVIEW, APPLICATION FORM, AND JOB OFFER

Demonstrating a professional attitude and appearance throughout the job search process will help you in your job search. The interview provides you an opportunity to discuss your skills, but also helps you to learn more about the company and the people with whom you may be working. Completing the application form and negotiating a job offer are also important steps in the job search process.

The Interview

When you go to your appointment remember that first impressions are vital. Dress neatly and look your best.

It is better to go alone to the interview. Bringing someone with you to the interview may give the impression that you are not able to make decisions alone.

Before you go to the interview, research all you can about the agency. (Check in the yellow pages to see what services they offer, ask employees about what type of clients they serve, etc.). It is also good to familiarize yourself with typical interview questions and decide how you will answer them. Practice answering typical interview questions. Some sample interview questions are:

- Have you had previous homemaker/home health aide work experience?
- Do you have any training related to home health care?
- Can you tell me about your previous employment?
- Explain any time gaps between jobs.
- Why did you leave your last job?
- Why are you interested in this job?
- What did you like most/least about past jobs?
- What are your strengths/weaknesses?

Determine what you will wear. Dress neatly and conservatively—remember you only have one chance to make a good first impression. Avoid excessive jewelry and makeup (Figure 27-1).

Arrive at least 15 minutes early. This will tell your prospective employer that you are prepared to arrive on time for your assignments if you are hired. Make sure you know the name of the interviewer and that you know how to get to the appropriate location.

Introduce yourself to the interviewer by name, with a smile and *firm* handshake and eye contact. Always be polite, speak clearly, sit or stand straight, and use correct grammar—no slang. Do not chew gum or smoke during the interview. Answer all questions truthfully and with more than one word. Be ready to talk about the training and experiences you have had. Be positive about former employers and working conditions. Be honest about the kind of cases you prefer. Take a copy of certification, Social Security card, and also an official ID. The interview is the employer's opportunity to get to

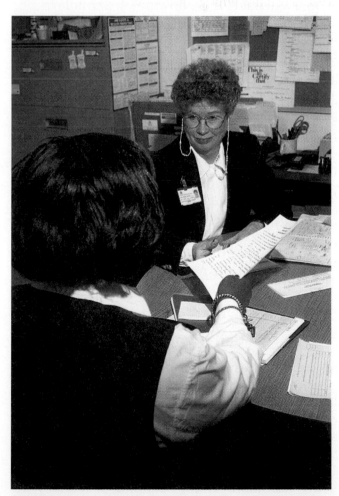

FIGURE 27-1   Dress neatly for the job interview.

know you. It is also the time for you to learn about the employer. Prepare a list of questions before going to the interview. The interviewer may ask if you have questions. It is good to ask questions; it shows that you prepared for the interview. Some suggested questions are:

- How far will I need to travel to and from each client? Is public transportation available or will I need to have an automobile?
- What shift or shifts will I be expected to work?
- If the position is part-time, is there a possibility of a full-time position soon?
- Is there a mechanism in place for advancement or additional training?
- Is overtime available?
- What are the fringe benefits? Is health insurance available and for what cost? Do I get holiday or vacation pay? Do I get sick days? Is there a pension plan available?
- Is child care available? If so, at what times and what is the cost? Do they take infants?
- If traveling is required between clients, is mileage paid? If so, how much per mile?

Listen carefully to your interviewer. Do not immediately ask about salary or benefits unless the employer brings it up first. This information is usually supplied by the interviewer toward the end of the interview. If you are unclear about information on the position, ask questions.

You should not anticipate receiving a definite indication of a job offer or rejection at the end of the interview. The interviewer will usually let you know when you will be contacted. Remember to thank the interviewer as you leave.

After the interview, send a thank-you letter and again express an interest in the position. Try to evaluate the interview to discover ways to improve for the next one. It is all right to call the agency in a few days to inquire about the status of the position.

The Application Form

Have an **information sheet** with you listing some facts that usually appear on an application form. This will save you time and you will not make foolish errors when you fill out the application. Some of the facts that you should have on your information sheet are listed in Figure 27-2.

If you do not have a telephone, you should leave the number of a neighbor or friend who has agreed to take messages for you. **Personal**

references may not be relatives, but may include your minister, doctor, or instructor(s). Be sure that you have permission from those people you list as references to use their names. If possible, obtain letters of recommendation from these people before you go for a job interview. This will save time for the agency, and the person who is giving the recommendation only has to write one letter of reference. The agency can then make a copy of your letters of reference and confirm them by telephone.

Each agency will have its own application form, but if you are prepared with the sample in Figure 27-2, you should not have any difficulty completing the agency application form. It is always a good idea to read the application form carefully before completing it. It may include special instructions, such as asking the applicant to type or print all information. Fill out each item neatly and completely. Do not leave any items blank; if the item does not apply to you, write "N.A." (not applicable). Take care to spell words and to punctuate sentences carefully. Bring a pocket dictionary if you have difficulty spelling. Do not write in spaces marked "office use only." Review your application before submitting it to the employer. Remember to bring your own black or blue pen.

You should have with you your Social Security card, your alien green card, a driver's license, your certificate, and, if at all possible, a copy of your most recent physical examination showing your immunizations, including hepatitis B, the results of a tuberculosis test, and other facts about your personal physical condition. Some agencies will have their own form to be given to the examining physician (Figure 27-3).

The Job Offer

If you are offered the job, you have the choice of accepting the agency's terms, thinking about it for a few days, or looking elsewhere for a position. Once you have accepted a position with an agency, be realistic in your goals. As in any kind of employment, this is a system of progression where the new employees must prove themselves. It is possible that an agency may test you by calling you for weekend or holiday part-time work. Many employers think it is a sign of dedication if you accept the assignments offered. After you have worked for a while, the agency will have a better idea of your abilities

CUSHMAN MANAGEMENT ASSOCIATES

EMPLOYER:

APPLICATION FOR EMPLOYMENT

We are an equal opportunity employer. Federal and state laws prohibit discrimination in employment practices based on race, color, religion, sex, age, handicap, disability, or national origin. No question on this application is asked for the purpose of limiting or excluding any applicant's consideration for employment because of his or her race, color, religion, sex, age, handicap, disability, or national origin.

Name: Last	First	Middle	Social Security No.	Telephone No.

Address: Street	City	State	Zip Code	Licensed Nurses Only	
				Mass. Reg. No.	Date Granted:

If your records may be under a name other than indicated above, please specify:	Last Renewal:	Expiration Date:

Are you a citizen of the United States? ☐ yes ☐ no	If you are not a U.S. Citizen, do you have the legal right to remain permanently in the United States? ☐ yes ☐ no	Explain

Are you between the ages of 18 and 70? ☐ yes ☐ no	Do you know of any fact that would limit or impair your ability to perform the functions of the job you are applying for? ☐ yes ☐ no	Describe

Date of last Physical Examination:	Family Physician:	I authorize my doctor to release to you the results of my pre-employment and subsequent medical examinations, and to discuss those results with you. ☐ yes ☐ no

Position desired:	Hours desired:	Salary expected:

Specialized training or experience not shown on other side of form:

Where now employed?	Reason for desiring change:

Have you ever pleaded guilty or been convicted of a felony? ☐ yes ☐ no   If yes to either, please explain:

or a misdemeanor other than a first conviction for drunkenness, simple assault, speeding, minor traffic violations, affray, or disturbance of the peace within the past 5 years? ☐ yes ☐ no

In case of emergency notify	name	relationship
	address	telephone

*I authorize the schools, employers, and individuals listed in this application to release any information regarding my previous employment, character, general reputation and personal characteristics. ☐ yes ☐ no

I certify that the statements I have made in this application are true and hereby grant the employer permission to verify the accuracy and completeness of this information and to investigate all references and educational records. I understand that any false or misleading statements made by me on this application or in conjunction with my physical examination will be sufficient cause for the rejection of this application or for immediate dismissal if such false or misleading information is discovered after my employment. If I am accepted for employment, I agree to abide by the rules and regulations of the employer.

Signed _____

Date _____

E-2   "It is unlawful in Massachusetts to require or administer a lie detector test as a condition of employment or continued employment. An employer who violates this law shall be subject to criminal penalties and civil liability".

FIGURE 27-2 On application forms, answer all questions to the best of your ability. Be sure the information is accurate. (Courtesy of Danvers Twin Oaks Nursing Home)

and strengths and will work you into a regular schedule.

When you are employed by an agency, you may be asked to sign a document similar to the one presented in Figure 27-4. This document will indicate the policies and rules of the agency and the consequences to employees for breaking the

rules (**infractions**) or for incidents of **misconduct.** Read it carefully and be willing to accept and abide by the conditions included in it.

Many states now require restrictive codes for agencies providing home health care services. To be qualified to operate, agencies must meet exacting standards set by both the Depart-

TO THE PHYSICIAN: Please fill out the following medical form as completely as possible. State law requires that our employees have a completed physical on file with a yearly update. Please forward this form immediately on completion of examination. Pending test results will be followed up by our office. Information required is indicated by a checkmark.

NAME OF PATIENT: _____ AGE: _____

ADDRESS: _____

           Street No.   Town (City)   State   Zip Code

PHYSICAL FINDINGS:

BP:_____ Pulse:_____ Resp:_____ Height:_____ Weight:_____

___ Cardiovascular   ___ Gastrointestinal   ___ Musculoskeletal
___ Respiratory   ___ Genitourinary   ___ Nervous

___ Above physical findings essentially normal.
___ Abnormal findings/limitations: _____

_____

HISTORY

Habituation/Addiction
___ Alcohol   ___ Depressants   ___ Stimulants   ___ Narcotics   ___ Other: _____
If any, please explain: _____

Illness/Injury — please indicate any past or present condition that would result in physical, mental, or behavioral limitations in normal functioning: _____

MANDATORY IMMUNIZATIONS/TESTS:

DIPHTHERIA/TETANUS — should have booster every 10 years.
Date of Last Immunization: _____

RUBELLA — *Must* show proof of immunity through direct immunization or *positive* antibody titer test.
Date of immunization: _____ Date of Antibody Titer Test: _____
                                    Results: _____

TUBERCULOSIS — *Must* have Mantoux (PPD) skin test every year and follow-up chest x-ray if test
    results positive.   Follow-up Chest
Date of Mantoux: _____ Results: _____ x-ray date: _____
Hepatitis B Vaccine: _____   Pos.   Neg.
ENTERIC PATHOGENS — stool examination and/or culture (only if indicated by checkmark)
Date of Examination/Culture: _____ Results: _____

This person (is is not) physically and mentally capable of performing the functions of an aide in the home setting, and is free from any condition that would endanger his/her safety or the safety and well-being of the clients to be cared for.

DATE: _____ PHYSICIAN'S SIGNATURE: _____

                ADDRESS: _____
                        Street No.   City   State   Zip Code
                PHONE NO.: _____

FIGURE 27-3 Some agencies have their own forms for physical examination.

TO THE EMPLOYEE

Because you are important to us, we want to help you develop a good work record. If we feel that you are violating any of our rules and policies, or that you have misunderstood the terms of employment, we will hold a conference with you. Continued *infractions* will cause your immediate dismissal. PLEASE READ THE FOLLOWING CAREFULLY.

1. *Attendance and tardiness record:* Recurring cancellations of promised scheduled workdays may result in dismissal. Absence without call in may result in immediate termination. No pay raises will be granted if attendance and tardiness records are unsatisfactory. We must be able to depend on you. You must call in if you are unable to meet your assignment.

2. *Unbecoming conduct:* Any of the following are considered to be gross *misconduct:* carelessness and inattention to client care; failure to perform duties; violation of safe practices; inefficiency and wasting of materials; refusal to obey direct orders; insubordination; rude, discourteous, or uncivil behavior; intoxication, drinking, or possession of intoxicating beverages while on duty; gambling on duty; sleeping on duty; unauthorized absence from assignment or leaving early without permission; failure to report an injury or accident concerning an employee or client; soliciting tips from clients or families; sale of services to clients or families; divulging confidential information about client and family; theft and/or dishonesty; *pilferage* of drugs or violation of any law on drug use including use or sale of same; damaging, defacing, or mishandling equipment or property; interfering with work performance of another employee; falsifying client or personnel records or any form of misrepresentation.

Employee's statement:

I have read the above rules and regulations and understand my responsibilities to the agency and client. I agree to abide by these terms of employment.

_____   _____
Employee Signature   Date

_____   _____
Supervisor's Signature   Date

FIGURE 27-4 Once you have decided to accept a position with an agency, you may be asked to sign a document that states that you have read and understand the rules of the agency.

ment of Health and the Department of Social Services. Included in the standards required by New York State are:

- A grievance procedure for an agency's employees
- A patient's bill of rights that *must* be explained to the client (or client's family) in the presence of a witness
- Documentation of certification of all employees
- Proof of an annual physical examination by employees
- Proof of employee's attendance at a minimum number of in-service programs each year
- Proof of citizenship or verified alien registration
- Satisfactory completion of an approved home health aide course of study
- No legal record of client abuse or misuses of client's property in a caregiver's situation
- Proof of being on the state registry for home health aide in the state in which you are applying for a position

REVIEW

1. A recent trend affecting home health care employment is:
   a. Hospitals are discharging sicker patients
   b. The focus of hospitals is now a community concept approach
   c. Millions of individuals who live in their own homes need assistance with daily living activities
   d. All of the above

2. When is the best time to arrive for an interview?
   a. An hour before the scheduled interview time
   b. Five minutes late to show you are not overly eager
   c. Exactly at the scheduled interview time
   d. Fifteen minutes before the scheduled interview time

3. T   F   You should bring someone with you to the interview.

4. T   F   You should practice interviewing before you go.

5. T   F   Do not ask any questions in the interview.

6. T   F   If you do not know how to answer a question on an application, leave it blank.

Use the following terms to fill in the blanks in questions 7–11.

information sheet   misconduct   personal references

infractions   newspaper

7. The employment section of the _____ is a good place to locate job leads.

8. Complete an _____ before the interview so you will be prepared to complete a job application.

9. Ministers, doctors, and instructors are considered _____ . Relatives are not.

10. Continued _____ could lead to immediate dismissal when employed.

11. Violation of safe work practices, carelessness, and inattention to client care, failure to perform duties, and insubordination are all examples of _____ .

12. You are in the waiting room of a prospective employer. A lady in the waiting room asks you to hold her 2-year-old child while she uses the bathroom. What should you do?

13. The interviewer offers you a job with her agency as soon as you walk in the door without asking you any questions or describing the position. What should you do?

14. You discover an ad in the newspaper for a job for which you are qualified and which is of interest to you. When you call about the position, the person answering the telephone says she does not know anything about it. What do you do?

Appendices

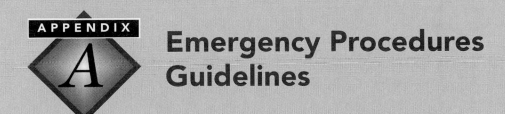

Emergency Procedures Guidelines

This appendix identifies emergency situations and the procedures that should be followed by the homemaker/home health aide in emergencies.

First aid is care given to clients who suffer from accidents or sudden illnesses until more help is available. A client should be treated physically and emotionally, and may need reassurance as well as physical care. The whole environment must be evaluated to prevent further injury. First aid is **immediate care** that must be given after the **emergency medical system (EMS)** in your area has been notified.

In the home, emergency phone numbers should be posted by the telephone. Include the local emergency squad, fire department, police, ambulance, poison control center, and family or friends the client wants contacted in case of an emergency. If someone needs immediate help, the homemaker/home health aide may need to evaluate the situation and give emergency care according to the priority of needs.

Do not leave someone who requires immediate help. Have someone else call for help. When clients need immediate help and there is no one in the home, homemaker/home health aides should assess each situation and respond based on their knowledge, abilities, training, and experience. Several emergency situations and the appropriate homemaker/home health aide responses will be covered in this appendix.

When a client needs help, but not **immediate** care to sustain life, the aide's responsibility is to prevent more injury, seek medical help, and keep the client calm. For example, if a client's skirt caught fire and burned her legs, you would put the fire out before getting help for the burns. **Good judgment** is needed to give good emergency care. The whole situation must be evaluated to see what help is needed first and what further problems could arise.

Because this appendix covers only some life-threatening situations, it is advisable to take a course in cardiopulmonary resuscitation (CPR) and have current first aid books readily available for handling emergencies. Check with your agency regarding its emergency procedure policies.

BLEEDING

1. Wear gloves and follow the principles of standard precautions for a client who is bleeding.
2. Cover wound using a clean cloth, gauze, or hand.
3. Place your hand over bandage. Apply firm pressure for approximately 5 minutes or until bleeding slows or stops.
4. Do not lift bandage to check bleeding. If blood soaks through, apply another bandage on top. Remember to keep pressure firm on wound.
5. Raise injured part above level of victim's heart (unless you suspect broken bones).
6. Stay with the client until help arrives.

BURNS

Burns are very painful and, in extreme cases, can even be life-threatening. To determine the severity of the burn, you will need to know the degree of injury involved.

1st degree—Red and painful, like a sunburn

2nd degree—Red and painful, with blistering

3rd degree—May be black or white; there may or may not be pain involved

What To Do

1. If at all possible, "stop the burning." This is done by removing the source of burn, i.e., hot iron.
2. Immerse burned area in cold water. If this is not possible, apply cold water directly to area with a cloth, sponge, etc.
3. *Do not* apply oil, butter, or ointments to burn (this holds heat in).
4. *Do not* break blisters.
5. Place clean wet dressing on area (use sterile cloth if available).
6. Call physician or emergency room for further instructions. Stay with the client until help arrives.

CHOKING

When a client is choking, you must act quickly; seconds count and can mean the difference between life or death. Figure 1 shows the universal sign for choking.

1. If the client can speak, wheeze, or moan, encourage him or her to cough out the object.
2. If client is coughing, encourage him or her to keep coughing until object is actually dislodged.
3. If client is unable to make any noise:
   - Stand directly behind client.
   - Place one hand on client's chest.
   - Give client four quick slaps to upper back area, between shoulder blades, using the palm of your hand.

If this attempt to dislodge the object fails, you must immediately begin to give abdominal

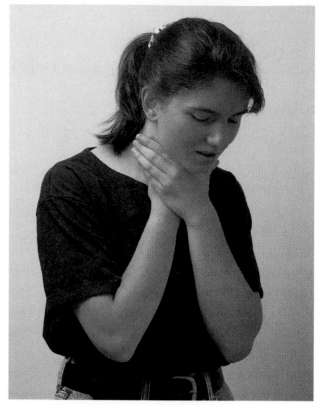

FIGURE 1 The person is choking. She cannot speak, cough, or breathe.

thrusts (Heimlich maneuver). (Again, check with your agency regarding their emergency policies before using certain procedures.)

Abdominal Thrusts (Heimlich Maneuver)

1. Stand directly behind client.
2. Reach both your arms around client's waist.
3. Make a fist with one hand, keeping thumb straight (Figure 2A). Place fist, thumb side in, against abdomen slightly above navel.
4. Grasp hold of fist with other hand (Figure 2B); press fist inward and upward, using short, quick movements.
5. Procedure should be repeated until object is dislodged or person becomes unconscious.

Obstructed Airway

If you suspect a blockage or obstruction of the airway and are not trained in the procedures of CPR, you may open the individual's

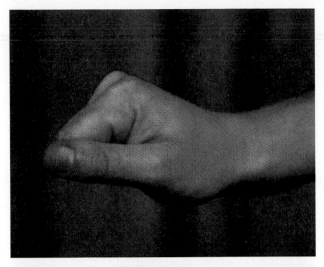

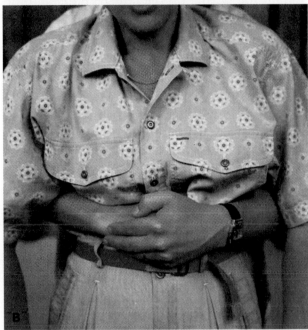

FIGURE 2 Abdominal thrust

airway until the emergency medical service or help arrives. This is done as follows:

1. Place fingers of one hand on forehead.
2. Place fingers of opposite hand just beneath chin area.
3. Hyperextend (or tilt neck upward).
4. Activate EMS.

Do not attempt this procedure if you suspect neck or spinal cord injury or see obvious fracture.

POISONING

Swallowed

When you suspect someone may have swallowed poison, the three most important things you can do are:

1. Find out exactly what was taken (you will need to know name, ingredients—if listed—and amount swallowed).
2. Call your local poison control center (PCC) or hospital emergency room.
3. Follow the instructions they give you.

(Do not give antidotes or induce vomiting unless specifically told by PCC to do so.)

Inhaled

1. Get fresh air for patient—preferably outdoors.
2. Call PCC or activate EMS.

Skin

1. Flush with water at least 10 minutes.
2. Call PCC or activate EMS.

SHOCK

Shock can be life-threatening, and requires immediate attention. Symptoms may include:

Pale, cool, moist, or sweaty skin. Patient may be restless or drowsy, may have rapid and irregular heartbeat and breathing, may complain of nausea and chills; may have bluish discoloration of lips and nailbeds. Pupils may be enlarged or dilated.

Activate EMS Immediately

1. Induce patient to lie down.
2. Elevate legs (unless you suspect fracture).
3. Cover with blanket if cold; provide shade if hot.
4. Keep patient quiet and comfortable (be reassuring).
5. Do NOT give anything by mouth.

SEIZURES

A convulsive seizure occurs when the whole brain is suddenly swamped with *extra electrical energy*. It may start out as a hoarse cry caused by air being suddenly forced out of the lungs. The person may fall to the ground unconscious. The body may briefly stiffen; this may be followed by the onset of jerky movements.

First aid for seizures is simple and designed to protect the safety of the person until the seizure stops naturally, by itself. These are the key things to remember:

1. Keep calm and reassure other people who may be nearby.
2. Clear the area around the person of anything hard or sharp.
3. Loosen constrictive clothing that may make breathing difficult, such as a necktie, shirt collar, or belt. Remove glasses if worn.
4. Put something flat and soft, like a folded jacket, under the person's head.
5. If there is excess saliva during the convulsion, turn the head (*and the head only*) gently to the side to facilitate drainage of mucus and saliva. This will help keep the airway clear. *Do not* try to force the mouth open with any hard object or with fingers. A person having a seizure *cannot swallow his tongue*, and efforts to hold the tongue down can injure teeth or jaw.
6. Do not hold the person down or try to stop his movements.
7. Do not attempt artificial respiration except in the unlikely event the person does not start breathing again after the seizure has stopped.
8. Stay with the person until the seizure ends naturally.
9. Be friendly and reassuring as consciousness returns.

HEART ATTACK/STROKE

Heart attacks and strokes are both serious medical conditions that require immediate attention.

Heart attack symptoms may include chest pain (described as pressure, or like something sitting on the chest), nausea, indigestion, vomiting, profuse sweating, or pain radiating into arm or jaw.

What To Do (if Victim is Conscious)

1. Activate EMS in your area.
2. Tell EMS your exact location.
3. Stay with client and remain calm.
4. Do not take client to hospital yourself or allow client to refuse treatment.
5. If you are trained in CPR, be prepared to start procedure immediately if symptoms require CPR.

Stroke symptoms may vary, but the most common symptoms are sudden weakness or numbness in the face or arm or one side of the body, loss or slurring of speech, difficulty understanding speech of others, consistently falling to one side, or unexplained unsteadiness.

Because stroke is diagnosed by history and physical examination, prompt medical treatment is necessary and should be sought immediately.

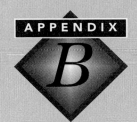
Temperature Conversion Chart

NOTE: The following table is provided as an aid for study and comparison of temperatures. Some homemaking duties and client care procedures refer to temperatures in Fahrenheit or Celsius.

DEGREES FAHRENHEIT TO DEGREES CELSIUS AND VICE VERSA											
°F	°C	°F	°C	°F	°C	°F	°C	°F	°C	°F	°C
96	35.6	118	47.8	140	60	162	72.2	184	84.4	206.6	97
96.8	36	118.4	48	141	60.6	163	72.8	185	85	207	97.2
97	36.1	119	48.3	141.8	61	163.4	73	186	85.6	208	97.8
98	36.7	120	48.9	142	61.1	164	73.3	186.8	86	208.4	98
98.6	37	120.2	49	143	61.7	165	73.9	187	86.1	209	98.3
99	37.2	121	49.4	143.6	62	165.2	74	188	86.7	210	98.9
100	37.8	122	50	144	62.2	166	74.4	188.6	87	210.2	99
100.4	38	123	50.6	145	62.8	167	75	189	87.2	211	99.4
101	38.3	123.8	51	145.4	63	168	75.6	190	87.8	212	100
102	38.9	124	51.1	146	63.3	168.8	76	190.4	88	213	100.6
102.2	39	125	51.7	147	63.9	169	76.1	191	88.3	213.8	101
103	39.4	125.6	52	147.2	64	170	76.7	192	88.9	214	101.1
104	40	126	52.2	148	64.4	170.6	77	192.2	89	215	101.7
105	40.6	127	52.8	149	65	171	77.2	193	89.4	215.6	102
105.8	41	127.4	53	150	65.6	172	77.8	194	90	216	102.2
106	41.1	128	53.3	150.8	66	172.4	78	195	90.6	217	102.8
107	41.7	129	53.9	151	66.1	173	78.3	195.8	91	217.4	103
107.6	42	129.2	54	152	66.7	174	78.9	196	91.1	218	103.3
108	42.2	130	54.4	152.6	67	174.2	79	197	91.7	219	103.9
109	42.8	131	55	153	67.2	175	79.4	197.6	92	219.2	104
109.4	43	132	55.6	154	67.8	176	80	198	92.2	220	104.4
110	43.3	132.8	56	154.4	68	177	80.6	199	92.8	221	105
111	43.9	133	56.1	155	68.3	177.8	81	199.4	93	225	107.2
111.2	44	134	56.7	156	68.9	178	81.1	200	93.3	230	110
112	44.4	134.6	57	156.2	69	179	81.7	201	93.9	235	112.8
113	45	135	57.2	157	69.4	179.6	82	201.2	94	239	115
114	45.6	136	57.8	158	70	180	82.2	202	94.4	240	115.6
114.8	46	136.4	58	159	70.6	181	82.8	203	95	245	118.3
115	46.1	137	58.3	159.8	71	181.4	83	204	95.6	248	120
116	46.7	138	58.9	160	71.1	182	83.3	204.8	96	250	121.1
116.6	47	138.2	59	161	71.7	183	83.9	205	96.1	255	123.9
117	47.2	139	59.4	161.6	72	183.2	84	206	96.7	257	125

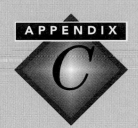

Sample of Weekly Time Sheet

064·40·0878	Name:	Judy Goldstein		W/E	00-00-00
SS #					Month - Day - Year

PRINT THIS TIME SHEET   USE A SEPARATE LINE FOR EACH CASE   SKIP A LINE BETWEEN DAYS

Agency	Case #	CLIENT Last Name–First initial	DATE Mo.	Day	Travel to 1st Case Hr.	Min.	Mi.	Fare	Arrived Hr.	Min.	Left Hr.	Min.	Svce. Hrs.	Miles on Case	Travel to next case Hr.	Min.	Mi.	Fare	Travel to Home Hr.	Min.	Mi.	Fare	Other Exp.	Signature
VNA	2303	Brown, J.	9	6	25	6			9	00	12	00	3						25	6			.10	J. Brown
		Holiday	9	7																				
ERDS·C	1963	Casillio, P.	9	8	20	8			8	30	12	30	4	6		30	10							P. Casillio
SOC.SERV	2036	Williams, S.	9	8					1	00	4	00	3						35	12			.30	Sam Williams
V.A.	1845	Kelly, A.	9	9	20	8			9	00	5	00	8	28					25					A. Kelly
VNA	2306	Garcia, M.	9	10	40	15			8	30	12	30	4											M. Garcia
SOC.SERV	1495	Garcia, M.	9	10	20	8			12	30	4	30	4						45	15				M. Garcia

Daily and Weekly Scheduling Chart

DAILY AND WEEKLY SCHEDULING

As a beginning home health aide, you may have some difficulty in scheduling your activities. The authors have prepared a time checklist, which they recommend be used until you have established a pattern of work. It provides a reminder of what is expected. An individual notebook, detailing the procedures done and the time required for each, can be kept instead of a checklist.

You should become accustomed to making a working schedule and putting it into prac-tice. Conferences with your instructor may be helpful in recognizing areas in which you can make adjustments leading to greater efficiency and ease of accomplishing goals. The need for personal flexibility should be stressed. You should be flexible to meet client needs and still maintain the home within reasonable bounds.

As each procedure is completed, note the time required. At the end of the day make a note of undone tasks, and see if the time spent could have been used more effectively.

Daily Checklist

Duties	Completed	Time Required
AM client care	_____	_____
Client unit—bedroom/bath	_____	_____
Breakfast made/served	_____	_____
Kitchen clean up	_____	_____
Shopping	_____	_____
House cleaned	_____	_____
Lunch made/served	_____	_____
Aide's lunch period	_____	_____
Kitchen clean up	_____	_____
Laundry/ironing	_____	_____
Major job—clean oven	_____	_____
refrigerator		
mop floor		
vacuum		
Other client care	_____	_____
List procedures		
_____	_____	_____
_____	_____	_____
_____	_____	_____
PM client care	_____	_____

Observations by home health aide_____

_____

_____

APPENDIX E
Living Will and Durable Power of Attorney

In 1991, the United States government mandated that individuals seeking health care complete an advance directives statement. The two common types of advance directives are living wills and durable power of attorney. One of these forms should be completed before the client's care is started and while the client is mentally competent.

LIVING WILL

DIRECTIVE MADE this _____ day of _____, 19__, to my physicians, my attorneys, my clergyman, my family or others responsible for my health, welfare or affairs.

BE IT KNOWN, that I, _____, of _____ State of _____, being of sound mind, willfully and voluntarily make known my desire that my life shall not be artificially prolonged under the circumstances set forth below and do hereby declare that, if at any time I should have an incurable injury, disease or illness certified to be a terminal condition by two physicians and where the application of life-sustaining procedures would serve only to artificially prolong the moment of my death and where my physician determines that my death is imminent or needlessly prolonged whether or not life-sustaining procedures are utilized, I direct that such procedures be withheld or withdrawn and that I be permitted to die naturally with only the merciful administration of medication to eliminate or reduce pain to my mind and body or the performance of any medical procedure deemed necessary to provide me with comfort care. In the absence of my ability to give directions regarding the use of such life-sustaining procedures, it is my intention that this directive shall be honored by my family and physician(s) as the final expression of my legal right to refuse medical or surgical treatment and I accept the consequences from such refusal. If I have bequeathed organs, I ask that I be kept alive for a sufficient time to enable the proper withdrawal and transplant of said organs.

Special provisions:

As a witness to this act I state the declarer has been personally known to me and I believe said declarer to be of sound mind.

Signed in the presence of:

_____   _____
Witness   Address

_____   _____
Witness   Address

State of

County of   SS.   , 19

      BE IT KNOWN, that the above named   ,
personally known to me as the same person described in and who executed the within Living Will acknowledged to me that said instrument was freely and voluntarily executed for the purposes therein expressed, and that said Living Will was duly executed in my presence.

_____
Notary Public

My Commission Expires:

DURABLE POWER OF ATTORNEY
FOR HEALTH CARE

BE IT KNOWN, that   ,
of   , the
undersigned Grantor, does hereby grant a durable power of attorney for health care to
                                                                    , of
, as my attorney-in-fact and Agent.

I hereby grant to my Agent full power and authority to make health care decisions for me to the same extent that I could make such decisions for myself if I had the capacity to do so. In exercising this authority, my Agent shall make health care decisions that are consistent with my desires as stated in this document or otherwise made known to my Agent, including, but not limited to, my desires concerning obtaining or refusing or withdrawing life prolonging care, treatment, services, and procedures.

I hereby authorize all physicians and psychiatrists who have treated me, and all other providers of health care, including hospitals, to release to my Agent all information contained in my medical records which my Agent may request. I hereby waive all privileges attached to physician-patient relationship and to any communication, verbal or written, arising out of such a relationship. My Agent is authorized to request, receive and review any information, verbal or written, pertaining to my physical or mental health, including medical and hospital records, and to execute any releases, waivers or other documents that may be required in order to obtain such information, and to disclose such information to such persons, organizations and health care providers as my Agent shall deem appropriate. My Agent is authorized to employ and discharge health care providers including physicians, psychiatrists, dentists, nurses, and therapists as my Agent shall deem appropriate for my physical, mental and emotional well-being. My Agent is also authorized to pay reasonable fees and expenses for such services contracted.

My Agent is authorized to apply for my admission to a medical, nursing, residential or other similar facility, execute any consent or admission forms required by such facility and enter into agreements for my care at such facility or elsewhere during my lifetime. My Agent is authorized to arrange for and consent to medical, therapeutical and surgical procedures for me including the administration of drugs. The power to make health care decisions for me shall include the power to give consent, refuse consent, or withdraw consent to any care, treatment, service, or procedure to maintain, diagnose, or treat a physical or mental condition.

I reserve unto myself the right to revoke the authority granted to my Agent hereunder to make health care decisions for me by notifying the treating physician, hospital, or other health care provider orally or in writing. Notwithstanding any provision herein to the contrary, I retain the right to make medical and other health care decisions for myself so long as I am able to give informed consent with respect to a particular decision. In addition, no treatment may be given to me over my objection, and health care necessary to keep me alive may not be stopped if I object.

This power of attorney shall not be affected by subsequent disability or incapacity of the principal. Notwithstanding any provision herein to the contrary, my Agent shall take no action under this instrument unless I am deemed to be disabled or incapacitated as defined herein. My incapacity shall be deemed to exist when so certified in writing by two licensed physicians not related by blood or marriage to either me or to my Agent. The said certificate shall state that I am incapable of caring for myself and that I am physically and mentally incapable of managing my financial affairs. The certificate of the physicians described above shall be attached to the original of this instrument and if this instrument is filed or recorded among public records, then such certificate shall also be similarly filed or recorded if permitted by applicable law. To the extent permitted by law, I herewith nominate, constitute and appoint my Agent to serve as my guardian, conservator and/or in any similar representative capacity, and, if I am not permitted by law to so nominate, constitute and appoint, then I request any court of competent jurisdiction which may be petitioned by any person to appoint a guardian, conservator or similar representative for me to give due consideration to my request.

Signed this   day of   , 19   .

Signed in the presence of:

_____   _____

State of

County of   SS.   , 19

Then personally appeared the foregoing   , as
Grantor, who known to me acknowledged the foregoing to be his or her free act and deed, before me.

_____
Notary Public
My Commission Expires:

Prefixes and Suffixes Commonly Used in Medical Terminology

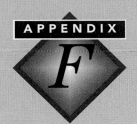

a-, *an-:* without, not
ab-: from, away
ad-: to, toward
adeno-, *aden-:* gland, glandular
-algia: pain
ambi-: both
angio-: vessel, duct
ante-, *pre-:* before
anti-, *contra-:* against
audio-: sound, hearing, dealing with the ear
auto-: self

bi-, *bis-:* twice, double
bio-: life
brady-: slow
bronch-, *bronchi-:* air tubes in the lungs, bronchi

cardi-, *cardia-*, *cardio-:* pertaining to the heart
-cide: causing death
crani-, *cranio-:* pertaining to the skull
cyst-, *cysto-*, *cysti-:* bladder, bag
-cyte, *cyt-:* cell

derm-, *derma-*, *dermo-*, *dermat-:* pertaining to skin
dia-: through, between, apart
dorsi-, *dorso-:* to the back, back
dys-: difficult, painful

ecto-, *ex-*, *exo-:* outside of, external
-ectomy: surgical removal of
endo-: within, innermost
entero-: intestine, pertaining to the intestine

gastro-, *gasti-:* stomach
-genetic, *-genic:* origin, producing
genito-: organs of reproduction
glyco-, *gly-:* sugar

gyn-, *gyno-:* women, female

hemi-: half
hema-, *hem-*, *hemo-*, *hemato-:* blood
hepato-: liver
hetero-: other, unlike, different
homo-, *homeo-:* same, like
hydro-: water
hyper-: over, increased, high
hypo-: under, decreased, low
hystero-, *hyster-:* uterus

inter-: between, among
intra-: within, into
-itis: inflammation, inflammation of

leuko-, *leuco-:* white
-logy, *-ology:* study of, science of

mal-: abnormal, disordered
mast-, *masto-:* breast
micro-: small
mono-: one, single
multi-: many, much, a large amount
myo-: muscle

neph-, *nephro-*, *ren-:* kidney
neuro-, *neur-:* nerve or nervous system

-ology: study of a science
ophthalm-, *ophthalmo-:* eye
-ostomy: creation of an opening by surgery
ot-, *oto-:* ear
-otomy: cutting into

path-, *patho-*, *pathy*, *-pathia:* disease, abnormal condition
ped-, *pedia-:* child
peri-: around
-plegia: paralysis
pnea-: respiration/breathing
pneum-: lung, pertaining to the lungs

post-: after
proct-, procto-: rectum, rectal
pseudo-: false
psych-, psycho-: pertaining to the mind
sep-, septic-: poison, rot
sub-: less, under, below
super-, supra-: above, upon, over

tachy: fast
therm-, thermo-: heat
-toxic, -tox: poison
tracho-: trachea, windpipe
uria: urine

Glossary

abuse mistreatment or improper treatment, including physical abuse, sexual abuse, emotional abuse, and confinement.

acidosis a condition in which the balance of acids and bases in the body is disturbed because of loss of salts, sodium and potassium, or the accumulation of acids.

acquired immune deficiency [or immunodeficiency] syndrome (AIDS) a crippling and fatal disease first diagnosed in 1981. The disease breaks down the body's natural immune system so that victims are vulnerable to almost any infection.

active listening a tool that allows total involvement in the communication process; techniques include paraphrasing, reflecting the speaker's feelings, asking for more information, and using nonverbal communication.

activities pursuits or pastimes that help a person who is disabled relearn skills that were lost due to illness or accident.

activities of daily living the activities necessary for the client to fulfill basic human needs, such as dressing, eating, and toileting.

acuity sensitivity or keenness.

acute sudden and severe; often followed by complete recovery.

acute illness a change from normal body functioning to a sudden pathological condition requiring immediate care.

adjustment changes a person makes in his or her behavior to deal with a situation.

adolescence the period of physical and emotional development from early teens to young adulthood (usually between the ages of 13 to 18).

advance directive document specifying the type of treatment individuals want or do not want under serious medical conditions in which they may be unable to communicate their wishes. Generally two forms: living will or durable power of attorney.

aged old or mature.

Alzheimer's disease a progressive, degenerative illness causing loss of memory and mental incapacity.

amyotrophic lateral sclerosis (ALS) a progressive degeneration of the nerve cells in the brain and spinal cord that control the voluntary muscles. Commonly known as Lou Gehrig's disease after the famous baseball player who died from this disease.

anemia deficiency of quality or quantity of red blood cells in the blood.

aneurysm localized enlargement of a blood vessel; may be due to a congenital defect or weakness of the vessel's wall.

angina pectoris mild heart condition that may cause pain in the chest region. Pain is usually relieved with a drug called nitroglycerin.

anticoagulant a drug that delays or prevents the formation of blood clots within the circulatory system. Anticoagulants are not effective in dissolving clots that have already formed.

anti-inflammatory medication used to decrease pain and swelling in joints and muscles.

aphasia impaired or lost ability to communicate through speech due to dysfunction of brain centers. There can be a loss of verbal understanding, word blindness, inability to understand the meaning of spoken or written words, or speech in meaningless phrases.

apnea absence of breathing or respirations.

arterial insufficiency a narrowing of the arteries that deliver blood to the lower extremities.

arteriogram series of x-ray pictures that show the flow of blood in the arteries after the injection of a dye or contrast substance into the artery.

arteriosclerosis a condition in which the arteries become hard and lose the elasticity needed for good blood circulation.

artery any of a branching system of muscular tubes that carry blood away from the heart.

arthritis inflammation of the joints causing pain, swelling, and enlargement of the joints. Usually associated with aging, but can attack young people as well.

articulates utters intelligible sounds; speaks.

aseptic free or freed from pathogenic microorganisms.

aseptic techniques strategies used to rid the environment of microorganisms and provide a sterile area.

asthma a disorder of the respiratory system. Symptoms may include labored breathing, wheezing, and coughing. There may be secretion of fluid from the bronchials. Condition may be caused by pollutants, infection, emotional stress, and/or allergies.

atherosclerosis fatty tissue (lipid) collected within or beneath the surface of blood vessels causing impaired circulation. Common cause of arterial occlusion (blocking).

auditory relating to hearing.

autopsy a detailed examination of the body to determine the exact cause of death.

bacteria one-celled microorganisms that are round, rod-shaped, or spiral in form. They can cause infections in the body or in the environment.

benign noncancerous.

biopsy surgical technique in which a sample of tissue is removed from an area where cellular change is suspected and examined under the microscope for signs of cancer.

bladder a muscular organ for storing urine.

bland diet food prepared with no spices and featuring easily digested items that are soothing to the digestive tract.

blood lancet small, pointed surgical instrument used to pierce the skin to obtain a blood sample.

blood pressure the force exerted by the blood on the walls of the blood vessels.

body language a form of communication that uses gestures and facial expressions instead of words.

body mechanics the techniques used to get the most effective and least taxing body movements. Bending the knees when lifting, to avoid unnecessary strain on the back and legs, is an example of good body mechanics.

bonding a process of attachment of mother, father, and infant, happening immediately after birth. Infant is placed on mother's abdomen and father feels and touches infant.

bony prominences areas of the body where bones protrude, such as the elbows, wrists, knees, pelvic bones, spinal column. Such bones have little natural padding and are areas where pressure sores can easily form.

bottle-feeding to feed a baby with a bottle.

bradycardia an extremely slow heartbeat.

breast engorgement swollen, hard, and painful breasts resulting from the milk let-down process after birth.

breast-feeding to feed a baby mother's milk from the breast.

bulk roughage foods needed by the body to prevent constipation and to keep the stool soft. High-bulk foods are fruits, green leafy vegetables, potatoes, and whole-grain cereals.

calorie-controlled diet diet in which calorie count is adjusted either to high for a malnourished client, or to low for an obese client.

cancer a disease characterized by rapid growth of abnormal cells that form a tumor; it often spreads to other sites.

carbohydrates any of a group of photosynthetically produced organic compounds that includes sugars, starches, celluloses, and gums; serves as a major energy source in the diet.

carcinogen a substance or agent that produces cancer; may be related to environment or heredity.

cardiac arrest heart stops beating.

career a chosen pursuit, occupation, or profession.

case manager member of the health care team who coordinates all the services the client may require in the home. Usually a social worker or registered nurse.

cataract opacity of the lens of the eye causing partial or total blindness.

catheterization process in which a thin tube is introduced into an artery or vein and passed through the heart; diagnostic test used to diagnose heart abnormality.

cerebral hemorrhage blood vessel burst in the brain. Common cause of a stroke.

cerebral infarction condition in which a portion of the brain dies when an artery becomes blocked and blood is prevented from reaching that part of the brain.

cerebral palsy condition in which there is impaired muscular power and coordination due to lack of oxygen to the brain before or during birth.

cerebral vascular accident (CVA) a disorder of the blood vessels of the brain due to a blockage caused by an embolus or hemorrhage.

cervix the mouth of the womb.

cesarean section surgical abdominal delivery of a fetus; performed when normal birth canal delivery would be dangerous to the mother or fetus.

chemotherapy a treatment for cancer in which chemicals are used to destroy or slow the growth of cancerous cells.

Cheyne-Stokes respiration term used to describe breathing in which periods of apnea are followed by periods of dyspnea.

child abuse emotional or physical abuse of an individual under the age of 18 by an adult.

chronic lasting a long time.

chronic bronchitis inflammation of the bronchi, causing symptoms of low-grade fever, productive cough, lethargy, and malaise.

chronic illness a long-term condition.

chronic obstructive pulmonary disease (COPD) disease of the respiratory system, marked by decreased ability of the lungs to perform their ventilation function; may result from a lung infection or chronic lung condition.

circumcision the removal of the foreskin of a male.

clean-catch specimen a procedure for obtaining a urine specimen for a diagnostic test; the specimen collected this way is as free of contamination as possible.

clear liquid diet a special diet consisting of only liquids that one can see through, such as apple juice, tea, broth, and gelatin.

collateral circulation when small blood vessels take over the circulation from nearby damaged or scarred blood vessels; the small vessels enlarge themselves to carry the blood to the body parts.

colostomy the removal of a diseased area of the gastrointestinal tract and the creation of an external opening on the abdomen called a stoma; may be a temporary solution in cases in which the intestine can be reattached to the bowel later, or may be permanent.

communication the sending and receiving of messages; may be verbal or nonverbal.

companion a person hired to keep a client company or maintain safety. Usually does not provide personal or homemaking services.

components the separate parts of a machine, procedure, or system that make up the whole.

conception formation of a viable zygote by the union of the male sperm and the female ovum.

confidentiality keeping a client's personal affairs private. A home health aide must not give out information about the client except to the nursing supervisor or doctor.

congestive heart failure a condition in which the heart cannot pump enough blood to the body; can start as an acute problem that leads to a chronic condition with slow deterioration and the possibility of complications to other body systems.

constipation infrequent or difficult bowel movements where the feces are usually hard.

contaminated dirty, containing pathogens that may cause infection.

contracture the abnormal shortening of muscle tissue.

convenience foods prepared foods that are ready to serve or require only cooking. These foods are often more expensive and may not be as tasty as foods prepared from fresh products.

culture the behavior patterns, arts, beliefs, institutions, and all other products of human work and thought as expressed in a particular community or period.

cyanosis lack of oxygen in the blood causing the client to appear bluish; indicates improper heart/lung function.

cyanotic a bluish skin tone due to some problem of the respiratory system preventing proper inspiration and exhalation; the result of lack of oxygen to the blood cells.

cystic fibrosis an inherited condition that affects children's sweat glands, pancreas, and respiratory system.

cystitis inflammation of the bladder.

degenerative disease a disease or condition causing tissues or organs to weaken and become abnormal. May be a progressive degeneration in which the condition becomes worse over time.

delicatessen a specialty store selling cheeses, cold cuts, sodas, sandwiches, and convenience foods.

delirium a mental disorder characterized by a disturbance of consciousness, making it difficult for a person to focus or shift his or her attention.

dementia progressive mental deterioration due to organic brain disease.

depression a mental state characterized by loss of hope, feelings of rejection, generalized sadness, and, in severe cases, the inability to function.

dermis the inner layer of the skin.

detrusor instability another term for unstable bladder.

developmentally disabled a mental and/or physical impairment, usually apparent at birth, that is likely to continue indefinitely and may result in substantial functional limitations and require lifelong or extended care.

diabetes a chronic disorder related to metabolism; caused by the inadequate functioning of the islets of Langerhans in the pancreas, which produce insulin. Insulin is needed for the proper metabolism of sugars in the body.

diabetic diet a measured and low- or no-sugar diet for diabetics.

diagnosis-related group system (DRG) a process developed in 1983 to contain health care payments by only reimbursing hospitals for a specific time or amount of service.

diastolic measurement of blood pressure when the heart is relaxing.

disability a physical or mental impairment that impedes normal functioning or achievement.

disinfection use of a medication or germ-fighting agent to destroy microorganisms.

disruptive behaviors behaviors such as screaming, cursing, threatening, hitting, or biting. Frequently exhibited by those with Alzheimer's disease.

diuretic   a drug used to reduce fluid accumulation in the body. Persons taking diuretics urinate frequently.

diversity   the quality of being diverse, different; referring to variety, having many shapes and forms.

documentation   to record on the proper form your observations and actions.

Down's syndrome   a birth defect caused by the presence of an extra 21st chromosome; the affected person has mild to moderate retardation, short stature, and a flattened facial profile.

duct   a tube-like structure that transports fluid or air from one part of the body to another.

durable power of attorney   legal document that designates another person to act as an "agent" or a "proxy" in making medical decisions if the individual becomes unable to do so.

dysmenorrhea   painful menstruation.

dyspnea   difficult or labored respiration.

early adulthood   period between 20–39 years of age.

ectopic pregnancy   implantation and subsequent development of a fertilized ovum outside the uterus.

edema   the swelling of legs and/or arms or other body parts when water is being retained unnaturally.

embalming   the process of removing blood and fluid from a dead body and replacing the fluids with a chemical preservative, to keep the body from decomposing before burial.

embolus   floating blood clot.

emesis   vomiting.

emotions   basic feelings common to all, such as love, fear, anger, sorrow, and anxiety.

empathy   the ability to observe and share the feelings of others in a supportive manner.

emphysema   an abnormal condition of the lung tissue in which the lungs lose their normal spongy and elastic character; causes poor exchange of the gases needed for normal respiration. The condition may be acute or chronic.

empty calories   foods high in carbohydrates and fats and low in proteins, minerals, and vitamins; "junk" food.

empty nest syndrome   the stage in a person's life when children leave home, often characterized by feelings of sadness and worthlessness.

endocrine glands   a body system made up of ductless glands that secrete hormones directly into the blood and lymph system.

enema   a technique of introducing fluid into the rectum to remove feces and flatus (gas) from the rectum and colon.

engagement   the state of pregnancy when the uterus drops into the pelvic cavity.

enzymes   proteins produced by the body that break down organic matter (food) within the body; necessary for digestion and metabolism.

epidermis   the outer layer of the skin.

estrogen   any of several hormones produced chiefly by the ovaries and responsible for promoting the development and maintenance of female secondary sex characteristics.

ethics   a code of behavior. Medical ethics is the standard of professional conduct by health care team members.

evacuate   to empty or remove the contents from.

evaluation   a determination of how well a given duty or demonstration of skill is performed.

expectorate   to spit.

expressive aphasia   unable to correctly express oneself verbally.

external stimulus   a message or impulse sent to the nervous system from outside the body that causes a mental or physical response.

fallopian tubes   either of a pair of slender ducts through which ova pass from the ovaries to the uterus in human beings and higher mammals.

feces   waste products eliminated from the bowels.

fermented   rotted.

fetal alcohol syndrome (FAS)   condition seen in infants and children due to mother's intake of alcohol during pregnancy.

fetus   the unborn young from the end of the eighth week after conception to birth, as distinguished from the embryo.

fiber   indigestible plant matter consisting of cellulose; stimulates intestinal peristalsis.

fire extinguisher   portable apparatus containing chemicals that can be discharged to put out a small fire.

flatulence   feelings of gassiness in the abdomen.

flexible   the ability to adapt to new situations or conditions; pliant.

food allergy   any negative reaction to a food, or a food component, that involves the immune system.

food guide pyramid   the six food groups making up good nutritional standards for humans.

foreskin   the loose fold of skin that covers the glans of the penis.

fracture   a break in a bone requiring an x-ray to determine the type and treatment.

full-liquid diet   special diet consisting of foods that are liquid at room temperature, such as milk, pudding, and ice cream.

fungi   two groups of microorganisms that can cause diseases such as athlete's foot and vaginitis.

gait belt see *transfer belt*.

gangrene the formation of large areas of dead tissue, which can become a serious complication.

genital herpes a highly contagious, sexually transmitted viral infection of the genital and anal regions caused by herpes simplex and characterized by small clusters of painful lesions.

genitalia the genitals.

germs microorganisms capable of causing disease.

gestation development of a fetus in the uterus.

gestation period the time required from conception until birth; in humans, the gestation period is nine months.

gestational refers to a type of diabetes that occurs only during pregnancy.

glans the head of the penis.

glaucoma an eye disease characterized by abnormally high intraocular fluid pressure, hardening of the eyeball, and partial to complete loss of vision.

glucometer instrument used to measure the level of blood sugar.

glucose a form of sugar required by the body.

gonorrhea a venereal disease that develops within 48 hours after sexual contact with an infected person. Causes painful burning sensation during urination among males; females have urinary burning and vaginal discomfort. Complications can lead to reproductive disorders, liver involvement, and blindness (more common among women). Immediate treatment is required.

gout form of arthritis caused by an increased amount of uric acid in the body.

grieving the physical and emotional response to a severe loss, and the process of accepting the loss.

gynecologist a physician who specializes in delivering health care to women, especially the diagnosis and treatment of disorders affecting the female reproductive organs.

hazard that which is dangerous or could cause a serious accident.

heartburn a burning sensation near the sternum, caused by the reflux of acidic stomach fluids into the lower end of the esophagus.

hemiplagia a weakness or paralysis confined to one side of the body.

hemophilia a hereditary blood disease characterized by spontaneous hemorrhages due to deficiency of a clotting factor in the blood.

hemorrhoids an itchy or painful mass of dilated veins in swollen anal tissue.

hepatitis B a serious form of infectious liver inflammation transmitted by blood that contains the hepatitis B virus. Signs and symptoms come on suddenly.

high-fiber diet diet including foods that are high in fiber in order to stimulate bowel action.

high-risk pregnancy a pregnancy marked by physical, emotional, or environmental situations that could potentially compromise the well-being of the mother and/or the child.

home care aide caregiver who works with a client with the goal of assisting the client with independent living under professional supervision.

home health aide person who performs personal and nursing care skills, such as bathing the client, under the supervision of a registered nurse.

home health care agencies agencies, some of which are hospital-affiliated, that focus on providing medical aspects of care in the home.

homemaker person who performs household duties such as laundry and cooking.

homemaker/home care agencies agencies that provide a variety of nonmedical home support services.

homemaker/home health aide person who assists with general household tasks, personal care and simple nursing duties, such as feeding and bathing the client.

hormones products of body glands that assist in healthy body function.

hospice group that provides specialized care for dying clients and their families. The primary concern of a hospice is the quality of life, not prolonging the length of life. The goal is to keep the client as pain-free and as comfortable as possible.

human immunodeficiency virus (HIV) a virus that causes AIDS; lives in the blood, semen, and body fluids of an infected person.

hygiene personal cleanliness of the human body.

hyperglycemia high blood sugar.

hypertension sustained, elevated blood pressure.

hyperthermia abnormally high body temperature (heat stroke).

hyperthyroidism condition resulting from excessive activity of the thyroid gland; symptoms may include rapid heartbeat, restlessness, and irritability.

hypoglycemia low blood sugar.

hypotension blood pressure that is lower than normal.

hypothermia abnormally low body temperature.

hypothyroidism a condition resulting from severe thyroid insufficiency; symptoms may include sluggishness and fatigue, cold hands and feet, constipation, pale and dry skin, and puffiness in the face.

hysterectomy   a major surgical procedure in which the uterus is removed. In a panhysterectomy, all the female reproductive organs are removed.

ileostomy   the surgical removal of a diseased portion of the small intestine and the preparation of an external abdominal stoma (usually permanent) from which a liquid stool is expelled.

immunity   the ability to resist a particular disease.

impacted   tightly wedged.

impaction   in reference to the stool, a condition in which the feces become hardened and lodged in the lower colon or rectum.

incontinence   the loss of voluntary control of the bladder muscles, causing uncontrolled voiding.

incontinent   unable to control voiding of the bladder.

incubation period   the time between entry of germs into the body and the appearance of the first signs of the disease.

infection   invasion of pathogenic organisms causing inflammation, discomfort, or illness. Infections may be caused by viruses, bacteria, fungi, or animal parasites.

infection control   measures used in client's care to prevent the spread of contagious diseases.

infectious disease   a disease that is readily passed from one person to another.

information sheet   a list of key facts and information that may be needed or requested for completion of a job application, including references, job history, names, and telephone numbers.

infraction   violation of a rule or law.

insulin   a hormone produced by the pancreas; essential for the maintenance of proper blood sugar levels. Insulin can be medically prepared from animal pancreases for use in treatment of human diabetes.

interaction   the reciprocating actions between two people or between members of a group.

intermittent claudication   cramping pain in the calf or thigh caused by a narrowing of the arteries that hampers blood flow.

internal stimulus   a message or impulse from within the body that is transmitted through the nervous system and causes a mental or physical response.

interpersonal relationships   the feelings and understanding that result from the interactions between two or more persons.

invalidate   to negate; to make unjustified.

irrigation   the use of a fluid to cleanse an area.

ischemia   lack of blood supply.

isolation   procedure whereby the client is kept away from others to prevent the spread of a contagious disease.

jaundice   a condition in which there is a yellowish color to the skin, mucous membranes, and eyes. It is associated with liver failure when excessive amounts of bilirubin enter the blood.

kidney   primary organ of the urinary system; its function is to filter waste material from the bloodstream.

kidney stones   buildup of crystallized urine in the kidneys, caused by an excess of calcium.

lactose   sugar found in milk.

laryngectomy   the surgical removal of the larynx (voice box) because of disease. Laryngectomy patients can be taught to speak through an artificial airway by gulping air through the external stoma into the esophagus.

larynx   the voice box.

leukemia   a condition in which too many immature white blood cells are produced, blocking the normal transport of oxygen to body tissues; also called cancer of the blood.

liability   something for which a person has a responsibility or duty.

licensed nurse agencies   home health agencies that provide private-duty registered nurses, licensed practical nurses, and/or skilled therapists.

licensed practical nurse (LPN)   provides direct care to client; may supervise home care workers.

ligaments   the tough elastic fibers that hold the bones in place.

listening   hearing with thoughtful attention.

living will   legal document that outlines the medical care an individual wants or does not want if he or she becomes unable to make decisions.

lobectomy   partial removal of a lung.

lochia   the normal uterine discharge of blood, tissue, and mucus from the vagina following childbirth.

low birthweight   weight of less than three pounds for a full-term infant.

low-residue diet   diet in which only foods low in fiber are allowed; used to lessen bowel activity.

low-sodium diet   diet containing foods with low salt content; no extra salt is to be added.

lumpectomy   surgical excision of a tumor from the breast with the removal of a minimal amount of surrounding tissue.

malignant   uncontrolled growth that is resistant to treatment and has a tendency to spread to surrounding areas; often said of cancerous growths.

malnutrition a condition resulting from poor diet that lacks needed nutrients to maintain health; early signs include muscle weakness.

mammogram x-rays of the female breasts used to determine if a tumor is present in the breasts.

managed care a method of health care delivery that attempts to cut costs by controlling access to and use of physicians, hospitals, nursing facilities, and other forms of care.

mastectomy a surgical removal of the female breast(s); may be total or partial.

Meals on Wheels program that prepares and delivers meals to homebound clients or to senior citizens' centers to help assure that the disadvantaged, handicapped, ill, or aged have at least one meal a day that is nutritionally sound.

Medicaid federally and state-funded program that pays medical costs for those whose income is below a certain level.

Medicare federal program that assists persons over 65 years of age with hospital and medical costs.

menopause cessation of the monthly menstrual cycle; normally occurs during a woman's middle years (late forties to late fifties). Following menopause, reproductive ability ceases.

menstruation the process, or an instance of, discharging the mensus.

mental disorder a disorder of the mind, characterized by difficulty in functioning satisfactorily in society as a result of changes in thoughts, behavior, personality, or emotion.

metabolism the complex of physical and chemical processes occurring within a living cell or organism that are necessary for the maintenance of life.

metastasis spreading of cancer cells away from the primary site of the cancer tumor.

microorganism organism that is not visible with the naked eye, such as bacterium or protozoan; some microorganisms cause serious illnesses.

middle adulthood period of time during which an individual is between 40-65 years of age.

mildew a fuzzy, grayish fungus growth that appears in damp, dark areas.

misconduct improper behavior; mismanagement of responsibilities.

multi-infart dementia a common form of dementia, the result of multiple strokes that damage brain tissue.

multiple sclerosis a progressive disease involving the nerves of the brain and spinal cord. It may start slowly and become worse throughout life, or there may be periods of remission when the condition seems to stay about the same. Signs and symptoms are tremors and inability to coordinate muscles.

muscular dystrophy a progressive degenerative disease of the muscles surrounding the skeleton; characterized by loss of strength, physical disability, and deformity.

myocardial infarction an acute coronary occlusion, commonly called a heart attack.

myocardium heart muscle.

negligence failure to give care that is reasonably expected of a home health aide.

neuropathy term usually used in relation to diabetic clients, but generally means any disease of the nerves.

nitroglycerin medication used in treatment of heart conditions.

nongonococcal urethritis a urethral inflammation caused by an infection other than gonorrhea.

nonjudgmental the quality of refraining from forming or expressing personal opinions, or otherwise determining the worth or quality of something; open and accepting.

nonverbal communication a way of communicating without words, using gestures, facial expressions, or other body language.

nutrition the sum of those processes using food for growth, development, and body maintenance.

observation gathering of information about any change in the client's condition or behavior by using any of your five senses.

occupational therapist a skilled professional who evaluates a client's ability to perform skills necessary to independent living (such as bathing, dressing, cooking, and the like) and who works with clients to improve these abilities.

Omnibus Budget Reconciliation Act (OBRA) law that regulates the education and certification of home health aides' work in home health agencies and certified hospices.

optimist one who expects a positive outcome to a situation.

oral hygiene care of the gums, lips, mouth, teeth, and tongue.

osteoarthritis degenerative joint disease caused by disintegration of the cartilage that covers the ends of the bones.

osteoporosis loss of bone density and strength; the bones become increasingly porous and brittle, which may lead to malformations such as a dowager's hump or hip fractures. Postmenopausal women are at high risk. An adequate intake of calcium helps to prevent the disease.

ostomy surgical construction of an artificial excretory opening.

ostomy bag (stoma bag) a sack or bag placed over the stoma (opening) to collect wastes for clients who have had a colostomy or ileostomy.

otosclerosis chronic, progressive deafness, especially to low tones.

ovaries the paired female reproductive organ that produces ova, and in vertebrates estrogen and progesterone.

over the counter any type of medicine that can be purchased without a prescription.

Pap smear a medical technique whereby a sample of the vaginal cells are tested for cancer; recommended for women annually to detect early signs of cancer.

paraphrase restate a text, passage, or communication in another form or in other words, often to clarify meaning.

paraplegia paralysis of the lower body involving both legs.

Parkinson's disease a progressive degeneration of nerve cells in the area of the brain that controls muscle movement.

passive listening listening without seeming interested in what a speaker has said and without checking to confirm the speaker's meaning.

pathogens microorganisms causing disease or infection in the body.

Patient Self-Determination Act law that gives each individual the right to make choices regarding specific types and kinds of medical care before he or she becomes seriously ill.

pelvic inflammatory disease (PID) inflammation of the female genital tract, especially of the fallopian tubes, caused by any of several microorganisms, chiefly chlamydia and gonococci, and marked by abdominal pain, fever, and vaginal discharge.

penis the male organ of copulation in higher vertebrates that in mammals also serves as the male organ of urinary excretion.

perineum in the male, the area between the anus and scrotum; in the female, the area between the anus and vagina.

peripheral vision the outer boundaries of vision; side vision.

perishable likely to spoil or decay.

peristalsis the progressive, wavelike movements that occur involuntarily to move food through the digestive system.

permanent press fabric with combination of natural and manmade threads that requires little or no ironing.

personal care worker person who assists with minimal level of daily living activities, such as companionship and meal preparation.

personal reference a person, other than a member of the individual's family, who can give a prospective employer a recommendation concerning the character and ability of an individual seeking employment.

pessimist one who expects a negative or bad outcome to a situation, or who looks on the gloomy side of life.

phlebitis inflammation of a vein.

physical therapist (PT) a skilled professional who evaluates a client's ability to stand, walk, climb stairs, transfer, and do other activities related to strength and endurance, and who works with clients to improve these abilities.

physician (MD) a person who has completed medical school and has licensure to practice medicine.

pivot turn or rotate the entire body, rather than twisting at the waist.

platitude a trite remark or saying.

pneumonectomy surgical removal of the entire lung.

pneumonia an acute inflammation of the lungs caused by bacteria, viruses, or fungi; characterized by high fever, chills, headache, cough, and chest pains.

polyester fabrics man-made fabrics.

postpartum after childbirth.

postpartum blues feelings of anxiety, fatigue, mood swings, and/or sadness following childbirth.

practice the actual performance of the procedure; the clientele of a doctor or medical practice.

premature born before full term (37 weeks gestation is considered full term for humans).

pressure sore dermal ulcer or bedsore.

preventive health measures use of inoculations, special diets, or other techniques to avoid illness before it starts.

procedure the steps taken to accomplish a particular task; a course or plan of action.

produce fresh fruits and vegetables.

progesterone a steroid hormone, secreted by the ovary and the placenta, that prepares the uterus for implantation of the fertilized ovum, maintains pregnancy, and promotes development of the mammary glands.

prognosis the probable outcome of an illness.

prosthesis artificial replacement for a body part.

protozoa tiny, one-celled microscopic animals.

psychology the study or science concerned with mental processes and behavior of an individual; the study concerned with mental health.

psychosis a serious mental condition in which the thinking process is distorted by hallucinations, delusions, or both.

puberty the time period following childhood, when the body matures and reproduction becomes possible.

pulmonary embolus a blood clot that has broken away and traveled to the lungs.

pulse the measurement of the number of heartbeats per minute.

pureed diet food prepared by processing through a blender or strainer.

quadriplegia paralysis of four extremities (arms and legs).

rales bubbling sound from the lungs when fluid or mucus is trapped in the air passages.

range of motion exercises the exercises designed to prevent contractures and loss of motion and function in the joints; usually planned by a physical therapist.

reality orientation techniques used to keep confused clients in touch with reality.

receptive aphasia communication problem whereby a person does not understand the words someone else says.

recyclable reusable.

registered nurse (RN) a graduate trained nurse who has passed a state registration examination and has been licensed to practice nursing.

registry service an agency that employs certified individuals to give home health care.

rehabilitation the restoring of physical and/or mental abilities following an accident or illness. Some patients can be fully restored to normal functioning; others are brought up to the best possible level through exercise and retraining.

reminiscence the act or process of recalling the past.

remission a period in an illness when the symptoms cease or become less severe.

report a written record or oral summary of care of a client.

respiration the sum total of the processes by which the body exchanges oxygen and carbon dioxide in the respiratory system.

respiratory system the nose, pharynx, larynx, trachea, bronchi, and lungs; system that helps maintain a constant balance in the body through effective air distribution and gas exchange.

restate to say again.

rheumatism any of several pathological conditions of the muscles, tendons, joints, bones, or nerves, marked by pain and disability.

rheumatoid arthritis autoimmune response that results in inflammation of the joints.

rickettsiae microorganisms that can cause disease; they live on lice, ticks, fleas, and mites.

sanitary of or relating to health and cleanliness.

scrotum the external sac of skin enclosing the testes in most mammals.

seizure a sudden attack; a convulsion.

self-esteem value one places on one's self as a person functioning in society.

sensory deficits lack or lessening of ability to receive stimuli in a particular sense (loss of hearing, weak eyes, weakened taste buds, inability to feel heat or cold, etc.).

sexually transmitted disease (STD) any of various diseases contracted through intimate sexual contact, including the HIV virus and AIDS.

sibling rivalry the normal jealousy and competition found between brothers and sisters in the family setting.

sickle cell anemia a hereditary and chronic blood anemia in which the red blood cells are crescent-shaped and look like a sickle; occurs mainly in African Americans.

sigmoidoscopy direct examination of the interior of the sigmoid colon.

sign in medicine, a change in the patient that can be observed or measured.

social service agency an organization that provides assistance in solving problems such as housing, living conditions, clothing, or food stamps for those unable to find jobs or support themselves.

social worker (MSW, LCSW, LSW) an individual who has received the formal education required to treat individuals, families, or groups with social and/or psychological problems.

soft diet diet in which soft, easily digested foods are ordered for clients recovering from surgery or who have ulcers; this diet causes little upset to the digestive system.

somaticize to develop physical symptoms that mask emotional problems.

speech therapist (ST) a skilled professional who assesses a client's ability to speak, hear, understand, write, and swallow, and works with clients to improve these abilities.

sphygmomanometer the instrument used to measure blood pressure.

standard precautions a system of infectious disease control which assumes that every direct contact with body fluids is infectious and requires every health care worker exposed to direct contact with body fluids or body substance to be protected.

staple items those foodstuffs normally kept in most homes, which are used in many ways and are the basics for preparing meals (e.g., flour, sugar, spices, herbs, canned goods).

sterile free of pathogens.

steroids hormonal medications used to treat many conditions. Major side effects are edema, weight gain, susceptibility to infections, and elevated blood pressure.

stoma the surgically formed opening between a body cavity or passage and the body's surface.

stoma bag see *ostomy bag*.

stool a bowel movement; evacuated fecal matter; feces.

stress a mentally or emotionally disruptive or upsetting condition that occurs in response to adverse external stimuli.

subcutaneously beneath the skin; usually used in reference to an injection.

sublingually under the tongue.

substance abuse the use of alcohol or drugs that results in poor treatment of the body.

sudden infant death syndrome (SIDS) the unexpected and sudden death of a healthy infant; occurs while the infant is sleeping.

suppository a small plug of medication designed to melt within a body cavity other than the mouth.

symptoms those changes reported by the patient, such as feeling pain, that may not be visible.

synchronize cause to occur at the same time.

syphilis an infectious, chronic venereal disease characterized by open lesions that can spread to the entire body and affect the nervous system.

systolic measurement of blood pressure when the heart is contracting.

tachycardia a very rapid heartbeat.

terminal final; life-ending stage.

terminal illness a fatal illness.

testes the reproductive gland in a male vertebrate; the source of sperm and androgens.

testosterone a crystalline steroid hormone, produced in the testes and responsible for male secondary sex characteristics.

theory the practical and necessary information one must learn about a particular topic or subject.

thrombophlebitis a condition in which a vein becomes inflamed and a blood clot forms in the lower extremities.

thrombus blood clot that forms inside an artery.

time organization organizing your work in order to complete the task or tasks in the allotted time period.

tophi outpouches or protruding lesions that contain abnormal amounts of uric acid. Seen in individuals with gout.

trachea the main tube running from the throat to the lungs to bring air in and out of the body; the windpipe.

tracheostomy a surgical procedure to create an opening in the trachea; an emergency operation in cases where the trachea is obstructed and the person cannot breathe.

transfer belt a sturdy cloth strap, about 3 inches wide and 3 feet long, tied around the client's waist and used by a care provider to assist in lifting a client in and out of a chair, or as added support when ambulating an unsteady client.

transient ischemic attack (TIA) temporary reduction of flow of blood to the brain.

transmission-based precautions special precautions taken in addition to standard precautions with clients who are known to have a contagious disease, to prevent transmission to others.

tuberculosis lung disease caused by a microorganism, easily transmitted to others by sneezing and/or coughing.

ureter one of the two long narrow ducts that transfer urine from the kidney to the bladder.

urethra mucus-lined tube conveying urine from the urinary bladder to the exterior of the body; in the male, the urethra also conveys the semen.

urinary catheter a tube inserted into the bladder to drain urine.

uterus an organ of the female reproductive system; contains and nourishes the embryo and fetus from the time the fertilized egg is implanted to the time of birth of the fetus.

vagina the passage leading from the opening of the vulva to the cervix of the uterus in female mammals.

vaginitis inflammation of the vagina.

validation therapy a communication technique designed to foster positive self-esteem by confirming the feelings of another.

varicose veins abnormally swollen or knotted veins.

vegetarian one who does not eat meat or meat products.

venous insufficiency damage to the veins that return blood to the heart, which causes pain and discoloration of the lower extremities.

virus microorganism that lives and grows by feeding on living cells; the cause of may infections.

vital signs measurements of temperature, pulse, respiration, and blood pressure.

vulva external female genitalia, including the labia, clitoris, and vestibule of the vagina.

wandering moving around purposelessly; often seen in clients with dementia.

Index

....

Note: Page numbers ending with "f" refer to a figure, those ending with "p" refer to a photo, and those ending with "t" refer to a table on the cited page.